# Clinical Decision Making in PSYCHIATRY

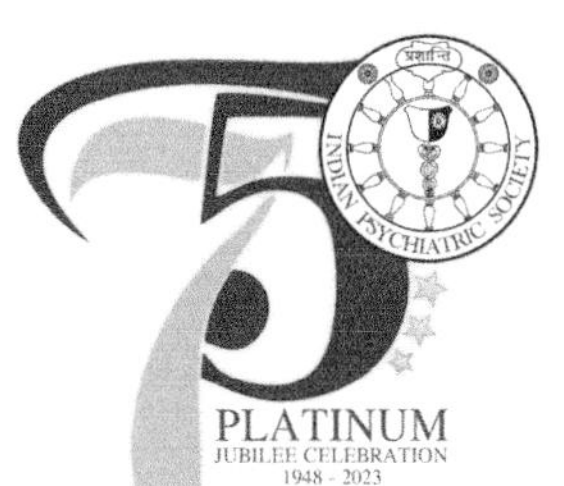


# Clinical Decision Making in PSYCHIATRY

*Editors*

**Samir Kumar Praharaj**
DPM MD (CIP Ranchi)
Professor
Department of Psychiatry
Kasturba Medical College, Manipal
Manipal Academy of Higher Education
Manipal, Karnataka, India

**Adarsh Tripathi**
MD MNAMS
Professor
Department of Psychiatry
King George's Medical University
Lucknow, Uttar Pradesh, India

**Vikas Menon**
MD DNB
Professor
Department of Psychiatry
Jawaharlal Institute of Postgraduate Medical Education and Research
Puducherry, India

**Sai Krishna Tikka**
DPM MD
Additional Professor and Head
Department of Psychiatry
All India Institute of Medical Sciences
Yadadri Bhuvanagiri, Telangana, India

*Foreword*

**Ramaswamy Viswanathan**

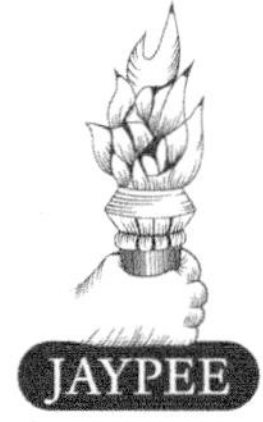


JAYPEE BROTHERS MEDICAL PUBLISHERS
*The Health Sciences Publisher*
New Delhi | London

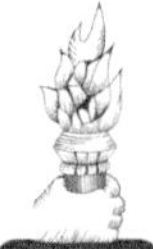

**Jaypee Brothers Medical Publishers (P) Ltd**

**Headquarters**
EMCA House
23/23-B, Ansari Road, Daryaganj
New Delhi 110 002, India
Landline: +91-11-23272143, +91-11-23272703
+91-11-23282021, +91-11-23245672
E-mail: jaypee@jaypeebrothers.com

**Corporate Office**
4838/24, Ansari Road, Daryaganj
New Delhi 110 002, India
Phone: +91-11-43574357
Fax: +91-11-43574314
E-mail: jaypee@jaypeebrothers.com

**Overseas Office**
J.P. Medical Ltd
83 Victoria Street, London
SW1H 0HW (UK)
Phone: +44-20 3170 8910
E-mail: info@jpmedpub.com

**EU GPSR** Authorised Representative
Logos Europe, 9 rue Nicolas Poussin
17000, La Rochelle, France
Phone: +33 (0) 6 67 93 73 78
E-mail: contact@logoseurope.eu

Website: www.jaypeebrothers.com
Website: www.jaypeedigital.com



**Inquiries for bulk sales may be solicited at:** jaypee@jaypeebrothers.com

***Clinical Decision Making in Psychiatry***

*First Edition:* **2026**

ISBN: 978-93-6616-753-4

*Printed in India*

# Contributors

**Aanushka Suklabaidya** MD
Senior Resident
Department of Psychiatry
All India Institute of Medical Sciences
Jodhpur, Rajasthan, India

**Adarsh Tripathi** MD MNAMS
Professor
Department of Psychiatry
King George's Medical University
Lucknow, Uttar Pradesh, India

**Aditya Agarwal** MD
Senior Resident
Department of Psychiatry
Dr Ram Manohar Lohia Institute
of Medical Sciences
Lucknow, Uttar Pradesh, India

**Aditya Somani** MD DNB
Associate Professor
Department of Psychiatry
All India Institute of Medical Sciences
Raipur, Chhattisgarh, India

**Alankrit Jaiswal** MD (Psychiatry)
Specialty Doctor
General Adult Psychiatry
Rotherham, Doncaster and South
Humber
NHS Foundation Trust
South Yorkshire, UK

**Alka Subramanyam** DPM MD DNB
Professor (Additional)
Department of Psychiatry
Topiwala National Medical College and
BYL Nair Hospital
Mumbai, Maharashtra, India

**Amit Singh** MD DM
Assistant Professor
Department of Psychiatry
King George's Medical University
Lucknow, Uttar Pradesh, India

**Anil Kakunje** DPM MD
Professor and Head
Department of Psychiatry
Yenepoya Medical College
Mangaluru, Karnataka, India

**Anindya Das** MD DPM MPH
Professor
Department of Psychiatry
All India Institute of Medical Sciences
Rishikesh, Uttarakhand, India

**Anirban Saha** MD
Senior Resident
Department of Psychiatry
All India Institute of Medical Sciences
Raipur, Chhattisgarh, India

**Anju Kuruvilla** MD
Professor
Department of Psychiatry
Christian Medical College
Vellore, Tamil Nadu, India

**Aparna Goyal** DPM DNB
Associate Professor
Department of Psychiatry
Institute of Human Behaviour and Allied
Sciences
New Delhi, India

**Arghya Pal** MD DNB
Assistant Professor
Department of Psychiatry
All India Institute of Medical Sciences
Raebareli, Uttar Pradesh, India

**Arghya Pal** MD DNB
Assistant Professor
Department of Psychiatry
All India Institute of Medical Sciences
Kalyani, West Bengal, India

**Arpit Parmar** MD DM
Assistant Professor
Department of Psychiatry
All India Institute of Medical Sciences
Bhubaneswar, Odisha, India

**Arvind Nongpiur** DPM MD
Additional Professor
Department of Psychiatry
North Eastern Indira Gandhi Regional
Institute of Health and Medical Sciences
Shillong, Meghalaya, India

**AM Ashfaq U Rahman** MD
Associate Professor
Department of Psychiatry
Government Medical College
Kozhikode, Kerala, India

**Babita Sharma** MD
Consultant Psychiatrist
RR Polyclinic Private Limited
Jhapa, Nepal

**Bandita Abhijita** MD
Senior Resident
Department of Psychiatry
Jawaharlal Institute of Postgraduate
Medical Education
and Research
Puducherry, India

**Barikar C Malathesh**
MBBS MD PDF Forensic Psy
Associate Professor
Department of Psychiatry
All India Institute of Medical Sciences
Hyderabad, Telangana, India

**Bhawna Yadav** MD
Senior Resident in Psychiatry
Centre for Cognitive Neurosciences,
Central Institute of Psychiatry
Ranchi, Jharkhand, India

**Biswa Ranjan Mishra** MD DPM
Professor and Head
Department of Psychiatry
All India Institute of Medical Sciences
Bhubaneswar, Odisha, India

**Chandrima Naskar** MD
Senior Resident
Fellow in Consultation-Liaison Psychiatry
Post Graduate Institute of Medical Education and Research
Chandigarh, India

**Chetan Anand** MS
Associate Professor
Department of General Surgery
All India Institute of Medical Sciences
Raipur, Chhattisgarh, India

**Dayal Narayan** MD
Professor and Head
Department of Psychiatry
Government Medical College
Wayanad, Kerala, India

**Deepak Kumar** MD DNB
Professor and Head
Department of Psychiatry
Institute of Human Behaviour and Allied Sciences
Delhi, India

**Dibyendu Mohanty** MD
Assistant Professor
Department of Psychiatry
Kalinga Institute of Medical Sciences
Bhubaneswar, Odisha, India

**Dinesh M** MD DNB
Senior Resident (DM Addiction Psychiatry)
Department of Psychiatry and National Drug Dependence Treatment Centre
All India Institute of Medical Sciences
New Delhi, India

**Ebin Joseph** MD
Senior Registrar
Western Mental Health Services
Melbourne, Australia

**Gajanan Ganapati Sabhahit** MD
Senior Resident
Apex Co-ordinating Centre for Tele MANAS
Department of Psychiatry
National Institute of Mental Health and Neurosciences
Bengaluru, Karnataka, India

**Ganesan Venkatasubramanian** MD PhD
Professor
Department of Psychiatry
National Institute of Mental Health and Neurosciences
Bengaluru, Karnataka, India

**Ganesh Kini** MD
Associate Professor
Department of Psychiatry
Yenepoya Medical College
Mangaluru, Karnataka, India

**Harsh Pathak** MD PDF
Assistant Professor
Clinical Research Centre for Neuromodulation
Department of Psychiatry
National Institute of Mental Health and Neurosciences
Bengaluru, Karnataka, India

**Heena Khanna** MD
Senior Resident
Department of Psychiatry
Surat Municipal Institute of Medical Education and Research
Surat, Gujarat, India

**Jagadisha Thirthalli** MD
Professor and Head
Department of Psychiatry
National Institute of Mental Health and Neurosciences
Bengaluru, Karnataka, India

**Jahnavi Kedare** MD
Professor (Additional)
Department of Psychiatry
Topiwala National Medical College and BYL Nair Charitable Hospital
Mumbai, Maharashtra, India

**Jibi Achamma Jacob** MD
Associate Professor
Department of Psychiatry
Christian Medical College
Vellore, Tamil Nadu, India

**Karthick Subramanian** MD
Professor
Department of Psychiatry
Mahatma Gandhi Medical College and Research Institute
Sri Balaji Vidyapeeth, Deemed-to-be University
Puducherry, India

**Kaustav Kundu** MD
Post Doc Fellow
Department of Psychiatry and Division of Sleep Medicine
All India Institute of Medical Sciences
Rishikesh, Uttarakhand, India

**Lokesh Kumar Saini** MD
Associate Professor
Department of Pulmonary Medicine and Division of Sleep Medicine
All India Institute of Medical Sciences
Rishikesh, Uttarakhand, India

**Lokesh Kumar Singh** MD
Additional Professor and Head
Department of Psychiatry
All India Institute of Medical Sciences
Raipur, Chhattisgarh, India

**Mamidipally Sai Spoorthy** MD
Assistant Professor
Department of Psychiatry
All India Institute of Medical Sciences
Hyderabad, Telangana, India

**Manjunatha Narayana**
DPM MD (Psychiatry)
Additional Professor
Department of Psychiatry
National Institute of Mental Health and Neurosciences
Bengaluru, Karnataka, India

**Manushree Gupta** MD
Professor (Central Health Services)
Department of Psychiatry
Vardhaman Mahavir Medical College and Safdarjung Hospital
New Delhi, India

**Midhun Sidharthan** MD
Assistant Professor
Department of Psychiatry
Government Medical College
Kozhikode, Kerala, India

**Muralidharan Kesavan** MBBS MD
Professor
Department of Psychiatry
National Institute of Mental Health and Neurosciences
Bengaluru, Karnataka, India

**Muthukrishnan Venkatesan** MD PDF (Child and Adolescent Psychiatry) MRCPsych
Specialty Registrar (CAMHS)
Cumbria, Northumberland
Tyne and Wear NHS Foundation Trust
Newcastle upon Tyne, UK

**NA Uvais** MBBS DPM
Consultant Psychiatrist
Iqraa International Hospital and Research Center
Kozhikode, Kerala, India

**Naresh Nebhinani** MD DNB
Professor and Head
Department of Psychiatry
All India Institute of Medical Sciences
Jodhpur, Rajasthan, India

**Nishant Goyal** MD DPM
Professor of Psychiatry, In-charge, fMRI Centre
Centre for Cognitive Neurosciences and Centre for Child and Adolescent Psychiatry
Central Institute of Psychiatry
Ranchi, Jharkhand, India

**P Lakshmi Nirisha** MD
Assistant Professor
Department of Psychiatry
All India Institute of Medical Sciences
Raipur, Chhattisgarh, India

**Panna Sharma** MD
Senior Resident
Department of Psychiatry
All India Institute of Medical Sciences
New Delhi, India

**Parag Shah** MD DNB PhD
Professor and Head
Department of Psychiatry
Surat Municipal Institute of Medical Education and Research
Surat, Gujarat, India

**Pavithra Jayasankar** MBBS MD
Assistant Professor
Centre for Brain and Mind
Department of Psychiatry
National Institute of Mental Health and Neurosciences
Bengaluru, Karnataka, India

**Pooja Sharma** MD (Psychiatry)
Former Senior Resident in Psychiatry
Centre for Child and Adolescent Psychiatry
Central Institute of Psychiatry
Ranchi, Jharkhand, India

**Pratap Sharan** MD PhD
Professor and Head
Department of Psychiatry
All India Institute of Medical Sciences
New Delhi, India

**Preethy Kathiresan** MD DM
Assistant Professor
Department of Psychiatry
All India Institute of Medical Sciences
New Delhi, India

**Prerna Khar**
MD PDF Child and Adolescent Psychiatry
Consultant Psychiatrist
Department of Psychiatry
Early intervention and Rehabilitation Cente
Topiwala National Medical College and BYL Nair Hospital
Mumbai, Maharashtra, India

**Prerna Kukreti** MD (Psychiatry)
Associate Professor
Department of Psychiatry
Lady Hardinge Medical College
New Delhi, India

**Rahul Patley** MD (Psychiatry) PDF in Community Psychiatry
Assistant Professor
Department of Psychiatry
National Institute of Mental Health and Neurosciences
Bengaluru, Karnataka, India

**Rajesh Gopalakrishnan** MD
Professor
Department of Psychiatry
Christian Medical College
Vellore, Tamil Nadu, India

**Rajshekhar Bipeta** MBBS DPM DNB
Professor and Head
Department of Psychiatry
Government Medical College
Medak, Telangana, India

**Rakshathi Basavaraju** MD
Consultant Psychiatrist
Manosuraksha Private Limited and Mental Health Foundation
Bengaluru, Karnataka, India

**Rashmi Arasappa** MBBS DPM MD
Associate Professor
Department of Psychiatry
National Institute of Mental Health and Neurosciences
Bengaluru, Karnataka, India

**Ravi Gupta** MD PhD
Professor
Department of Psychiatry and Division of Sleep Medicine
All India Institute of Medical Sciences
Rishikesh, Uttarakhand, India

**Ravi Philip Rajkumar** MD (Psychiatry)
Professor
Department of Psychiatry
Jawaharlal Institute of Postgraduate Medical Education and Research
Puducherry, India

**Ravindra Neelakanthappa Munoli** MD
Additional Professor
Department of Psychiatry
Kasturba Medical College, Manipal
Manipal Academy of Higher Education
Manipal, Karnataka, India

**Raviteja Innamuri** MD DPM DNB MBBS
Consultant Psychiatrist
Ananda Mind Care
Nizamabad, Telangana, India

**Rohit Verma** MD
Professor
Department of Psychiatry
All India Institute of Medical Sciences
New Delhi, India

**Sachin Baliga** MD DNB Post-Doctoral Fellowship in Non Invasive Brain Stimulation of Psychiatric Disorders
Consultant Psychiatrist
Department of Mental Health and Behavioral Sciences
Fortis Hospital
Bengaluru, Karnataka, India

**Sai Krishna Tikka** DPM MD
Additional Professor and Head
Department of Psychiatry
All India Institute of Medical Sciences
Yadadri Bhuvanagiri, Telangana, India

**Sai Sreeja Vullanki** MD
Senior Resident
Department of Psychiatry
All India Institute of Medical Sciences
Guntur, Andhra Pradesh, India

**Saloni Seth** MD (Psychiatry)
Senior Resident
Department of Psychiatry
Lady Hardinge Medical College
New Delhi, India

**Samir Kumar Praharaj**
DPM MD (CIP Ranchi)
Professor
Department of Psychiatry
Kasturba Medical College, Manipal
Manipal Academy of Higher Education
Manipal, Karnataka, India

**Sandeep Grover** MD
Professor
Department of Psychiatry
Postgraduate Institute of Medical Education and Research
Chandigarh, India

**Santanu Nath** MD DNB
Associate Professor
Department of Psychiatry
All India Institute of Medical Sciences
Deoghar, Jharkhand, India

**Shahul Ameen** MD
Consultant Psychiatrist
St Thomas Hospital
Kottayam, Kerala, India

**Shaily Mittal** MD
Assistant Professor
Department of Psychiatry
GS Medical College and Hospital
Hapur, Uttar Pradesh, India

**Shalini Kumari** MD
Assistant Professor
Department of Psychiatry
SKS Hospital Medical College and Research Centre
Mathura, Uttar Pradesh, India

**Shanti Mohan Kethawath** MBBS MD
Consultant Psychiatrist
Yashoda Hospital
Secunderabad, Telangana, India

**Shashwath Sathyanath** MD
Assistant Professor
Department of Psychiatry
Yenepoya Medical College
Mangaluru, Karnataka, India

**Shivani Sivaramakrishnan** MD
Psychiatry Registrar
Victorian Institute of Forensic Mental Health (Forensicare), Australia

**Shobit Garg** MD DPM
Professor
Department of Psychiatry
Shri Guru Ram Rai Institute of Medical and Health Sciences
Dehradun, Uttarakhand, India

**Shyam Sundar Arumugham** MD DNB
Professor
Department of Psychiatry
National Institute of Mental Health and Neurosciences
Bengaluru, Karnataka, India

**Siddharth Sarkar** MD
Additional Professor
National Drug Dependence Treatment Centre
All India Institute of Medical Sciences
New Delhi, India

**Siddharth Sethi** MBBS MD
Senior Resident
Department of Psychiatry
Vardhaman Mahavir Medical College and Safdarjung Hospital
New Delhi, India

**Snehil Gupta** MD (Psychiatry) DNB
Associate Professor
Department of Psychiatry
All India Institute of Medical Sciences
Bhopal, Madhya Pradesh, India

**Sonia Shenoy** MD PDF
Associate Professor
Department of Psychiatry
Kasturba Medical College, Manipal
Manipal Academy of Higher Education
Manipal, Karnataka, India

**Sreya Mariyam Salim** MD
Specialty Doctor
Powys Teaching Health Board
Ystradgynlais Community Hospital
Ystradgynlais, Wales, UK

**Srilakshmi Pingali** MD
Professor of Psychiatry
Department of Psychiatry
Government Medical College
Sangareddy, Telangana, India

**Subashree Kathatharan** MD (Psychiatry) DNB (Psychiatry)
Senior Resident
Department of Psychiatry
Jawaharlal Institute of Postgraduate Medical Education and Research
Puducherry, India

**Subhash Das** MD
Professor and Head
Department of Psychiatry
North Eastern Indira Gandhi Institute of Health and Medical Sciences
Shillong, Meghalaya, India

**Suchandra Harihara** MD (Psychiatry)
PDF in Emergency Psychiatry
Assistant Professor
Department of Psychiatry
National Institute of Mental Health
and Neurosciences
Bengaluru, Karnataka, India

**Sujit Sarkhel** MD (Psychiatry) DPM
Professor
Department of Psychiatry
Institute of Psychiatry
Institute of Postgraduate Medical
Education and Research
Kolkata, West Bengal, India

**Sujita Kumar Kar** MD
Additional Professor
Department of Psychiatry
King George's Medical University
Lucknow, Uttar Pradesh, India

**Sukanto Sarkar**
MBBS DPM MD (Psychiatry)
Professor
Department of Psychiatry
All India Institute of Medical Sciences
Kalyani, West Bengal, India

**Sukriti Mukherjee**
MBBS MD (Psychiatry)
Senior Resident
Department of Psychiatry
All India Institute of Medical Sciences
Kalyani, West Bengal, India

**Sumegha Mittal** MBBS MD (Psychiatry)
Associate Consultant Psychiatrist
Saarthak Mental Health Services
New Delhi, India

**Surendra Paliwal** MD (Psychiatry)
Associate Professor
Department of Psychiatry
Central Institute of Psychiatry
Ranchi, Jharkhand, India

**Suresh Bada Math** MD DNB PGDMLE
PGDHRL PhD in Law (NLSIU)
Professor of Psychiatry
Department of Psychiatry
Head of Forensic Psychiatry Unit
Head of Telemedicine Centre
Head of the Unit-5 (Adult Psychiatry)
Officer-in-Charge of NIMHANS Digital
Academy
Nodal Officer, NMCN
National Institute of Mental Health
and Neurosciences
Bengaluru, Karnataka, India

**Suriya Kumar** MD
Associate Professor
Department of Psychiatry
Mahatma Gandhi Medical College
and Research Institute
Sri Balaji Vidyapeeth
(Deemed-to-be University)
Puducherry, India

**Swarna Buddha Nayok** DPM MD PhD
Assistant Professor and Clinician
Scientist
Centre for Brain and Mind
Department of Psychiatry
National Institute of Mental Health and
Neurosciences
Bengaluru, Karnataka, India

**Tess Maria Rajan** MD DNB DM (Child and
adolescent Psychiatry) MRCPsych
Specialty Registrar (CAMHS)
Cumbria, Northumberland
Tyne and Wear NHS Foundation Trust
Newcastle upon Tyne, UK

**Umesh Shreekantiah**
MD (Psychiatry) DPM
Professor
Department of Psychiatry
Center for Cognitive Neurosciences
and fMRI Center
Central Institute of Psychiatry
Ranchi, Jharkhand, India

**Urvakhsh Meherwan Mehta** MD
Additional Professor
Department of Psychiatry
National Institute of Mental Health
and Neurosciences
Bengaluru, Karnataka, India

**Vaibhav Patil** MD
Associate Professor
Department of Psychiatry
All India Institute of Medical Sciences
New Delhi, India

**Vanteemar S Sreeraj** DPM DNB PDF
Associate Professor
Department of Psychiatry
National Institute of Mental Health
and Neurosciences
Bengaluru, Karnataka, India

**Varun S Mehta** MD DNB (Psychiatry)
MRCPsych
Associate Professor
Department of Psychiatry
Central Institute of Psychiatry
Ranchi, Jharkhand, India

**Venkata Lakshmi Narasimha**
MD PDF DM
Assistant Professor
Centre for Addiction Medicine
Department of Psychiatry
National Institute of Mental Health
and Neurosciences
Bengaluru, Karnataka, India

**Vikas Menon** MD DNB
Professor
Department of Psychiatry
Jawaharlal Institute of Postgraduate
Medical Education and Research
Puducherry, India

**Vinyas Nisarga** MD PDF Child and
Adolescent Psychiatry
Assistant Professor
Department of Psychiatry
Early Intervention and Rehabilitation
Centre
Topiwala National Medical College
and BYL Nair Hospital
Mumbai, Maharashtra, India

**Yatan Pal Singh Balhara** MD DNB
MNAMS MSc
Professor
Department of Psychiatry
National Drug Dependence
Treatment Center
All India Institute of Medical Sciences
New Delhi, India

# Foreword

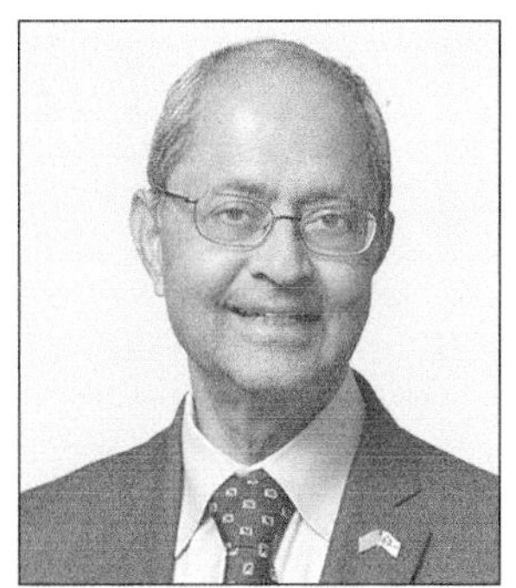

Decision-making is where the rubber meets the road. It is a single act that has enormous consequences, but a number of considerations need to go behind it. The field of psychiatry is not only one of the most challenging areas of medicine in this regard, but also one of the most rewarding. It requires a delicate balance of scientific knowledge, clinical expertise, and compassionate care. The effectiveness of many psychiatric interventions is better than many treatments for many other medical conditions. But the field suffers from paucity of reliable and valid biomarkers to guide treatment for many disorders. There is overwhelming scientific literature out there, of different qualities, sometimes contradictory or indefinite, often done in ideal research settings which may overlook some practical issues in dealing with actual clinical situations in various settings. Many cases a practitioner confronts are complex. The psychiatric clinician at the frontline needs a clear set of recommendations on how to approach common complicated clinical conditions. Such a guide needs to be evidence-informed and provide easy-to-apply, practical approaches. This book *Clinical Decision Making in Psychiatry* by Dr Samir Kumar Praharaj and colleagues does exactly that.

The chapters of this book cover a broad array of topics that are essential for understanding and managing complex mental health conditions. From "difficult-to-treat depression" to "drug-induced sedation," each chapter delves into the intricacies of these conditions, offering insights into their assessment, treatment, and management. It is to the editors' credit that they have kept in mind that clinicians deal with humans and not simply diagnoses, and address problems that are often vexing to our patients, such as sexual dysfunction due to antidepressants, management of lithium-induced cognitive dysfunction, and management of drug-induced constipation.

One of the standout features of this book is its focus on practical, evidence-informed, clinically useful approaches. The authors have meticulously compiled the latest research and clinical guidelines, and added their own clinical expertise, to provide readers with up-to-date information that can be directly applied in clinical practice. From decade-old effective medications such as the still gold standard antimanic agent lithium to avant-garde treatments such as when and how to use ketamine in depressive disorders, a number of treatments are discussed. The use of tables, algorithms, and flowcharts throughout the book further enhances its usability, allowing readers to quickly navigate complex decision-making processes.

A common reason our patients do not adhere to effective and important medications is because of unpleasant side effects, such as gastrointestinal, endocrine, metabolic, or cognitive adverse effects. These can significantly impact a patient's quality of life. Justifiably several chapters are devoted to addressing these issues. When to stop using medications and avoiding irrational pharmacotherapy are also discussed. Depressive and anxiety disorders being so prevalent, several chapters are rightfully devoted to these topics. I commend the authors for incorporating effective nonpharmacologic interventions also, as exemplified by the chapters on management of insomnia and drug-induced sedation.

In sum, *Clinical Decision Making in Psychiatry* is an essential resource for anyone involved in the care of patients with psychiatric conditions. The book's evidence-informed, practical approach, combined with its clear and concise presentation, makes it a timely and invaluable tool for clinicians and students. The authors have done an outstanding job of combing research and clinical literature and their own clinical experience and knowledge of human factors, providing readers with the knowledge and tools they need to make informed, effective decisions in their practice.

I am confident that this book will be a valuable addition to the field of psychiatry and will greatly benefit the patients we serve.

**Ramaswamy Viswanathan**
MD DrMedSc DLFAPA
Professor and Interim Chair
Department of Psychiatry and Behavioral Sciences
Senator, SUNY Faculty Senate
State University of New York Downstate Health Sciences University
Brooklyn, New York
Past President (2024 May–2025 May), American Psychiatric Association

# Preface

In the dynamic and ever-evolving field of psychiatry, clinicians are routinely confronted with complex decisions that demand a nuanced understanding of individual patient contexts, clinical variability, and the expanding body of psychiatric research. *Clinical Decision Making in Psychiatry* emerges as a vital and timely resource, designed to support practitioners in navigating these challenges with confidence and clarity. This book serves not only as a compendium of clinically relevant topics but also as a practical guide that introduces structured, algorithm-driven frameworks to enhance the decision-making process across diverse psychiatric scenarios.

What distinguishes this volume from traditional psychiatric texts is its deliberate integration of evidence-based practices with the experiential insights of frontline clinicians. Each chapter is thoughtfully developed to address the most pressing and commonly encountered challenges in psychiatric diagnosis, treatment planning, and long-term management. Whether dealing with treatment-resistant conditions, comorbidities, or ambiguous symptom profiles, readers will find clear, actionable guidance grounded in the latest scientific literature and real-world clinical experience.

A defining feature of this book is the inclusion of universal decision-making algorithms tailored to each topic. These algorithms offer systematic, step-by-step pathways to help clinicians synthesize information, weigh clinical variables, incorporate patient values, and make informed, personalized choices. They not only provide structure and consistency in clinical reasoning but also support flexibility and individualization—recognizing that every patient presents a unique clinical picture.

*Clinical Decision Making in Psychiatry* is designed to be a practical, go-to reference for psychiatrists, clinical psychologists, psychiatric nurses, social workers, trainees, and other mental health professionals who strive for excellence in patient care. By combining rigorous research, clinical acumen, and adaptable algorithms, this book aspires to be a cornerstone of effective, evidence-informed, and compassionate psychiatric practice.

**Samir Kumar Praharaj**
**Vikas Menon**
**Adarsh Tripathi**
**Sai Krishna Tikka**

# Acknowledgments

We extend our heartfelt gratitude to the President, Secretary, and all the esteemed office bearers of the Indian Psychiatric Society (IPS) for their unwavering support, encouragement, and guidance throughout the development of this book. Their commitment to advancing psychiatric education and practice has been instrumental in bringing this initiative to fruition.

We owe a special debt of appreciation to Dr Vinay Kumar, Past President of the Indian Psychiatric Society, whose vision and initiative laid the foundation for this book. His insightful foresight and dedication to strengthening clinical decision-making in psychiatry inspired this endeavor and provided the initial impetus that made it possible.

This work is a reflection of the collective spirit and commitment of the Indian Psychiatric Society to excellence in mental health care and education.

# Contents

CHAPTER 1

# Assessment of Difficult-to-Treat Depression

*Bandita Abhijita, Vikas Menon*

## INTRODUCTION

Current evidence suggests a high burden of treatment nonresponse in major depression. According to the Sequenced Treatment Alternatives to Relieve Depression (STAR*D) trial, only two-thirds of patients achieved remission even after four sequential treatments.[1] These outcomes and similar research findings formed the basis for the concept of treatment-resistant depression (TRD), typically defined by multiple failed acute phase treatment trials.[2]

However, the TRD construct has been critiqued for its over-reliance on the biomedical model and its definition of treatment response based on pharmacotherapy, without considering potential contributors such as nonadherence, treatment delays, current social circumstances, and comorbidities. Owing to these conceptual issues with TRD, an alternative term was proposed: "Difficult-to-treat depression (DTD)". The consensus definition of DTD, or suspected DTD, is "depression that continues to cause significant burden despite usual treatment efforts".[3] A key feature of DTD is the collaborative biopsychosocial approach to the illness to optimize symptom control, reduce relapse risk, and enhance functional recovery as opposed to the classical approach of focusing on symptom remission.

## ASSESSMENT OF DIFFICULT-TO-TREAT DEPRESSION

An algorithm for assessing DTD and its differential diagnosis are shown in **Flowchart 1**.

### Illness-related Factors

#### *Consideration of Differential Diagnoses*

In all cases of DTD, it is crucial to regularly revisit the diagnosis and rule out common etiologies, particularly affective illness secondary to medical conditions such as dementia or epilepsy. In such cases, the treatment of depression will proceed in parallel with the treatment of underlying medical condition. Cognitive screening using the Mini-Mental State Examination or Montreal Cognitive Assessment should be done, especially in the elderly, as it is well acknowledged that depressive symptoms in this group may herald a diagnosis of dementia. An important differential diagnosis that must always be considered is bipolar depression which can be hard to distinguish from unipolar depression but requires alternate pharmacologic treatment strategies. Primary psychiatric disorders such as eating disorders, substance use, gender identity disturbances, or nonaffective psychosis presenting with secondary depressive symptoms must be considered. In such cases, the resolution of depression is likely contingent upon treatment of the primary condition.

#### *Medical/Psychiatric Comorbidity*

Common psychiatric comorbidities, including, but not limited to, anxiety disorders, post-traumatic stress disorder, attention-deficit hyperactivity disorder, substance use disorders, psychotic disorders, and personality disorders, should be specifically assessed. A peculiar comorbidity in major depression is dysthymia (called "double depression"), where treatment outcomes often involve a return to a "premorbid" dysthymic state. Medical conditions and depression may commonly co-occur; hence, assess for conditions such as asthma, coronary heart disease, diabetes, hypertension, thyroid disorders, pain, and Parkinson's disease through a comprehensive physical examination. These conditions may have a bearing on the prognosis and influence the selection of antidepressant agents from a safety perspective.

#### *Past Medical/Psychiatric History*

Assess the history of past depressive episodes and responses to treatments. This may not only help

**Flowchart 1:** Assessment of difficult-to-treat depression (DTD).

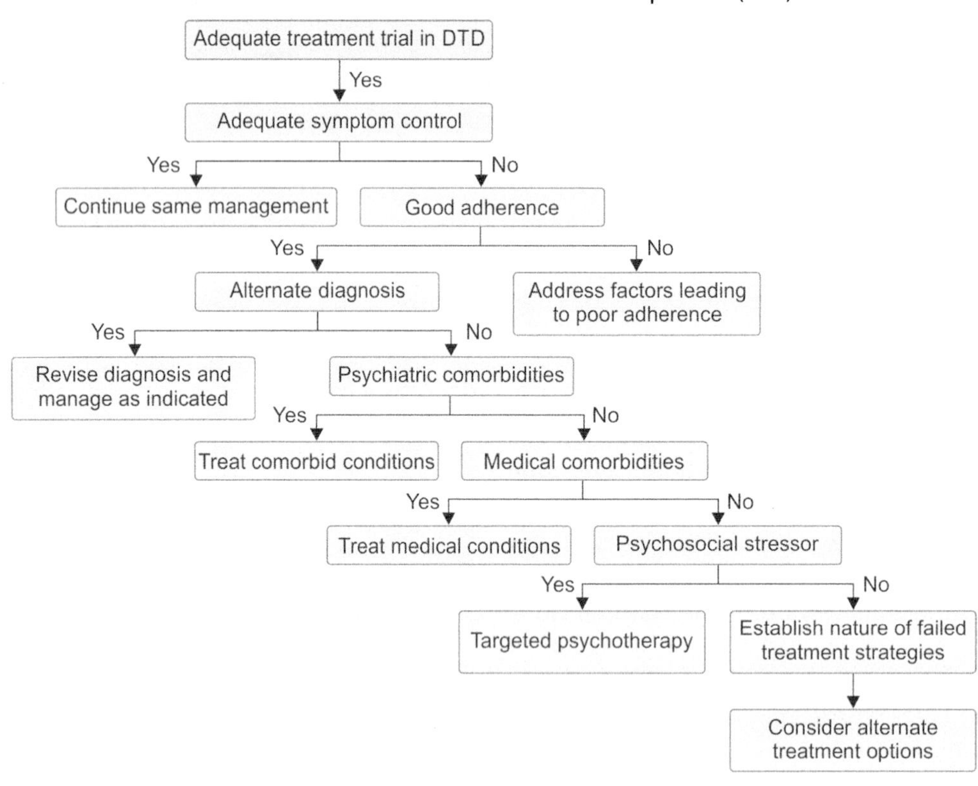


confirm the diagnosis but also provide clues to selecting pharmacologic agents for the current episode, based on past treatment response.

### Symptom Profile

The evidence linking symptom profile, treatment selection, and response remains inconclusive. Some post hoc analyses show a relationship between atypical symptoms and response to monoamine oxidase inhibitors; however, the evidence is not robust enough for definitive recommendations. Nonetheless, critical symptoms, such as suicidality and psychosis, must be diligently examined and may require additional treatments such as antipsychotics for effective management.

## Patient-related Factors

### Role of Stressor

Numerous stressors, such as childhood trauma, stressful life events, or marital separation, are associated with poorer outcomes in depression. If present, they are associated with poorer outcomes and must be addressed adequately by incorporating them into the management plan using additional psychosocial treatments, as indicated.

### Adherence

Suboptimal treatment adherence to physician recommendations, including lifestyle modifications and irregular follow-up, often contribute to many cases of DTD. Wherever feasible, obtaining therapeutic blood levels of medications can help verify medication adherence. If blood tests are unavailable or unaffordable, other adherence measures such as pill counts and pharmacy refill records, although less robust, may be used for verification.

### Assessment of Personality

Certain personality traits have been associated with the risk of depression and the likelihood of treatment response or relapse. For instance, traits such as optimism, but not pessimism, may influence the susceptibility to depression, while both can influence clinical and functional treatment outcomes. Similarly, dependent traits may affect service utilization and treatment outcomes in depression.[3]

## Treatment-related Factors

Key questions pertain to the adequacy of prior treatment trials throughout the course of the illness, including pharmacological, psychological, or neurostimulatory approaches. Has the patient undergone trials of only one class of antidepressants, or have drugs with different mechanisms of action also been considered? What has been the nature, extent, and durability of responses to previous trials? Consistent with staging models for treatment resistance, a patient who has failed multiple classes of antidepressants and electroconvulsive therapy trials might be considered more difficult to treat than a patient who failed a single drug trial. A key caveat is that a partial treatment response with a negative impact on functioning should be considered a treatment failure. At present, evidence is inadequate to advocate for routine therapeutic blood level monitoring or pharmacogenetic testing in DTD.

## Laboratory Evaluation

### *Common Investigations*

Though the utility of laboratory tests for patients with DTD without comorbid physical conditions has not been established, there may be value in performing common laboratory tests. These include complete blood counts, liver and renal function tests, blood biochemistry and metabolic panel, urine screening (routine and toxicology), and thyroid function tests. A baseline electrocardiogram may be helpful in older adults.

### *Additional Investigations*

Additional investigations such as serum vitamin B12, folate, ferritin, magnesium or C-reactive protein levels may be considered as indicated by the patient's history and review of systems.

### *Neuroimaging*

Neuroimaging investigations are indicated for patients with grounds to suspect structural brain disease, including localizing signs, focal neurological deficits, or persistent cognitive deficits. In late-life depression, neuroimaging is an important part of safety assessment for electroconvulsive therapy intended to rule out contraindications such as space-occupying lesions. In this group, it is also used to identify conditions such as neoplasms or structural brain changes (e.g., marked atrophy) that may attenuate response to conventional antidepressant therapy.

## REFERENCES

1. Rush AJ, Trivedi MH, Wisniewski SR, Nierenberg AA, Stewart JW, Warden D, et al. Acute and longer-term outcomes in depressed outpatients requiring one or several treatment steps: a STAR*D report. Am J Psychiatry. 2006;163:1905-17.
2. Fava M. Diagnosis and definition of treatment-resistant depression. Biol Psychiatry. 2003;53:649-59.
3. McAllister-Williams RH, Arango C, Blier P, Demyttenaere K, Falkai P, Gorwood P, et al. The identification, assessment and management of difficult-to-treat depression: An international consensus statement. J Affect Disord. 2020;267:264-82.

# Management of Difficult-to-treat Depression

*Vikas Menon, Subashree Kathatharan*

## INTRODUCTION

Difficult-to-treat depression (DTD) has been defined as "*depression that continues to cause significant burden despite usual treatment efforts*".[1] The term represents a semantic and conceptual change from the earlier concept of treatment-resistant depression, which was critiqued for being nihilistic in outlook and lacking empathy. Fundamentally, the change in terminology represents an attempt to broaden the treatment approach from mainly a physician-oriented biological/biomedical one emphasizing cure to a more collaboratively oriented biopsychosocial approach focusing on optimizing symptom control and minimizing the impact of symptoms on functioning and quality of life.[2] **Flowchart 1** shows management of DTD.

## GENERAL PRINCIPLES AND GOALS OF MANAGEMENT OF DIFFICULT-TO-TREAT DEPRESSION

There are three main principles in the management of DTD:

1. *Formulating treatment goals based on "shared decision-making" with the patient:* This is based on the understanding that a greater convergence between physician and patient expectations results in better treatment outcomes. Further, this approach facilitates the communication of "self-help strategies" designed to empower patients and families to manage their illnesses in the long run.
2. *Implementing measurement-based care:* This involves regularly monitoring the severity of different domains

**Flowchart 1:** Management of difficult-to-treat depression.

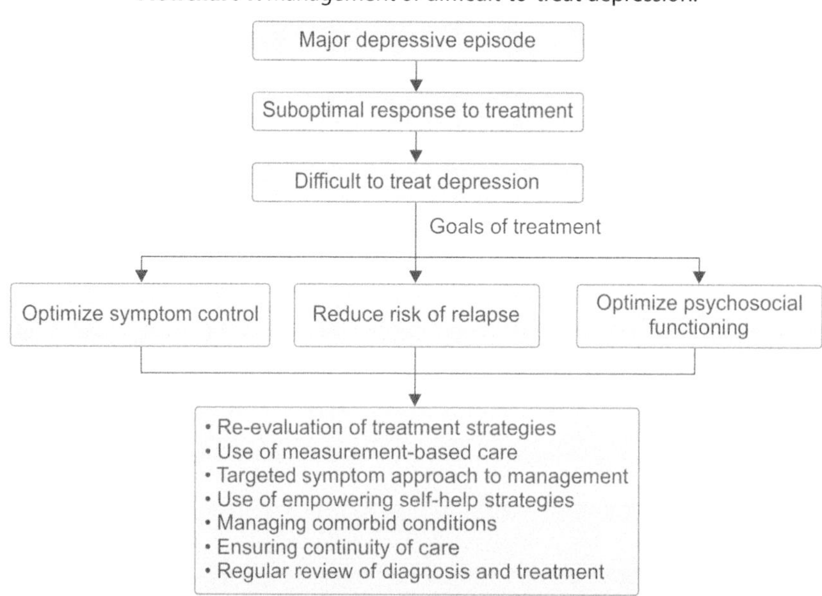

of depression using structured assessment tools to improve outcomes, similar to managing chronic medical illnesses such as diabetes and hypertension.

3. *Periodic reassessment and consideration of treatment direction:* The aim is to balance over- and under-treatment of the patient. This involves periodic reassessment of contributory psychological (e.g., hopelessness) and psychosocial factors (e.g., strained interpersonal relationships) and changes in their nature, and whether these changes necessitate use of additional treatment modalities such as cognitive behavior therapy or interpersonal therapy, or considering alternate treatments such as neuromodulation.

There are two main goals of the management of DTD:

1. *Optimizing symptom control:* Acknowledging the fluctuating nature of symptoms, the goal is to achieve symptom control, recognizing that complete resolution may not be feasible for all patients. It focuses on balancing the burden of symptoms versus treatment, aligning with the principle of maintaining a balance between over- and under-treatment of depression.
2. *Reducing the burden of symptoms and risk of relapse:* Regardless of levels of persistent depressive symptoms, management aims to minimize symptoms' impact on day-to-day functioning, improve quality of life, and curtail risk of relapse.

## HOW TO ACHIEVE THE ABOVE GOALS? A ROADMAP FOR MANAGING DIFFICULT-TO-TREAT DEPRESSION

- *Re-evaluation of treatment strategies:* Numerous consensus guidelines are available for managing major depression. However, a key question arises regarding whether to augment or switch when faced with poor treatment response. As a guiding principle, augmenting in partial response cases and switching in nonresponse cases is a reasonable approach. Clinicians must also recognize when it is appropriate to consider options such as neuromodulation, typically done when reaching a point of diminishing returns in trial-and-error process with different pharmacotherapies.
- *Measuring treatment response:* This includes not only the use of standard rating measures for depression, such as Patient Health Questionnaire 9 (PHQ-9) or Quick Inventory of Depressive Symptomatology 16 (QIDS-16), but also encourages the use of instruments designed to measure disability, functioning and quality of life, such as the Sheehan Disability Scale to capture impairments that more accurately reflect real-world functioning.
- *Targeted symptom-based approach to management:* For instance, focusing on symptoms such as anxiety and pain that are associated with poorer outcomes in depression can be a more efficient and potentially effective approach. This may involve the use of targeted treatments for these symptoms (e.g., quetiapine or gabapentin for anxiety). Likewise, targeting patient-reported symptoms such as fatigue and daytime cognitive impairment, which may contribute to poor functioning, using adjunctive stimulants could be a viable strategy.
- *Managing comorbid conditions to reduce symptom burden:* This not only involves managing comorbid physical conditions but also being mindful of concomitant medications that may either aggravate underlying mood symptoms (e.g., propranolol), or reduce the efficacy of ongoing treatments due to drug interaction (e.g., carbamazepine). There is a bidirectional relationship between conditions such as diabetes and depression; effectively addressing one may positively impact the other. Additionally, psychiatric comorbidities can significantly worsen outcomes in depression and should be considered while managing DTD.
- *Promoting the use of self-help strategies:* There can be times when depression becomes overwhelming, and a feeling of hopelessness creeps in regarding treatment. This is where self-help strategies must be proactively encouraged, aside from encouraging healthy questioning about the basis of maladaptive cognitions. The strategies include healthy lifestyle measures such as good diet and sleep habits, physical exercise, relaxation strategies, and behavioral activation, including activity scheduling. Additionally, the use of online symptom monitoring tools is encouraged.
- *Ensuring access to and continuity of care:* A guiding tenet of the DTD management is the acceptance of the waxing and waning nature of symptoms. Coupled with the inherent patient-centered approach, this implies ensuring continuous access to care, including

primary and secondary health care, as appropriate. It also entails working with the patient's support system to enhance support for both the patient and the caregivers; the latter faces considerable strain while caring for a patient with DTD. These efforts serve to instill a sense of hope and containment in the patient.

- *Regular review of diagnosis and treatment:* In all patients with DTD, planning for regular review is critical to long-term care. Key questions to consider are: What is the level of treatment response across different symptom clusters of depression? Is there any recent worsening of depression? Are there new psychosocial stressors that demand attention? What is the level of treatment adherence? Is there any scope to rationalize the medication regimen? If the response is suboptimal, should the next step involve a switch or augmentation of medications? Should alternate treatment options, such as neuromodulation, be considered? Should a second opinion be obtained, or a referral to a higher center be considered? Due consideration should be given to personalized relapse signatures, increasing resilience and protective factors, and reducing risk factors in preventing relapse for patients with well-controlled symptoms.

In this chapter, we have provided a general roadmap for managing DTD. Recently published evidence-based guidelines for DTD that reviewed six specific interventions found weak evidence for repetitive transcranial magnetic stimulation and cognitive behavioral analysis system of psychotherapy (CBASP). In contrast, insufficient evidence was noted for using bright light therapy, intravenous ketamine/esketamine, rumination-focused psychotherapy, or cognitive remediation for patients with DTD.[3]

To conclude, the management of DTD is predicated upon the twin goals of optimizing symptom control and functioning and reducing the risk of symptom relapse through a collaborative, patient-centered approach while recognizing that full remission may not be achievable for all patients with major depression. Using measurement-based care, a targeted symptom approach to management, empowering patients through self-help strategies, and regular review of diagnosis and treatment are central to managing DTD.

## REFERENCES

1. McAllister-Williams RH, Arango C, Blier P, Demyttenaere K, Falkai P, Gorwood P, et al. The identification, assessment and management of difficult-to-treat depression: An international consensus statement. J Affect Disord 2020;267:264-82.
2. Rush AJ, Aaronson ST, Demyttenaere K. Difficult-to-treat depression: A clinical and research roadmap for when remission is elusive. Aust N Z J Psychiatry. 2019;53:109-18.
3. Moeller SB, Gbyl K, Hjorthøj C, Andreasen M, Austin SF, Buchholtz PE, et al. Treatment of difficult-to-treat depression—clinical guideline for selected interventions. Nord J Psychiatry. 2022;76:177-88.

# How to Choose which Antidepressant to Initiate?

*Rajshekhar Bipeta, Shanti Mohan Kethawath, Raviteja Innamuri*

## INTRODUCTION

Depression is a common mental health disorder with varying presentations. Clinicians choose antidepressants based on presenting symptoms. Symptom severity is an important factor for guiding treatment options. For mild depression, first-line management typically involves nonpharmacological approaches such as psychoeducation, self-management, and psychological therapies. However, antidepressants may be considered in certain cases, such as previous positive response or failure of nonpharmacological treatments.[1] For moderate to severe depression, globally all the guidelines recommend initiating antidepressants with or without nonpharmacological interventions.

Antidepressants effective in reducing depressive symptoms, but response rates vary. In one study, 50% of patients with moderate-to-severe depression responded to antidepressants, compared to 20% with no treatment.[2] However, the first antidepressant is effective in only 50–60% of cases.[3] The sequenced treatment alternatives to relieve depression (STAR*D) study found that over 40% of patients with major depressive disorder (MDD) did not achieve remission even after two optimal antidepressant trials.[4] These findings highlight that multiple factors can influence antidepressant response.

## SELECTING AN ANTIDEPRESSANT

The Canadian Network for Mood and Anxiety Treatments (CANMAT) guidelines[1] provide an antidepressant selection algorithm **(Flowchart 1)** and summarize available treatment options **(Table 1)**. While many medications are suitable for initiating treatment, selecting the right antidepressant in clinical practice can be challenging. Key factors influencing this decision are outlined in **Table 2** and discussed.

## SOME KEY QUESTIONS TO BE ANSWERED BEFORE INITIATING ANTIDEPRESSANTS

### Did the Patient Previously Respond to a Certain Antidepressant?

Both International and Indian Clinical Practice Guidelines recommend using the same antidepressant if the patient previously responded well.[5,6] Hence, it is recommended

**Flowchart 1:** Antidepressant selection algorithm.[4]

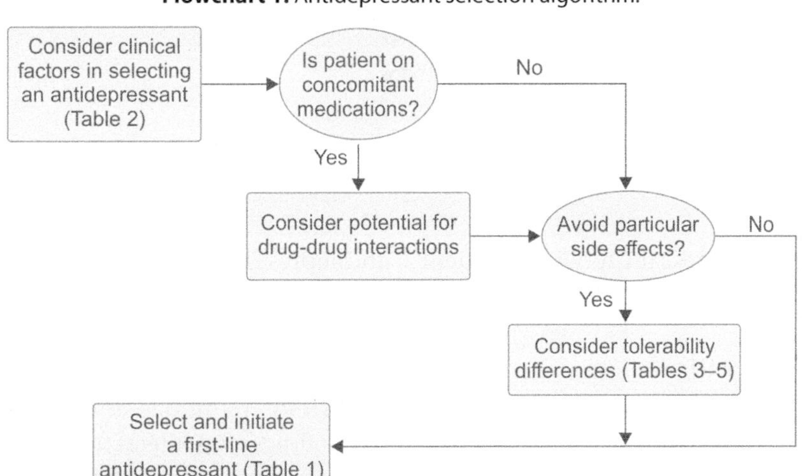

**TABLE 1:** Summary of recommended antidepressants.

| *Antidepressant* | *Mechanism* | *Dose range* |
|---|---|---|
| *First-line antidepressants* | | |
| Desvenlafaxine | SNRI | 50–100 mg |
| Duloxetine | SNRI | 60 mg |
| Escitalopram | SSRI | 10–20 mg |
| Fluoxetine | SSRI | 20–60 mg |
| Fluvoxamine | SSRI | 100–300 mg |
| Mianserin | α2-Adrenergic agonist; 5-HT2 antagonist | 60–120 mg |
| Milnacipran | SNRI | 100 mg |
| Mirtazapine | α2-Adrenergic agonist; 5-HT2 antagonist | 15–45 mg |
| Paroxetine | SSRI | 20–50 mg<br>25–62.5 mg for CR version |
| Sertraline | SSRI | 50–200 mg |
| Venlafaxine | SNRI | 75–225 mg |
| Vortioxetine | Serotonin reuptake inhibitor; 5-HT1A agonist; 5-HT1B partial agonist; 5-HT1D, 5-HT3A, and 5-HT7 antagonist | 10–20 mg |
| Agomelatine | MT1 and MT2 agonist; 5-HT2 antagonist | 25–50 mg |
| Bupropion | NDRI | 150–300 mg |
| Citalopram | SSRI | 20–40 mg |
| *Second-line antidepressants* (higher side effect burden) | | |
| Amitriptyline, clomipramine, and others | TCA | Various dosages |
| Levomilnacipran (lack of comparative and relapse-prevention data) | SNRI | |
| Moclobemide | Reversible inhibitor of MAO-A | 300–600 mg |
| Selegiline transdermal | Irreversible MAO-B inhibitor | 6–12 mg daily transdermal |
| Trazodone | Serotonin reuptake inhibitor; 5-HT2 antagonist | 150–300 mg |
| Vilazodone (lack of comparative and relapse prevention data, need to titrate and taken with food) | Serotonin reuptake inhibitor; 5-HT1A partial agonist | 20–40 mg (titrate from 10 mg) |
| *Third-line antidepressants* (higher side effect burden, potential serious drug, and dietary interactions) | | |
| Phenelzine | Irreversible MAO inhibitor | 45–90 mg |
| Tranylcypromine | Irreversible MAO inhibitor | 20–60 mg |
| Reboxetine (lower efficacy) | Noradrenaline reuptake inhibitor | 8–10 mg |

(5-HT: 5-Hydroxy Tryptamine (Serotonin); MAO: monoamine oxidase; MT: melatonin; NDRI: noradrenaline and dopamine reuptake inhibitor; SNRI: serotonin and noradrenaline reuptake inhibitor; SSRI: selective serotonin reuptake inhibitor; TCA: tricyclic antidepressant)

to reinitiate the same antidepressant to which patient responded previously.

## Is There a Family History of Antidepressant Response?

Genetic variation significantly affects antidepressant response.[7] A positive family history of response to a specific antidepressant can guide treatment choice, making it reasonable to consider the same medication.

## Is the Patient Taking Several Drugs?

Comorbid conditions and polypharmacy increase the risk of drug-drug interactions. It is prudent to remember the adverse pharmacokinetic and pharmacodynamic

**TABLE 2:** Factors to consider while initiating an antidepressant.

| *Clinical Profile* | *Comorbid conditions* | *Medication-related factors* | *Other factors* |
|---|---|---|---|
| • Clinical features such as loss of appetite/increased appetite, decreased sleep/over sleepy (clinical specifiers as per DSM-5)<br>• Age<br>• Pregnancy/postpartum<br>• Previous drug response<br>• Family history of drug response | • Comorbid psychiatric conditions<br>• Comorbid medical conditions | • Drug efficacy<br>• Drug tolerability (side effects)<br>• Potential drug-drug interactions<br>• Easiness of availability<br>• Cost effective | • Patient preference<br>• Doctors' preference |

(DSM-5: Diagnostic and Statistical Manual of Mental Disorders, 5th edition)

interactions of some antidepressants, not only while initiating but also during switching. Certain selective serotonin reuptake inhibitors (SSRIs)—fluoxetine, fluvoxamine, and paroxetine—are more likely to cause interactions due to enzyme inhibition. In patients with chronic health issues, sertraline or escitalopram may be safer options due to their lower interaction potential. Additionally, SSRIs can increase bleeding risk, especially in older adults; gastroprotective agents should be considered when coprescribed with nonsteroidal anti-inflammatory drugs (NSAIDs) or aspirin.

## Is there Persistent Pain?

Chronic pain is common and often linked to depression, with musculoskeletal pain (e.g., back pain) being the most prevalent, followed by headaches, orofacial, and visceral pain.[8] Serotonin and noradrenaline reuptake inhibitors (SNRIs) such as duloxetine and venlafaxine show moderate certainty of evidence of efficacy in treating chronic back pain, postoperative pain, fibromyalgia, and neuropathic pain.[9] Tricyclic antidepressants (TCAs) are effective for conditions such as irritable bowel syndrome,[10] neuropathic pain,[11] and chronic tension-type headaches.[12]

## Is there Existing Cardiovascular Disease?

Sertraline is considered relatively safe for patients with cardiovascular disease. In contrast, antidepressants such as bupropion, citalopram, escitalopram, moclobemide, lofepramine, and venlafaxine should be used cautiously—or avoided—in those at risk of arrhythmias, such as patients with heart failure, left ventricular hypertrophy, prior arrhythmia, or myocardial infarction.[13]

The TCAs (except lofepramine) have established arrhythmogenic potential due to sodium and potassium channel blockade[14] and are best avoided in such patients. Other non-TCAs have a very low risk of inducing arrhythmia. The risk is dose-dependent. If use is unavoidable, ECG monitoring is recommended at baseline, after dose increases, and periodically.

Regarding overdose risk, TCAs (excluding lofepramine) have the highest fatal toxicity index (FTI), while venlafaxine and moclobemide have moderate toxicity. SSRIs, mirtazapine, and reboxetine have lower FTI scores.[15,16]

## Is there a Lack of Sleep, a Decrease of Appetite, or Weight Loss?

**Table 3** outlines the relative sedative and weight gain effects of various antidepressants. Sometimes, these side effects can be therapeutically beneficial. For example, TCAs cause sedation and weight gain due to their antihistaminic (H1) activity, but are generally not first-line treatments due to significant anticholinergic side effects such as blurred vision, constipation, dry mouth, confusion, urinary retention, and tachycardia.[17]

Mirtazapine, a noradrenergic and specific serotonergic antidepressant (NaSSA), blocks adrenergic alpha-2 autoreceptors, and alpha-2 heteroreceptors as well as 5HT1, 5-HT2, and 5-HT3 receptors. It has fewer anticholinergic effects than TCAs and is better tolerated. Its strong antihistaminic action causes sedation and weight gain, making it useful for patients with insomnia, poor appetite, or weight loss associated with depression.

## Is Patient Sleeping Excessively?

Insomnia is a common symptom of depression and may also result from medications, substance use, poor sleep hygiene, or a combination of factors. Some antidepressants, such as mirtazapine and TCAs, have sedative properties, while others, such as SSRIs, can be activating **(Table 4)**. These effects can be strategically used

**TABLE 3:** Relative sedative and weight gain properties of antidepressants.

| | *Medication* | *Sedation* | *Weight gain* | *Remarks* |
|---|---|---|---|---|
| SSRI | Escitalopram | 0 | 2+ | |
| | Fluoxetine | 0 | 1+ | |
| | Fluvoxamine | 1+ | 1+ | |
| | Paroxetine | 1+ | 2+ | |
| | Sertraline | 1+ | 1+ | |
| Others | Vilazodone | 1+ | 1+ | |
| SNRI | Desvenlafaxine | 1+ | 0 | |
| | Duloxetine | 0 | 1+ | |
| | Venlafaxine-XR | 1+ | 1+ | |
| NDRI | Bupropion-XL | 0 | 0 | Comorbid nicotine use disorder |
| NaSSA | Mirtazapine | 4+ | 4+ | |

(NaSSA: noradrenergic and specific serotonergic antidepressant; NDRI: noradrenaline and dopamine reuptake inhibitor; SSRI: selective serotonin reuptake inhibitor; SNRI: serotonin and noradrenaline reuptake inhibitor; TCA: tricyclic antidepressant; XR: extended-release; XL: extended-release)

**TABLE 4:** Tendency of the antidepressant medication to cause insomnia.

| | *Medication* | *Insomnia* |
|---|---|---|
| SSRI | Escitalopram | 1+ |
| | Fluoxetine | 2+ |
| | Fluvoxamine | 1+ |
| | Paroxetine | 1+ |
| | Sertraline | 2+ |
| Others | Vilazodone | 1+ |
| SNRI | Desvenlafaxine | 2+ |
| | Duloxetine | 2+ |
| | Levomilnacipran | 2+ |
| | Venlafaxine-XR | 2+ |
| NDRI | Bupropion-XL | 2+ |

(NaSSA: noradrenergic and specific serotonergic antidepressant; NDRI: noradrenaline and dopamine reuptake inhibitor; SSRI: selective serotonin reuptake inhibitor; SNRI: serotonin and noradrenaline reuptake inhibitor; XR: extended-release; XL: extended-release)

to match the patient's symptom profile and improve sleep when needed.

## Is the Patient Concerned about Sexual Adverse Effects?

Sexual dysfunction, such as reduced libido or erectile dysfunction, can be a symptom of depression or a side effect of antidepressants—particularly at higher doses. In such cases, medications such as mirtazapine, bupropion, or vilazodone **(Table 5)** may be preferred due to their lower risk of sexual side effects. Conversely, certain SSRIs (e.g., fluoxetine and sertraline) may delay ejaculation even at low doses, which can be beneficial in patients presenting with premature ejaculation.

**TABLE 5:** Tendency of antidepressant medication to cause sexual dysfunction.

| *Category* | *Medication* | *Sexual* |
|---|---|---|
| Others | Vilazodone | 0 to 1+ |
| | Vortioxetine | 0 to 3+ |
| NDRI | Bupropion-XL | 0 |
| NaSSA | Mirtazapine | 1+ |

(NDRI: noradrenaline and dopamine reuptake inhibitor; NaSSA: noradrenergic and specific serotonergic antidepressant; XL: extended-release)

## Is the Patient a Child or Adolescent (Under the Age of 18)?

The NICE guidelines, along with Treatment of Adolescents with Depression Study (TADS) and Treatment of Resistant Depression in Adolescence (TORDIA) studies, support combining antidepressants with psychological interventions for treating depression in children and adolescents. For moderate-to-severe depression, SSRIs are first-line agents. In the U.S., fluoxetine and escitalopram are Food and Drug Administration (FDA) approved for this age group, with fluoxetine licensed for prepubertal children (over 8 years). Treatment should follow the "start low, go slow" approach, with twice-daily dosing due to faster metabolism in children. Careful monitoring is essential for activating effects, suicidal behaviors, and hostility.

## Is the Patient Pregnant or Postpartum?

Antidepressant use in pregnancy—primarily SSRIs—is more common than often assumed. Concerns include risks of miscarriage, preterm birth, low birth weight, neonatal respiratory distress, low APGAR scores, neonatal intensive care unit (NICU) admission, and increased rates of gestational hypertension, preeclampsia, and postpartum hemorrhage. Women already stable on antidepressants and at risk of relapse should usually continue the same medication. For untreated cases, sertraline is preferred, with mirtazapine as an option if sleep disturbance is prominent. Breastfeeding is encouraged to reduce the risk of neonatal withdrawal symptoms after delivery.

## Is Price a Concern? If so, Have a Glance at Less Expensive Drugs

Psychiatric treatment is typically long-term, and medication costs represent a recurring, direct expense—often a key factor influencing adherence, especially in low- and middle-income populations.[18,19] Despite this, cost considerations are frequently overlooked in clinical training and practice. It is essential to discuss medication affordability with patients and caregivers before initiating treatment. Clinicians should recommend the most affordable brands ensuring quality, while avoiding low cost, unregulated alternatives.[20]

**Table 6** presents the approximate monthly cost of the minimum effective doses of commonly prescribed antidepressants, based on Maudsley Prescribing Guidelines and prescription patterns reported by Tripathi et al. (2016).[21] Prices are average online costs, with ceiling prices applied for fluoxetine, escitalopram, amitriptyline, and clomipramine as set by the National Pharmaceutical Pricing Authority (https://www.nppaindia.nic.in/wp-content/uploads/2022/09/Compendium-Prices-2022.pdf).

**TABLE 6:** Cost incurred per month for minimum effective dosage of antidepressant.

| *Antidepressant medication* | *Recommended minimum effective dosage of antidepressants* | *Average cost per tablet* | *Cost of the average dosage incurred per month (price per tablet × 30 days) in INR* |
|---|---|---|---|
| *SSRIs* | | | |
| Fluoxetine | 20 mg/day | 4* (DPCO) | 120 |
| Escitalopram | 10 mg/day | 9* (DPCO) | 270 |
| Sertraline | 50 mg/day | 10 | 300 |
| Fluvoxamine | 50 mg/day | 16 | 480 |
| Paroxetine | 20 mg/day | 24 | 720 |
| *Others* | | | |
| Amitriptyline | 75 mg/day | 6* (DPCO) | 180 |
| Desvenlafaxine | 50 mg/day | 15 | 450 |
| Mirtazapine | 30 mg/day | 15 | 450 |
| Vortioxetine | 10 mg/day | 15 | 450 |
| Trazodone | 150 mg/day | 16 | 480 |
| Vilazodone | 20 mg/day | 18 | 540 |
| Duloxetine | 60 mg/day | 25 | 750 |

*Note:*
**DPCO: Drugs (Prices Control) Order ceiling price 2022 (rounded figure)*

## Favored by the Patient

Patient preference often stems from informed, collaborative decision-making between the psychiatrist and patient, which enhances adherence and overall quality of life. Preferences are shaped by the therapeutic relationship and past experiences with antidepressants, including efficacy and side effects. Clinicians can support this process by reviewing the patient's treatment history in a structured format **(Table 7)**, helping identify the medication that provided the best balance of symptom relief and quality of life.

**TABLE 7:** Parameters to help choose the patient favored antidepressant through collaborative decision making.

| *Medication name* | *Drug 1* | *Drug 2* | *Drug 3* | *Drug 4* |
|---|---|---|---|---|
| Maximum dosage | | | | |
| Adherence | | | | |
| Duration | | | | |
| Response | | | | |
| Augmentation | | | | |
| Side effects | | | | |
| Adverse drug reaction (ADR) | | | | |
| Quality of life | | | | |

## OTHERS FACTORS TO BE CONSIDERED

Depression presents heterogeneously and often includes emotional and behavioral disturbances. To better classify these variations, the Diagnostic and Statistical Manual of Mental Disorders, 5th edition (DSM-5)[22] uses episode and course specifiers for MDD, while clinical dimensions such as cognitive dysfunction, sleep disturbance, and

**TABLE 8:** Recommendations for clinical specifiers and dimensions of major depressive disorder.

| *Specifiers/dimensions* | *Recommendations (level of evidence)* | *Comments* |
|---|---|---|
| With anxious distress[a] | Use an antidepressant with efficacy in generalized anxiety disorder (Level 4) | No differences in efficacy between SSRIs, SNRIs, and bupropion (Level 2) |
| With catatonic features[a] | Benzodiazepines (Level 3) | No antidepressants have been studied |
| With melancholic features[a] | No specific antidepressants have demonstrated superiority (Level 2) | TCAs and SNRIs have been studied |
| With atypical features[a] | No specific antidepressants have demonstrated superiority (Level 2) | Older studies found MAO inhibitors superior to TCAs |
| With psychotic features[a] | Use antipsychotic and antidepressant cotreatment (Level 1) | Few studies involved atypical antipsychotics |
| With mixed features[a] | • Lurasidone[b] (Level 2)<br>• Ziprasidone[b] (Level 3) | No comparative studies |
| With seasonal pattern[a] | • No specific antidepressants have demonstrated superiority (Level 2 and 3) | SSRIs, agomelatine, bupropion, and moclobemide have been studied |
| With cognitive dysfunction | • Vortioxetine (Level 1)<br>• Bupropion (Level 2)<br>• Duloxetine (Level 2)<br>• SSRIs (Level 2)[b]<br>• Moclobemide (Level 3) | Limited data available on cognitive effects of other antidepressants and on comparative differences in efficacy |
| With sleep disturbances | • Agomelatine (Level 1)<br>• Mirtazapine (Level 2)<br>• Quetiapine (Level 2)<br>• Trazodone (Level 2) | Beneficial effects on sleep must be balanced against potential for side effects (e.g., daytime sedation) |
| With somatic symptoms | • Duloxetine (pain) (Level 1)<br>• Other SNRIs (pain) (Level 2)<br>• Bupropion (fatigue) (Level 1)<br>• SSRIs[b] (fatigue) (Level 2)<br>• Duloxetine[b] (energy) (Level 2) | • Few antidepressants have been studied for somatic symptoms other than pain<br>• Few comparative antidepressant studies for pain and other somatic symptoms |

(MAO: monoamine oxidase; SNRI: serotonin and noradrenaline reuptake inhibitor; SSRI: selective serotonin reuptake inhibitor; TCA: tricyclic antidepressant)

*Notes:*

[a]*DSM-5 specifiers*

[b]*Comparisons only with placebo*

*Level of evidence:* (1) Meta-analysis with narrow confidence intervals and/or 2 or more randomized controlled trials (RCTs) with adequate sample size, preferably placebo controlled; (2) meta-analyses with wide confidence intervals and/or 1 or more RCTs with adequate sample size; (3) small-sample RCTs or nonrandomized, controlled prospective studies or case series or high-quality retrospective studies; and (4) expert opinion/consensus.

somatic symptoms (e.g., pain and fatigue) have also been proposed.[4] Although many antidepressants have been evaluated for these subtypes, most studies compare them to placebo, with limited evidence on differential efficacy. The CANMAT guidelines recommend specific antidepressants based on subtypes and specifiers (summarized in **Table 8**). Age is another key factor—fluoxetine is the only antidepressant consistently shown to be effective in children,[23] while a broader range of options is suitable for adults and older adults.

## CONCLUSION

The SSRIs remain the first-line treatment for depression, with escitalopram and sertraline ranking highest in efficacy, tolerability, and acceptability—supported by evidence-based medicine, cost-effectiveness, and prescribing trends. The main concern is a higher incidence of sexual dysfunction. However, the overall benefits outweigh the risks, including in populations such as pregnant women, where the small risk of postpartum hemorrhage or neonatal behavioral syndrome is outweighed by the benefit of treatment.

Few clinical dictums that may help in routine practice are mentioned below.

- Though SSRIs are well tolerated, drug-drug interactions with fluoxetine and fluvoxamine need to be considered in people on multiple medications/comorbidities. Fluoxetine can be stopped abruptly with lesser risks of discontinuation syndrome.
- TCAs and desvenlafaxine/venlafaxine may have marginally higher efficacy.
- The choice of antidepressant can be determined by subtype of depression:
  - Atypical depression—SNRI/monoamine oxidase inhibitor (MAOI)
  - Bipolar depression—bupropion (lesser risk of switch)
  - Melancholic/biological depression—TCA/SNRI
  - Resistant depression—mirtazapine + venlafaxine/TCA
- The choice of antidepressant can be determined by comorbidity:
  - If comorbid obsessive-compulsive disorder (OCD)—prefer SSRI (higher dose)
  - Insomnia—mirtazapine
  - Panic symptoms—TCA/SNRI
  - Substance use—SSRI/bupropion
- The choice of antidepressant can be determined by comorbidity as well. For example, in case of sexual dysfunction—mirtazapine/bupropion/vilazodone can be preferred.

## REFERENCES


1. Lam RW, Kennedy SH, Parikh SV, MacQueen GM, Milev RV, Ravindran AV; CANMAT Depression Work Group. Canadian Network for Mood and Anxiety Treatments (CANMAT) 2016 Clinical Guidelines for the Management of Adults with Major Depressive Disorder: Introduction and Methods. Can J Psychiatry. 2016;61(9):506-9.
2. Anderson IM, Ferrier IN, Baldwin RC, Cowen PJ, Howard L, Lewis G, et al. Evidence-based guidelines for treating depressive disorders with antidepressants: a revision of the 2000 British Association for Psychopharmacology guidelines. J Psychopharmacol. 2008;22:343-96.
3. Frodl T. Recent advances in predicting responses to antidepressant treatment. F1000Res. 2017;6:F1000 Faculty Rev-619.
4. Nierenberg AA, Fava M, Trivedi MH, Wisniewski SR, Thase ME, McGrath PJ, et al. A comparison of lithium and T3 augmentation following two failed medication treatments for depression: a STAR*D report. Am J Psychiatry. 2006;163(9):1519-30.
5. Gautam S, Jain A, Gautam M, Vahia VN, Grover S. Clinical Practice Guidelines for the management of Depression. Indian J Psychiatry. 2017;59(Suppl 1):S34-S50.
6. Bosman RC, Waumans RC, Jacobs GE, Oude Voshaar RC, Muntingh ADT, Batelaan NM, et al. Failure to Respond after Reinstatement of Antidepressant Medication: A Systematic Review. Psychother Psychosom. 2018;87(5):268-75.
7. Pain O, Hodgson K, Trubetskoy V, Ripke S, Marshe VS, Adams MJ, et al; GSRD Consortium; Major Depressive Disorder Working Group of the Psychiatric Genomics Consortium; McIntosh AM, Lewis CM. Identifying the Common Genetic Basis of Antidepressant Response. Biol Psychiatry Glob Open Sci. 2022;2(2):115-26.
8. Ferreira GE, Abdel-Shaheed C, Underwood M, Finnerup NB, Day RO, McLachlan A, et al. Efficacy, safety, and tolerability of antidepressants for pain in adults: overview of systematic reviews. BMJ. 2023;380:e072415.
9. Ferreira GE, McLachlan AJ, Lin CC, Zadro JR, Abdel-Shaheed C, O'Keeffe M, et al. Efficacy and safety of anti-depressants for the treatment of back pain and osteoarthritis: systematic review and meta-analysis. BMJ. 2021;372:m4825.
10. Ford AC, Lacy BE, Harris LA, Quigley EMM, Moayyedi P. Effect of Antidepressants and Psychological Therapies in Irritable Bowel Syndrome: An Updated Systematic Review and Meta-Analysis. Am J Gastroenterol. 2019;114:21-39.
11. Finnerup NB, Attal N, Haroutounian S, McNicol E, Baron R, Dworkin RH, et al. Pharmacotherap for neuropathic pain in adults: a systematic review and meta-analysis. Lancet Neurol. 2015;14:162-73.
12. Jackson JL, Mancuso JM, Nickoloff S, Bernstein R, Kay C. Tricyclic and Tetracyclic Antidepressants for the Prevention of Frequent Episodic or Chronic Tension-Type Headache in Adults: A Systematic Review and Meta-Analysis. J Gen Intern Med. 2017;32:1351-8.
13. Taylor DM, Barnes TR, Young AH. The Maudsley prescribing guidelines in psychiatry. Philadelphia: John Wiley & Sons; 2021.
14. Thanacoody HK, Thomas SH. Tricyclic antidepressant poisoning: cardiovascular toxicity. Toxicol Rev 2005;24:205-14.

15. Buckley NA, McManus PR. Fatal toxicity of serotoninergic and other antidepressant drugs: analysis of United Kingdom mortality data. BMJ. 2002;325:1332-3.
16. Morgan O, Griffiths C, Baker A, Majeed A. Fatal toxicity of antidepressants in England and Wales, 1993-2002. Health Stat Q. 2004;(23):18-24.
17. Güloglu C, Orak M, Ustündag M, Altunci YA. Analysis of amitriptyline overdose in emergency medicine. Emerg Med J. 2011;28(4):296-9.
18. Roy R, Jahan M, Kumari S, Chakraborty P. Reasons for Drug Non-Compliance of Psychiatric Patients: A Centre Based Study. J Indian Acad Appl Psychol. 2005;31(1-2):24-8.
19. Taj R, Khan S. 2005. A Study of Reasons of Non-Compliance to Psychiatric Treatment. J Ayub Med Coll Abbottabad: 2005;17(2):26-8.
20. Lal A, ML S. A calm look at cost of drugs in psychiatric practice. Indian J Psychiatry. 1992;34(1): 18-20.
21. Tripathi A, Avasthi A, Desousa A, Bhagabati D, Shah N, Kallivayalil RA, et al. 2016. Prescription Pattern of Antidepressants in Five Tertiary Care Psychiatric Centres of India. Indian J Med Res. 2016;143 (4):507-13.
22. American Psychiatric Association (APA). Diagnostic and statistical manual of mental disorders. 5th ed. Arlington (VA): APA; 2013.
23. Cipriani A, Zhou X, Del Giovane C, Hetrick SE, Qin B, Whittington C, Coghill D, et al. Comparative efficacy and tolerability of antidepressants for major depressive disorder in children and adolescents: a network meta-analysis. Lancet. 2016;388:881-90.

# Pharmacological Management of Depression: How to Decide for Switching or Augmentation?

*Pratap Sharan, Sumegha Mittal*

## INTRODUCTION

Unipolar major depression [major depressive disorder (MDD)] is diagnosed in patients who have experienced at least one major depressive episode without a history of mania or hypomania. Pharmacological treatment remains the primary approach for managing unipolar depression. Despite advances in antidepressant therapy, initial response rates are moderate (40–60%), and full remission is achieved in about 30–45% of patients. Treatment-resistant depression (TRD) is defined as having failed at least two prior treatment attempts in adequate dose and duration (typically, six weeks at a recognized minimum dose).[1,2]

## TREATMENT APPROACHES IN CASE OF NO OR POOR RESPONSE TO FIRST ANTIDEPRESSANT

The Canadian Network for Mood and Anxiety Treatment (CANMAT Guidelines) suggests that if there is no response to initial antidepressant dose within 2–4 weeks, the next step is to increase the dose of the same antidepressant. But if there is still no or insufficient response to optimally dosed antidepressants medications, consider one of the following treatment strategies:

- Pharmacotherapy with another antidepressant "(switching strategies)"
- Adding another antidepressant "(combination strategy)"
- Adding other psychotropic medications "(augmentation strategies)"

No single strategy is universally preferred over others in treatment guidelines.

### Switching Strategies

The switching approach involves discontinuing an ineffective antidepressant and initiating a new antidepressant from a similar (*in-class* switch) or different (*out-of-class* switch) class for patients who do not respond to the first or subsequent trials of antidepressants. In-class switching usually occurs after the initial trial fails to produce a response (<35% improvement) or when the first antidepressant needs to be discontinued due to intolerable side effects or drug interactions in patients with nonpsychotic major depression.

Switching is often chosen over augmentation or combination therapy for patients with mild-to-moderate depression and lesser functional impairment. Switching antidepressants is preferable because of better adherence and lower costs associated with monotherapy than combination treatment.

Antidepressants with a short half-life, such as paroxetine or venlafaxine, should not be stopped abruptly. Typically, these medications are cross-tapered with another antidepressant when switching. However, if patients experience intolerable or serious side effects, the ongoing antidepressant can be stopped abruptly, and the new antidepressant can be started the following day. For patients on antidepressants with a long-half life like fluoxetine, it is recommended to wait for an adequate washout period before starting the next antidepressant, to decrease the risk of serotonin syndrome.

Switching to non-serotonin-specific reuptake inhibitor (SSRI) antidepressant, such as serotonin–norepinephrine reuptake inhibitor (SNRI) or tricyclic antidepressant (TCA), may be a better switching strategy in patients with severe or melancholic nonpsychotic major depression due to their broader receptor profile. However, broad-spectrum antidepressants are often associated with higher discontinuation rates than SSRI, because of their increased side effects.

The Sequenced Treatment Alternatives to Relieve Depression (STAR-D) study reported that switching to either mirtazapine or nortriptyline were comparable after two unsuccessful trials of antidepressants.

## Combination Strategy

Combination strategies involve adding two or more antidepressants together. Combining with another antidepressant is preferred for patients who had partial response to an initial trial of antidepressant. Combining antidepressants with different mechanisms of action can enhance the efficacy of the initial antidepressant; for example, combining mirtazapine and bupropion. Strong evidence supports combining SSRIs/SNRIs with noradrenergic and specific serotonergic antidepressants (NaSSAs)/serotonin antagonist and reuptake inhibitors (SARIs), as this combination often has a synergistic effect.

Combination approaches can also improve the tolerability of an initial antidepressant. For example, adding bupropion, an noradrenaline and dopamine reuptake inhibitor/releaser (NDRI) to SSRI/SNRI can help mitigate side effects such as sedation, weight gain, or sexual dysfunction. Boosting noradrenergic neurotransmission is beneficial for some depressed patients, especially those with fatigue, apathy, and mental or physical slowing. Antidepressants like desipramine and bupropion are used for this purpose.

Bupropion is effective and well-studied in early-stage TRD, but its use in this context is not reflected in most guidelines.

## Augmentation Strategies

Augmentation strategies involve adding a non-antidepressant medication to an antidepressant that is usually partially effective. These strategies are typically indicated for patients with TRD. Patients who have tolerated their initial antidepressant but experienced a partial response (>25% improvement) may benefit from the addition of another psychotropic medication.[3] Augmenting an antidepressant with a second drug may provide faster, complimentary, or synergistic effects, compared to switching antidepressants, as the added agent works through a different mechanism of action.

Augmentation with second-generation antipsychotic drugs (SGAs) is well established as a first-line medication in TRD. In patients with psychotic depression, adding an antipsychotic medication is preferred. Antipsychotics with evidence as an augmentation treatment for depression include aripiprazole, olanzapine (in combination with fluoxetine), quetiapine (extended release), brexpiprazole, and risperidone. Aripiprazole is particularly recommended atypical antipsychotic for TRD. Recommended dose for SGAs in unipolar depression are typically lower than those used in schizophrenia management.

Augmentation with lithium is effective, specifically in patients at high risk of suicide, or with a family history of bipolar disorder, or MDD patients with signs of bipolarity. It is extensively studied augmenting agent in patients with TRD, although its use in clinical practice is less frequent because of poor-quality evidence, adverse effects, and a delayed onset of action.

Thyroid hormones have been recommended as effective augmentation strategies based on recent network meta-analysis, yet this does not reflect in most of the guidelines.[4]

Dopaminergic agents such as modafinil and lisdexamfetamine have been proposed for use in both unipolar and bipolar depression to target specific symptoms like sedation and fatigue. However, clinical guidelines such as CANMAT and some meta-analyses advise caution regarding the use of stimulant and stimulant-like substances in depression treatment.

For patients needing a rapid response, esketamine has shown superior efficacy, producing faster reductions in depression severity and achieving higher response rates within 2 weeks of treatment initiation; however, long-term data beyond 2 weeks are not available.

## Evidence on Switching versus Augmentation Strategies

The STAR-D study was conducted to determine the best strategy after initial nonresponse to SSRI treatment. It found that only 49% and 37% of adult patients with MDD achieved response and remission, respectively, after their first treatment step.[5]

Patients who had fared better in the previous treatment step and experienced minimal intolerance typically preferred augmentation strategies. In contrast, patients who had little benefit and significant side effect preferred to switch treatment. Both within-class (from citalopram to sertraline) and out-of-class (from citalopram to bupropion) switch were effective strategies. Among augmentation approaches, thyroid hormone augmentation was found to be as effective as lithium augmentation.

A study by the Veterans Affairs Office of Research and Development compared three strategies for MDD treatment after one failed antidepressant trial: Switching to bupropion, combination with bupropion, and augmentation with aripiprazole.[6] The results indicated that augmentation with aripiprazole was more effective than combination or switching with bupropion in achieving remission. Response rates were also higher with aripiprazole augmentation compared to switching or augmentation with bupropion.

## CONCLUSION

Both switching and augmentation strategies are considered viable options for patients who do not respond to initial antidepressant treatment. Evidence supports both switching and augmentation strategies, and the decision should be individualized. Symptom severity, cost, treatment complexity, and patients' level of disability can help guide clinicians the treatment choice. Electroconvulsive therapy (ECT) and repetitive transcranial magnetic stimulation (rTMS) are also available and can be considered in cases where pharmacotherapy alone is insufficient or not well tolerated.

## REFERENCES

1. Strawbridge R, Carter B, Marwood L, Bandelow B, Tsapekos D, Nikolova VL, et al. Augmentation therapies for treatment-resistant depression: systematic review and meta-analysis. Br J Psychiatry. 2019;214(1):42-51.
2. Scott F, Hampsey E, Gnanapragasam S, Carter B, Marwood L, Taylor RW, et al. Systematic review and meta-analysis of augmentation and combination treatments for early-stage treatment-resistant depression. J Psychopharmacol. 2023;37(3):268-78.
3. Nierenberg D, DeCecco LM. Definitions of antidepressant treatment response, remission, nonresponse, partial response, and other relevant outcomes: a focus on treatment-resistant depression. J Clin Psychiatry. 2001:62 Suppl 16:5-9.
4. Nuñez NA, Joseph B, Pahwa M, Kumar R, Resendez MG, Prokop LJ, et al. Augmentation strategies for treatment resistant major depression: A systematic review and network meta-analysis. J Affect Disord. 2022;302: 385-400.
5. Rush JA. STAR*D: What Have We Learned? Am J Psychiatry. 2007;164(2):201-4.
6. Mohamed S, Johnson GR, Chen P, Hicks PB, Davis LL, Yoon J, et al. Effect of Antidepressant Switching vs Augmentation on Remission Among Patients with Major Depressive Disorder Unresponsive to Antidepressant Treatment: The VAST-D Randomized Clinical Trial. JAMA. 2017;318(2): 132-45.

# How to Choose a Tricyclic Antidepressant

*Manushree Gupta, Siddharth Sethi*

## INTRODUCTION

Major depressive disorder (MDD) is a leading cause of morbidity worldwide, with an estimated lifetime risk ranging from 15 to 18%, affecting approximately 264 million people globally.[1] MDD is commonly treated with selective serotonin reuptake inhibitors (SSRIs), tricyclic antidepressants (TCAs), and serotonin-norepinephrine reuptake inhibitors (SNRIs), among other agents. Imipramine, a TCA, was the first antidepressant on which a written public report was presented at the World Psychiatric Association conference in Zurich in 1957.[2]

The SSRIs and SNRIs have been established as first-line agents in the management of MDD in recent decades, primarily due to their favorable adverse drug reaction profiles and lower risk of lethal overdose.[3,4] However, TCAs continue to be prescribed for MDD in cases where SSRIs or SNRIs have shown inadequate response or for other specific considerations.

Named for their chemical structures, TCAs contain three rings and a side chain. These drugs are further divided into secondary and tertiary amines **(Table 1)**.[5]

## TRICYCLIC ANTIDEPRESSANT PHARMACOLOGY

The TCAs are absorbed in the small intestine and undergo first-pass metabolism in the liver. They are highly protein bound, which can lead to interactions with other protein-bound drugs. Due to their lipophilic nature, TCAs circulate extensively throughout the body. The peak plasma concentration of TCAs occurs within 2–6 hours after administration, and their elimination half-life is about 24 hours for most of these drugs. Clearance of TCAs is primarily dependent on cytochrome P450 enzymes.[5]

**TABLE 1:** Classification of TCAs.

| | |
|---|---|
| Secondary amine TCAs | • Desipramine<br>• Maprotiline<br>• Nortriptyline |
| Tertiary amine TCAs | • Amitriptyline<br>• Clomipramine<br>• Doxepin<br>• Imipramine |

TCA: Tricyclic antidepressant

The TCAs act by inhibiting the reuptake of norepinephrine and serotonin, which increases the concentration of these neurotransmitters in the synaptic cleft. Additionally, TCAs block postsynaptic histamine, alpha-adrenergic, and muscarinic receptors.[1] TCAs help in pain relief by two mechanisms—(1) centrally, they inhibit pain signal transmission in the spinal cord, and (2) peripherally, through complex antineuroimmune actions.[6]

Among TCAs, secondary amine TCAs primarily inhibit the reuptake of norepinephrine more than serotonin, leading to higher levels of norepinephrine in the synaptic clefts, whereas, tertiary amine TCAs tend to inhibit the reuptake of serotonin more than norepinephrine, with the exception of doxepin and imipramine, which inhibit the reuptake of both neurotransmitters equally.[5]

Due to their effects on postsynaptic histamine receptors, TCAs can cause sedation, and their action on alpha-adrenergic receptors may lead to weight gain, dizziness, and orthostatic hypotension. TCAs also affect muscarinic receptors, which can cause urinary retention, constipation, dry mouth, and blurred vision. TCAs weakly block voltage-sensitive sodium channels in the heart and brain. This action is particularly important in cases of TCA overdose, where it can cause seizures and coma due to CNS actions, and cardiac arrhythmias, potentially leading to cardiac arrest and death.[7]

## CHOOSING AN ANTIDEPRESSANT

When selecting an antidepressant, both patient-related and drug-related factors are crucial. Key patient-related factors include patient preference, age, previous response or tolerability in patient or family member, past side effects, comorbid medical and psychiatric illnesses, potential drug interactions, intellectual capacity, and gender issues. Important drug-related factors include side effect profile, cost, dosing strategy, and safety in overdose.[8]

## Choosing a Tricyclic Antidepressant Based on Comorbidity

The TCAs have been used to treat various conditions other than MDD. These conditions can occur independently or alongside depression. When MDD is comorbid with these conditions, the use of TCAs may be warranted **(Table 2)**.

- *Headache and migraine:* Amitriptyline is the most studied TCA for chronic daily and episodic migraine headaches, comparable in efficacy to propranolol, venlafaxine, and SSRIs. Most treatment guidelines recommend using amitriptyline for migraine prophylaxis, particularly in those with comorbid depression, at a doses of 25–300 mg per day.[9]
- *Neuropathic pain:* Neuropathic pain, secondary to lesions in the somatosensory nervous system, is common in conditions such as central poststroke pain, multiple sclerosis-associated pain, postherpetic neuralgia, spinal cord injury pain, and diabetic and nondiabetic painful polyneuropathy.[5] A recent meta-analysis showed that TCAs, mainly amitriptyline, are effective for treating neuropathic pain, with a number needed to treat (NNT) of 3.6.[9]
- *Chronic low back pain:* A double-blind randomized controlled trial (RCT) found that maprotiline significantly reduced chronic low back pain compared to paroxetine and placebo.[10] However, a meta-analysis later indicated there is little evidence to support the efficacy of TCAs over placebo for this condition.[11]
- *Fibromyalgia:* TCAs have shown a large effect size for pain reduction, improved sleep quality, reduced stiffness and tenderness, and fatigue reduction in fibromyalgia.[12] The NNT to treat for amitriptyline in fibromyalgia is 4.9.[13]
- *Insomnia:* Doxepin, maprotiline, and amitriptyline have been effective in treating insomnia. They increase somnolence, improve total sleep time and sleep efficiency, and reduce sleep latency and wake time after sleep onset.[14,15]

**TABLE 2:** Choosing a TCA based on the patient's clinical presentation.

| *Clinical presentation* | *TCA* |
|---|---|
| MMD with comorbid migraine, headache, neuropathic pain, fibromyalgia | Amitriptyline (25–300 mg/day ) |
| MDD with low back pain | Maprotiline (75–150 mg/day) |
| MDD with insomnia | Doxepin (3–6 mg/day ) |
| Obsessive-compulsive symptoms | Clomipramine (75–300 mg/day) |

(MDD: major depressive disorder; TCA: tricyclic antidepressant)

## Choosing a Tricyclic Antidepressant Based on Adverse Drug Profile

The adverse drug profile for TCAs is a major factor that influences the choice of drug **(Table 3)**.[5] Tertiary amines have greater serotonin reuptake inhibition, while secondary amines display greater norepinephrine reuptake inhibition. These differences contribute to varied adverse effects of TCAs.

Secondary amines (desipramine, nortriptyline, and protriptyline), which have moderate to high norepinephrine reuptake blockade, cause low to moderate

**TABLE 3:** Adverse drug profile of Tricyclic antidepressants.

| *Drug name* | *Sedation* | *Hypotension* | *Seizures* | *Weight gain* | *Cardiac* |
|---|---|---|---|---|---|
| Amitriptyline | +++ | +++ | ++ | ++ | +++ |
| Clomipramine | ++ | ++ | +++ | + | ++ |
| Doxepin | ++++ | + | ++ | ++ | + |
| Imipramine | ++ | +++ | ++ | ++ | +++ |
| Desipramine | + | + | + | + | ++ |
| Maprotiline | ++ | + | + | ++ | + |
| Nortriptyline | + | + | + | + | ++ |

*Note:* Plus sign indicates the potential severity of adverse drug reaction.

orthostatic hypotension. In contrast, tertiary amines (amitriptyline, clomipramine, doxepin, imipramine, and trimipramine), which have low to no norepinephrine reuptake blockade, cause greater orthostatic hypotension. This can be a major concern while treating the elderly.

## CONCLUSION

The TCAs, introduced seven decades ago, were widely used until drugs with fewer adverse reactions became available. However, TCAs are still used today in depression where there is a partial or no response to other drug classes, there is comorbid pain syndromes or insomnia, based on patient preference, or there is an earlier good response to TCAs. The choice of TCA for drug-naïve patients depends on patient preference, co-morbidities, and the drug's side effect profile.

## REFERENCES

1. Vos CF, Aarnoutse RE, Op de Coul MJ, Spijker J, Groothedde-Kuyvenhoven MM, Mihaescu R, et al. Tricyclic antidepressants for major depressive disorder: A comprehensive evaluation of current practice in the Netherlands. BMC psychiatry. 2021;21(1):481.
2. Pereira VS, Hiroaki-Sato VA. A brief history of antidepressant drug development: from tricyclics to beyond ketamine. Acta Neuropsychiatrica. 2018;30(6):307-22.
3. Chockalingam R, Gott BM, Conway CR. Tricyclic antidepressants and monoamine oxidase inhibitors: are they too old for a new look?. Handb Exp Pharmacol. 2019; 250:37-48.
4. Abbing-Karahagopian V, Huerta C, Souverein PC, De Abajo F, Leufkens HG, Slattery J, et al. Antidepressant prescribing in five European countries: application of common definitions to assess the prevalence, clinical observations, and methodological implications. Eur J Clin Pharmacol. 2014;70:849-57.
5. Schneider J, Patterson M, Jimenez XF. Beyond depression: Other uses for tricyclic antidepressants. Cleve Clin J Med. 2019;86(12):807-14.
6. Kremer M, Yalcin I, Goumon Y, Wurtz X, Nexon L, Daniel D, et al. A dual noradrenergic mechanism for the relief of neuropathic allodynia by the antidepressant drugs duloxetine and amitriptyline. J Neurosci. 2018; 38(46):9934-54.
7. Stahl SM. Stahl's essential psychopharmacology: Prescriber's guide. Cambridge: Cambridge university press; 2014.
8. Gautam S, Jain A, Gautam M, Vahia VN, Grover S. Clinical practice guidelines for the management of depression. Indian J Psychiatr. 2017;59(Suppl 1):S34.
9. Jackson JL, Cogbill E, Santana-Davila R, Eldredge C, Collier W, Gradall A, et al. A comparative effectiveness meta-analysis of drugs for the prophylaxis of migraine headache. PloS one. 2015;10(7):e0130733.
10. Atkinson JH, Slater MA, Wahlgren DR, Williams RA, Zisook S, Pruitt SD, et al. Effects of noradrenergic and serotonergic antidepressants on chronic low back pain intensity. Pain. 1999;83(2):137-45.
11. Urquhart DM, Hoving JL, Assendelft WW, Roland M, van Tulder MW. Antidepressants for non-specific low back pain. Cochrane Database Syst Rev. 2008;2008(1):CD001703.
12. Arnold LM, Keck PE, Welge JA. Antidepressant treatment of fibromyalgia: a meta-analysis and review. Psychosomatics. 2000;41(2):104-13.
13. Häuser W, Wolfe F, Tölle T, Üçeyler N, Sommer C. The role of antidepressants in the management of fibromyalgia syndrome: a systematic review and meta-analysis. CNS Drugs. 2012;26:297-307.
14. Liu Y, Xu X, Dong M, Jia S, Wei Y. Treatment of insomnia with tricyclic antidepressants: a meta-analysis of polysomnographic randomized controlled trials. Sleep Med. 2017;34:126-33.
15. McCall C, McCall WV. What is the role of sedating antidepressants, antipsychotics, and anticonvulsants in the management of insomnia?. Curr Psychiatry Rep. 2012;14:494-502.

CHAPTER 6

# Rational Antidepressant Polypharmacy

*Anil Kakunje, Shashwath Sathyanath, Ganesh Kini*

## INTRODUCTION

Major depressive disorder (MDD) is primarily treated with antidepressants, which are the cornerstone of management. However, treatment outcomes for individuals with depression are often far from satisfactory. In the context of treating depression, the term "response" refers to achieving at least 50% reduction in depressive symptoms as assessed using valid assessment tools such as Hamilton Depression Rating Scale (HAM-D) or Montgomery–Asberg Depression Rating Scale (MADRS).[1] Approximately 30% of individuals experiencing a major depressive episode will not exhibit a satisfactory response to appropriate standard treatment.[2] As a result, this poses a significant challenge for clinicians in the management of treatment resistant depression. A relatively recent approach involves the use of *"antidepressant polypharmacy"*, which entails the simultaneous administration of two or more antidepressant medications. However, when combining antidepressants, our objective should be to use *"rational polypharmacy"*, grounded in evidence-based trials.

Polypharmacy refers to the situation where two or more medications are employed either to treat the same illness or to treat different conditions using similar medications.[3] An instance of the first situation is the use of mirtazapine to ameliorate depressive symptoms in a patient who is already undergoing treatment with an specific selective serotonin reuptake inhibitor (SSRI). The second instance is exemplified by a patient who concurrently takes an SSRI for depression and bupropion for smoking cessation. Another instance of combining medication may be to counter the adverse effect caused by the first antidepressant. For example, mirtazapine combined with SSRI to ameliorate sexual dysfunction caused by SSRIs.

The limitations of monotherapy are:

- Single antidepressants may not treat all symptoms, resulting in residual symptoms such as insomnia, cognitive impairment, pain, and anxiety even after improvements in other domains of depression.
- Unforeseen genetic variations among patients might lead to nonresponsiveness to specific pharmacological agents, potentially causing a delay in achieving remission.
- Comorbid conditions can alter the neurochemistry in diverse ways, and a single agent may not modify all the associated neurochemical imbalances.
- Some patients may not tolerate specific side effects of some medications compared to others, which could lead to poor adherence and consequently reduce the effectiveness of the treatment.

Drugs can be combined in a rational manner using certain criteria:[4] (1) the drugs should not interact pharmacokinetically and pharmacodynamically; (2) the drugs should not have same or opposing mechanisms of action; (3) the drugs should have a simple metabolism with linear pharmacokinetics and an intermediate half-life; and (4) the combination should have a positive effect on the disorder, with more effectiveness than monotherapy, without any additional safety risks.

Large database analyses have shown that combination of antidepressants is associated with a lower risk of treatment discontinuation.[5] A myth that is widely accepted as a fact is that polypharmacy leads to more side effects. However, findings from the STAR*D trial indicated that there were no clinically significant differences in the adverse event profiles between patients treated with monotherapy and those receiving a combination of antidepressants.[6]

Some antidepressant combinations are not considered rational. In the past, the combination of tricyclic antidepressants (TCAs) with monoamine oxidase inhibitors (MAOIs) was used. However, this practice is no longer recommended due to the potential risk of severe reactions, such as serotonin syndrome.[7] Similarly, MAOIs are avoided when combined with SSRIs for the same reason.

## HOW COMMON IS ANTIDEPRESSANT POLYPHARMACY?

Existing literature suggests that the practice of polypharmacy in depression is widespread globally, although the exact prevalence remains uncertain. From the available data, it is evident that polypharmacy in depression is prevalent and shows a rising trend. The overall prevalence of patients with unipolar depression receiving polypharmacy, including antidepressants, was recorded as 24%.[8] The potential surge in polypharmacy could be attributed to clinicians' increasing confidence in the tolerability of the current medications, along with the availability of drugs targeting multiple neurotransmitters.

## WHEN TO INITIATE ANTIDEPRESSANT POLYPHARMACY?

Approximately, one-third of patients do not achieve an adequate response to their initial single antidepressant treatment, underscoring the relevance of using antidepressant combinations in the management of MDD, particularly in treatment resistant cases. However, clinicians must recognize that the ability to safely combine two treatments does not necessarily imply additive or synergistic effects. It is important to note that the practice of combining antidepressants lacks strong empirical grounding.[9,10] The STAR*D study, involving 565 patients, is the sole published trial with adequate funding that explored the use of combination antidepressants.[11] There is growing body of evidence from numerous case reports and small-sized trials suggesting the potential benefits of combining antidepressants.[12]

The following needs to be considered while combining antidepressants—(1) reduction of the primary symptoms of depression; (2) achieving synergy and a swift response to treatment; (3) managing and mitigating potential side effects; (4) addressing associated symptoms such as anxiety and cognitive impairment; (5) enhancing social functioning and overall quality of life; and (6) preventing relapse.

## RATIONAL COMBINATIONS OF ANTIDEPRESSANTS

### Serotonergic Approach

The SSRIs are the preferred first-line choice of antidepressants. The combined action of inhibiting 5HT reuptake and antagonizing $5HT_2$ receptors with another antidepressant holds promise in the treatment of resistant depression. Dual SSRIs given for treatment of depression could enhance reuptake inhibition by increasing the active S-enantiomer of citalopram compared to R-enantiomer.[10] However, there are only limited studies on dual SSRI combination treatment.[11] One needs to be cautious while combining SSRIs due to the potential risk of serotonin syndrome.

Another strategy used is combining SSRIs with trazodone. While SSRIs raise serotonin levels by stimulating $5HT_{1A}$ receptors for therapeutic effects, they also stimulate $5HT_{2A}$ and $5HT_{2C}$ receptors leading to side effects such as insomnia, agitation, and sexual dysfunction. Trazadone, possessing $5HT_{2A}$ blocking properties alongside serotonin reuptake inhibition (SARI), could mitigate these side effects by blocking $5HT_{2A}$ and $5HT_{2C}$ receptors.

Additionally, SSRIs have been combined with buspirone as an augmenting agent for the treatment of depression, specifically when it is associated and anxiety symptoms. Buspirone, acting as a $5HT_{1A}$ receptor agonist, when combined with SSRIs, could potentially enhance 5HT neuronal activity. However, there are limited trials evaluating the efficacy and tolerability of this combination.[12]

### Noradrenergic Approach

Reduced noradrenergic activity correlates with decreased alertness, low energy, impaired attention, concentration, and reduced cognitive ability. Hence, antidepressants increasing noradrenergic activity could alleviate these symptoms of depression. In nonresponders, a powerful strategy used is combining serotonin-norepinephrine reuptake inhibitors (SNRIs) with mirtazapine, known as California Rocket Fuel.[13] This combination takes advantage of the pharmacological synergy achieved by inhibition of both 5HT and NE reuptake through SNRI use, while also increasing the release of serotonin and norepinephrine facilitated by the $\alpha_2$ antagonist actions of mirtazapine. Venlafaxine functions as a dual inhibitor of serotonin and noradrenaline reuptake. In contrast, mirtazapine not only affects both neurotransmitter systems but also has $a_2$-adrenergic, $5HT_2$, and $5HT_3$ serotonergic receptor antagonism.[14] This combination may be preferred over tranylcypromine owing to reduced side effect profile and absence of dietary restrictions, as observed in STAR-D study.[15]

Combining SSRIs with mirtazapine (a NASSA), is a common antidepressant strategy. Mirtazapine, an antidepressant with dual action, enhances both serotonergic and noradrenergic activity by blocking the $\alpha_2$ adrenergic auto- and heteroreceptors. Additionally, it inhibits the serotonergic $5HT_2$ and $5HT_3$ receptors. This is useful in improving treatment response and addressing symptoms such as insomnia and weight loss. An open study done on SSRI nonresponders showed a good response to a combination of mirtazapine (15–30 mg/day) and SSRI.[16]

The combination of TCAs with SSRIs is a common practice in treating depression. While most tricyclics block serotonin and norepinephrine to some extent, few exhibit more selective norepinephrine transporter (NET) inhibition such as desipramine, nortriptyline, and maprotiline. Combining SSRI with TCAs can lead to higher blockade ratio of norepinephrine and serotonin receptors. However, there is a risk of serotonin syndrome associated with these combinations. Additionally, CYP450 inhibition by SSRIs can elevate TCA plasma levels, potentially enhancing clinical efficacy. A double-blind randomized controlled study comparing TCA monotherapy with a combination of TCA and SSRI showed combined treatment achieved better remission rates.[17]

### Serotonergic, Noradrenergic, and Dopaminergic Approach

Symptoms of depression such as reduced energy levels, poor motivation, anhedonia, and loss of sex drive may be due to decreased dopaminergic activity. Some treatment resistant individuals may benefit from stimulation of multiple neurotransmitter systems to achieve response. For example, SSRI plus bupropion combination targets both dopamine and norepinephrine in addition to serotonin. Bupropion is a norepinephrine-dopamine reuptake inhibitor (NDRI), usually prescribed as an augmenting agent for depression and for the treatment of smoking cessation. A large randomized controlled trial involving 565 patients compared citalopram monotherapy with bupropion extended release as an augmentation treatment. The study found augmentation strategy useful in reducing the severity of symptoms and better tolerated compared to monotherapy.[18] Another naturalistic open cohort study, conducted on 61 patients showed that SSRI plus bupropion combination proved more effective than monotherapy.[19]

## CONCLUSION

There are limited large, empirically validated, and well-controlled studies, as well as a paucity of standard guidelines on combination treatment for depression. However, existing studies suggest that combination treatments offer advantages over monotherapy, particularly for nonresponders, owing to multiple mechanisms of action and effectiveness in addressing additional symptoms such as anxiety and anhedonia. Antidepressant polypharmacy remains a complex and controversial topic. As clinicians, it is imperative to practice "rational polypharmacy", considering the mechanisms of action and potential side effect profile. Active patient involvement, with informed consent, is essential in the complex decision-making process, to achieve the best possible outcomes. Hence, antidepressant polypharmacy should be used cautiously and restricted to selected patients after considering both risks and benefits.

## REFERENCES

1. Frank E, Prien RF, Jarrett RB, Keller MB, Kupfer DJ, Lavori PW, et al. Conceptualization and rationale for consensus definitions of terms in major depressive disorder. Remission, recovery, relapse, and recurrence. Arch Gen Psychiatry. 1991;48:851-5.
2. Bauer M, Bschor T, Pfennig A, Whybrow PC, Angst J, Versiani M, et al. World Federation of Societies of Biological Psychiatry (WFSBP) guidelines for biological treatment of unipolar depressive disorders in primary care. World J Biol Psychiatry. 2007;8:67-104.
3. Kingsbury SJ, Yi D, Simpson GM. Psychopharmacology: Rational and irrational polypharmacy. Psychiatr Serv. 2001;52:1033-6.
4. Preskorn SH, Lacey RL. Polypharmacy: when is it rational? J Psychiatr Pract. 2007;13:97-105.
5. Milea D, Guelfucci F, Bent-Ennakhil N, Toumi M, Auray JP. Antidepressant monotherapy: A claims database analysis of treatment changes and treatment duration. Clin Ther 2010;32:2057-72.
6. Hansen RA, Dusetzina SB, Ellis AR, Stürmer T, Farley JF, Gaynes BN. Risk of adverse events in treatment-resistant depression: propensity-score-matched comparison of antidepressant augment and switch strategies. Gen Hosp Psychiatry. 2012;34:192-200.
7. White K, Simpson G. The combined use of MAOIs and tricyclics. J Clin Psychiatry. 1984;45:67-9.
8. Frye MA, Ketter TA, Leverich GS, Huggins T, Lantz C, Denicoff KD, et al. The increasing use of polypharmacotherapy for refractory mood disorders: 22 years of study. J Clin Psychiatry. 2000;61:9-15.
9. Thase ME. Antidepressant combinations: widely used, but far from empirically validated. Can J Psychiatry. 2011;56:317-23.
10. Bondolfi G, Lissner C, Kosel M, Eap CB, Baumann P. Fluoxetine augmentation in citalopram non-responders:

pharmacokinetic and clinical consequences. Int J Neuropsychopharmacol. 2000;3:55-60.

11. Dodd S, Horgan D, Malhi GS, Berk M. To combine or not to combine? A literature review of antidepressant combination therapy. J Affect Disord. 2005;89:1-11.
12. Landén M, Björling G, Agren H, Fahlén T. A randomized, double-blind, placebo-controlled trial of buspirone in combination with an SSRI in patients with treatment-refractory depression. J Clin Psychiatry. 1998;59: 664-8.
13. Stahl SM. Essential Psychopharmacology: Neuroscientific Basis and Practical Applications, 2nd edition. New York: Cambridge University Press; 2000.
14. Stahl SM. Basic psychopharmacology of antidepressants, part 1: Antidepressants have seven distinct mechanisms of action. J Clin Psychiatry. 1998;59 Suppl 4:5-14.
15. McGrath PJ, Stewart JW, Fava M, Trivedi MH, Wisniewski SR, Nierenberg AA, et al. Tranylcypromine versus venlafaxine plus mirtazapine following three failed antidepressant medication trials for depression: a STAR*D report. Am J Psychiatry. 2006;163:1531-41.
16. Carpenter LL, Jocic Z, Hall JM, Rasmussen SA, Price LH. Mirtazapine augmentation in the treatment of refractory depression. J Clin Psychiatry. 1999;60:45-9.
17. Nelson JC, Mazure CM, Jatlow PI, Bowers MB, Price LH. Combining norepinephrine and serotonin reuptake inhibition mechanisms for treatment of depression: a double-blind, randomized study. Biol Psychiatry. 2004;55:296-300.
18. Trivedi MH, Fava M, Wisniewski SR, Thase ME, Quitkin F, Warden D, et al. Medication augmentation after the failure of SSRIs for depression. N Engl J Med. 2006;354:1243-52.
19. Lam RW, Hossie H, Solomons K, Yatham LN. Citalopram and bupropion-SR: combining versus switching in patients with treatment-resistant depression. J Clin Psychiatry. 2004;65:337-40.

# How and When to Stop Treatment in Depressive Disorders

*Muralidharan Kesavan, Pavithra Jayasankar, Rashmi Arasappa*

## INTRODUCTION

Depression is one of the most prevalent and disabling psychiatric disorders. According to India's National Mental Health Survey 2016, the lifetime prevalence of depressive disorders was estimated to be 5.25%.[1] Antidepressants are the main stay of management in depression, with the goal of achieving and maintaining full remission for as long as possible.[2] Research suggests that long-term use of antidepressants can protect against relapse and recurrence of depressive symptoms.[3,4]

This chapter will provide an overview of when and how to stop antidepressants in depressive disorders, while briefly discussing the risks associated with discontinuation **(Flowchart 1)**.

**Flowchart 1:** How and when to stop treatment in depressive disorder.

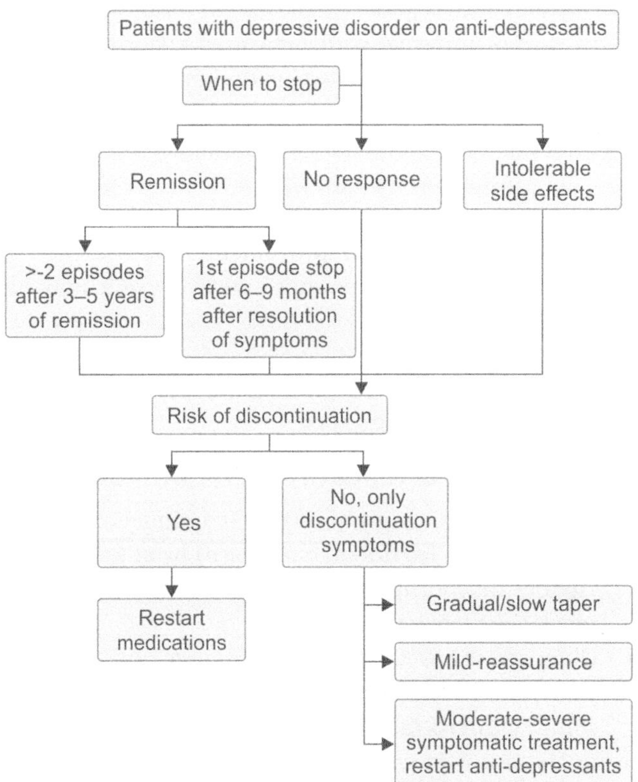


## WHEN TO STOP ANTIDEPRESSANTS?

The question of stopping antidepressants can arise in various situations. It can be broadly divided into discontinuation in maintenance phase, intolerability, or poor response to the drug. Since achieving true remission rather than partial symptomatic response is the therapeutic goal, it is essential to determine if remission has occurred before stopping treatment. The remission in a depressive episode is defined as follows:

- *Remission of depressive episode:* The remission criteria[5] require Hamilton Rating Scale for Depression (HAM-D) score of ≤7 and a Clinical Global Impression-Improvement (CGI-I) score of 1. The Sheehan Disability Scale may be used to assess functioning with a score of ≤1 indicates return to normal functioning in all three domains of life. These and similar scales can be used in clinical practice to determine return to normal functioning.
  - Antidepressants should be continued long enough to sustain remission and avoid relapse or recurrences. Patients with single episode of depression need to be maintained on the same dose of antidepressants given in acute phase for at least 6–9 months after the symptoms have resolved (continuation phase) to prevent relapse of symptoms.
  - Patients with history of multiple episodes (two or more) need to be given long-term treatment[6] (maintenance phase), possibly for life, to prevent recurrences.

The decision to discontinue antidepressants in maintenance phase may be based on factors such as probability of recurrence, frequency, and severity of past episodes, the persistence of depressive symptoms after recovery, comorbid disorders, and patient preferences.[7] When the decision is made to discontinue antidepressants in the maintenance phase, it must be done over the course of several weeks to months. Such gradual tapering can help detect emerging symptoms or recurrences and can be returned to full therapeutic intensity. Also, gradual tapering of antidepressants helps minimize the risks of discontinuation symptoms. During discontinuation, patients should be made aware of the potential risk of relapse and early warning signs.

- *Intolerable side effects:* When side effects are intolerable or do not improve with measures taken to reduce them, and when they outweigh the benefits of the drug, discontinuation may be necessary. In such cases, the drug must be tapered and discontinued. The tapering can be faster based on the nature of adverse effects.
- *Partial or poor or no response of the drug:* When there is no or partial improvement of the symptoms, cross-tapering with another antidepressant may be considered.

**TABLE 1:** Antidepressant discontinuation symptoms.

| *Antidepressant class* | *Discontinuation symptoms* |
|---|---|
| MAO inhibitors | • Aggressiveness, agitation<br>• Ataxia<br>• Catatonia<br>• Cognitive impairment<br>• Suicidality, labile affect<br>• Myoclonic jerks<br>• Paranoid delusions, hallucinations<br>• Pressured or slowed speech |
| SSRIs/TCAs | • Somatic—sweating, chills, flu-like symptoms<br>• Gastrointestinal—nausea, vomiting, anorexia, abdominal pain<br>• Sleep disorders—insomnia, vivid or excessive dreaming<br>• Affective disorders—anxiety, depression, agitation<br>• Balance—vertigo, ataxia, akathisia, parkinsonism<br>• Sensory disturbances—numbness, paresthesia, shock like sensations |

(MOA: monoamine oxidase; SSRI: selective serotonin reuptake inhibitor; TCAs: tricyclic antidepressant)

## RISKS ASSOCIATED WITH DISCONTINUATION OF ANTIDEPRESSANTS

### Relapse or Recurrence after Discontinuation

- Antidepressants prevent relapse (continuation phase) or recurrence (maintenance phase) by at least 50%.[8] Hence, discontinuation always carries the risk of relapse or recurrence.
- Older age of onset, comorbid substance use or anxiety disorders, and the presence of residual symptoms are some of the risk factors for relapse or recurrence.
- In the event of relapse or recurrence, the previous antidepressant that showed a good response is usually considered for reinitiation. A depressive relapse is more likely in the first weeks to months after recovery, with the risk declining with time.[9]

### Discontinuation Symptoms

- Antidepressant discontinuation symptoms are a constellation of physical and psychological symptoms that emerge soon after discontinuing antidepressants. These symptoms can occur across all classes of antidepressants and may vary in nature depending on the class of antidepressants and the individual drugs **(Table 1)**.
- Some of the risk factors associated with discontinuation symptoms include abrupt stoppage of drug, concurrent long-term medications such as antihypertensives, young age, and longer duration of treatment.[10]
- Berber[11] proposed the mnemonic *"FINISH"* for discontinuation symptoms: "flu-like symptoms, insomnia, nausea, imbalance, sensory disturbances, and hyperarousal". Some of the class specific discontinuation symptoms have been tabulated mentioned in **Table 1**.

### Management of Discontinuation Symptoms

- Prevention is the first-line strategy for avoiding or minimizing discontinuation symptoms. This includes educating patients regarding medication adherence, the need to continue medication during the continuation/maintenance phase, and the potential for withdrawal symptoms.[12]
- For mild symptoms, education and reassurance may be adequate. For moderate-to-severe symptoms, restarting the same antidepressant can provide relief. However, if the same antidepressant cannot be restarted due to intolerability or poor response, an alternative antidepressant may be initiated.

- Other drugs also can be used to relieve discontinuation symptoms. The choice of drug depends on the type of symptom. Anticholinergic agents such as trihexyphenidyl can improve gastrointestinal symptoms, sleep disturbances, and dystonia. Benzodiazepines can be prescribed for anxiety, and propranolol can be used to relieve akathisia.

## HOW TO STOP ANTIDEPRESSANTS?

### Antidepressant Discontinuation—Recommendations for Dose Tapering

- A *slow taper* is uniformly recommended.[13] Recently, *hyperbolic taper* is gaining evidence, involving progressively smaller dose reductions as the overall dose decreases.[14]
- While tapering, it is important to consider the drug's pharmacological profile, the duration of treatment, and the patient's response. Discontinuation syndromes are more frequent with antidepressants that have shorter half-lives, which therefore require longer and more gradual tapering.
- Since published recommendations for taper rates are often vague, the magnitude and speed of dose taper is often left to clinical judgement.[15] Some specific recommendations have been tabulated below in **Table 2.**[16]

**TABLE 2:** Recommendations for antidepressant dose tapering.

| *Antidepressant* | *Recommended taper rate* |
|---|---|
| *Monoamine oxidase inhibitors* | |
| Tranylcypromine | 10 mg/day every 2 weeks or 10% weekly |
| Phenelzine | 15 mg/day every 2 week or 10% weekly |
| Tricyclic antidepressants | Gradual taper up to 3 months |
| *Selective serotonin reuptake inhibitors* | |
| Fluoxetine | Gradual taper generally unnecessary (long half-life) |
| Fluvoxamine | 50 mg/day every 5–7 days with a final dose 25 mg/day before discontinuation |
| Paroxetine | 10 mg/day every 5–7 days with a final dose of 5–10 mg/day before discontinuation |
| Sertraline | 50 mg/day every 5–7 days with a final dose of 25–50 mg/day before discontinuation |
| Venlafaxine | 25 mg/day every 5–7 days with a final dose of 25–50 mg/day before discontinuation |

## CONCLUSION

Antidepressant discontinuation can occur due to various factors such as intolerability, poor response, or after remission. Stopping of antidepressant at any stage of illness/treatment can result in various physical and psychological symptoms more so if discontinuation is abrupt. The nature of symptoms may vary depending on the class of antidepressants. Discontinuation reactions are often seen in cases of abrupt withdrawal, nevertheless it can also be seen in gradual dose tapering/missing doses.

## REFERENCES


1. Murthy RS. National mental health survey of India 2015–2016. Indian J Psychiatry. 2017;59(1):21.
2. Judd LL, Akiskal HS. Delineating the longitudinal structure of depressive illness: beyond clinical subtypes and duration thresholds. Pharmacopsychiatry. 2000;33(1):3-7.
3. Hansen R, Gaynes B, Thieda P, Gartlehner G, Deveaugh-Geiss A, Krebs E, et al. Meta-analysis of major depressive disorder relapse and recurrence with second-generation antidepressants. Psychiatr Serv. 2008;59(10):1121-30.
4. Hollon SD, Thase ME, Markowitz JC. Treatment and Prevention of Depression. Psychol Sci Public Interest. 2002;3:39-77.
5. Kennedy S. Full remission: a return to normal functioning. J Psychiatry Neurosci. 2002;27(4):233-4.
6. National Institute for Clinical Excellence. (2018). Depression in adults: treatment and management. NICE Guideline: Short Version Draft for Second Consultation. [online] Available from https://www.nice.org.uk/guidance/ng222/documents/short-version-of-draft-guideline [Last accessed June, 2025).
7. American Psychiatric Association. Practice guideline for the treatment of patients with major depressive disorder, 3rd edition. Philadelphia: American Psychiatric Association; 2010.
8. Thase ME. Preventing relapse and recurrence of depression: a brief review of therapeutic options. CNS spectrums. 2006;11(S15):12-21.
9. Keller MB, Lavori PW, Lewis CE, Klerman GL. Predictors of relapse in major depressive disorder. Jama. 1983;250(24):3299-304.
10. Haddad PM. Antidepressant discontinuation syndromes: clinical relevance, prevention and management. Drug Safety. 2001;24(3):183-97.
11. Berber MJ: FINISH: remembering the discontinuation syndrome: flu-like symptoms, insomnia, nausea, imbalance, sensory disturbances, and hyperarousal (anxiety/agitation). J Clin Psychiatry. 1998;59:255

12. Jha MK, Rush AJ, Trivedi MH. When discontinuing SSRI antidepressants is a challenge: management tips. Am J Psychiatry. 2018;175(12):1176-84.
13. Bauer M, Pfennig A, Severus E, Whybrow PC, Angst J, Möller HJ; World Federation of Societies of Biological Psychiatry. World Federation of Societies of Biological Psychiatry (WFSBP) guidelines for biological treatment of unipolar depressive disorders, part 1: update 2013 on the acute and continuation treatment of unipolar depressive disorders. World J Biol Psychiatry. 2013;14:334-85.
14. van Os J, Groot PC. Outcomes of hyperbolic tapering of antidepressants. Therapeutic Advances in Psychopharmacology. 2023;13:20451253231171518.
15. Maund E, Stuart B, Moore M, Dowrick C, Geraghty AW, Dawson S, Kendrick T. Managing antidepressant discontinuation: a systematic review. Ann Fam Med. 2019;17(1):52-60.
16. Shelton RC. Steps following attainment of remission: discontinuation of antidepressant therapy. Prim Care Companion J Clin Psychiatry. 2001;3(4):168.

CHAPTER 8

# When and How to Use Ketamine in Clinical Practice?

*Jahnavi Kedare, Sachin Baliga*

## INTRODUCTION

Resistant depression is defined as an unsuccessful trial of two antidepressant medications. According to the STAR*D trial, over 50% of patients achieve remission after two treatment steps, with a cumulative remission rate of 67% after four acute treatment steps.[1] There is a delay in the onset of action of antidepressants, which is attributed to adaptive changes in receptor sensitivity, and it takes about 3–4 weeks for the antidepressant action.[2] Hence, there is a need for an antidepressant that is efficacious and has a faster onset of action.

Ketamine and its S-enantiomer, esketamine, are novel antidepressants with a faster onset of action. Additionally, their role in reducing suicidal ideas and suicidal behavior has been recognized. While ketamine has long been used as an anesthetic agent, research conducted in the last 20 years has explored its potential in subanesthetic dosages. At these lower doses, ketamine exhibits antidepressant properties. It has also been used as an analgesic agent in acute pain conditions.[3]

## MECHANISM OF ACTION OF KETAMINE

Ketamine acts as an antagonist on N-methyl-D-aspartate receptor (NMDA) receptors. At subanesthetic doses, ketamine selectively blocks NMDA receptor function specifically on inhibitory gamma-aminobutyric acid (GABA)-ergic interneurons. This blockage leads to an increase in glutamate release and the phasic activation of postsynaptic aminomethylphosphonic acid (AMPA) receptors. This NMDA receptor action leads to an increased local protein and brain-derived neurotrophic factor (BDNF) expression. The AMPA receptor activation also leads to enhanced neuroplasticity and synaptogenesis. This has been a proposed mechanism of action of ketamine as an antidepressant. Apart from NMDA receptors, ketamine also has action on opioid receptors, which leads to mood elevation. The diverse actions of ketamine on multiple receptors contribute to its varied side effects.[4]

## REGULATORY APPROVAL

Use of ketamine in subanesthetic dosages is mainly "off-label" usage. It has not yet received approval by any regulatory body for use in subanesthetic dosages. Due to its classification as a controlled substance and potential for abuse, it can only be administered under the observation of a licensed medical practitioner and is prohibited for self-administration. Intranasal esketamine, to be used along with an antidepressant, was approved by the US Food and Drug Administration (FDA) for adults with treatment-resistant depression in March 2019, and the European Medicines Agency approved it in December 2019. Furthermore, in August 2020, it received approval for use in patients with major depressive disorder with suicidal ideas and behavior.[3]

## INDICATIONS, CONTRAINDICATIONS, AND ADMINISTRATION

**Box 1** provides indications for the use of ketamine (in subanesthetic dosages, off-label). A few studies have indicated the usefulness of ketamine in bipolar depression, PTSD, and other anxiety disorders.[4]

Ketamine has a plasma protein binding of approximately 10–15%. Its elimination half-life is 2–4 hours,

**BOX 1:** Indications for ketamine.

- Treatment-resistant depression[3]
- Major depressive disorder with suicidal thoughts and behavior[3]
- Treatment-resistant bipolar depression[5]
- Earlier recovery and lower seizure threshold used with ECT (small studies)[6]
- Acute pain in sickle cell crises, renal colic, and trauma[7]
- In painful surgeries on opioid dependent or opioid tolerant patients[7]

whereas it is 5 hours for esketamine. The bioavailability is approximately 100% for intravenous ketamine and approximately 30–50% for intranasal esketamine. Notably, 0.5 mg/kg of ketamine is considered equivalent to 56 mg of esketamine.[3]

*Relative contraindications* against considering ketamine as a treatment modality include:[7]

- Known hypersensitivity to ketamine or its components
- Moderate to severe hepatic dysfunction
- Uncontrolled hypertension and/or high-risk coronary artery disease
- Evidence of elevated intracranial or intraocular pressure
- Pregnancy
- Active psychotic or manic symptoms or history of a primary psychotic disorder such as schizophrenia.

*Settings for administration:* Administration of ketamine-based treatments is preferably conducted in facilities that have secure storage provisions, physiological monitoring instruments, and medications to manage adverse events. The clinician administering the treatment, or a member of the team, should be qualified to manage neurological, cardiorespiratory, and psychiatric adverse events. Particularly, in outpatient settings, the administering professional or team members should be qualified for airway support and resuscitation.[8]

## IMPLEMENTATION CHECKLIST

- *Baseline assessment:*
  - Detailed clinical assessment including rating of severity of depression with instruments such as the Montgomery–Åsberg Depression Rating Scale (MADRS), the Beck's Depression Inventory-II (BDI-II), and Beck Anxiety Inventory (BAI).
  - Rating of severity of suicidality using instruments such as the Beck Suicidality Scale (BSS).
  - Establishment of clear indication (treatment-resistant unipolar or bipolar depression without psychotic symptoms, acute suicidality in the background of depression).
  - Evaluation and documentation of other concurrently prescribed treatments to rule out drug-drug interactions.
  - Rule out any comorbid substance use disorder.
  - Rule out prior hypersensitivity reaction to ketamine
  - Baseline medical assessment including physical examination, heart rate, blood pressure, complete blood count, blood sugar levels, electrocardiogram, liver function test, and kidney function test.
  - Written informed consent that mentions the risks and benefits and the off-label nature of the treatment.
  - Weight (for dose calculation).
- *On the day of the session:*
  - No solid food for at least 4 hours prior to the administration of ketamine; no clear liquids for 2 hours prior.
  - Abstinent from any substance of abuse for at least 48 hours (especially alcohol).
  - Antihypertensives and antidiabetic medications have been taken. The dose of insulin may require adjustment in view of dietary restrictions on that day.
  - Patient should be vitally stable (infusion to be avoided if baseline blood pressure is >140/90 mm Hg).[8]

**Table 1** provides various routes of administration and corresponding dosages for the use of ketamine and esketamine:

**TABLE 1:** Routes of administration and corresponding dosages of ketamine.

| *Route* | *Dose range* | *Method of administration* |
|---|---|---|
| Intravenous ketamine[3] | 0.5–1.0 mg/kg | Infused over 40–60 minutes twice weekly for 2 weeks |
| Oral ketamine[9] | 2–3 mg/kg | Required quantity mixed with around 100 mL of purified water (flavors may be added); sipped over 10–15 minutes for the first session and a little more rapidly in subsequent sessions |
| Sublingual[9] | Not established, however, to start with 10 mg | To place under the tongue without swallowing for 2 minutes |
| Intranasal[3] | • *Esketamine:* 56–84 mg intranasally twice weekly for 4 weeks<br>• *Ketamine:* 50–150 mg intranasally twice weekly | Nasal spray (comes with a proprietary dispenser that administers fixed doses) |

In some studies, esketamine has been shown to be effective for long-term use and for relapse prevention. 56–84 mg of esketamine can be administered every 1–2 weeks for this.[3] Intramuscular and transdermal routes of administration for ketamine have been explored, but their efficacy and safety profiles have not yet been firmly established. A single dose of intravenous ketamine 0.5 mg/kg has been shown to be effective in reducing suicidal thoughts. However, this effect is typically short-term, lasting up to 7 days according to some studies.[10,11] Notably, some studies have shown a reduction in suicidal thoughts for up to 6 weeks in persons receiving repeat-dose intravenous racemic infusion (0.5 mg/kg).[3]

The *following are the adverse effects that might be seen while using ketamine:*

- *Allergic reaction:* Anaphylactic reaction and rash
- *Cardiovascular:* Dizziness, elevation of heart rate and blood pressure, arrhythmias, and cardiac arrest
- *Gastrointestinal:* Dry mouth, nausea, vomiting, and anorexia.
- *Respiratory:* Apnea, rarely respiratory depression, and laryngospasm.
- *Neurological:* Headache, confusion, impaired coordination, and concentration.
- *Ophthalmic:* Blurred vision, increased intraocular pressure
- *Psychiatric:* Restlessness, confusion, disorientation, dysphoria, anxiety, and dissociative experiences (unusual thoughts, dream-like feeling of unreality, unawareness of self and environment, illusions, and hallucinations), treatment-induced affective switch, precipitation of psychosis, rarely emergence of delirium.

## MONITORING DURING TREATMENT[8]

Due to its psychotomimetic effects and changes on cardiorespiratory system, it is advised to monitor the level of consciousness, heart rate, blood pressure, respiratory rate and oxygen saturation at baseline and periodically (e.g., every 15 minutes) throughout the session and continuing for up to 2–3 hours after termination of the session. Instruments such as the Clinician Administered Dissociative States Scale (CADSS) can be used for a structured assessment of the dissociative/psychotomimetic experiences. Patients who are considered at risk for adverse effects may require more frequent and longer monitoring of vital signs.

## FREQUENCY AND DURATION OF TREATMENT

It has been seen that patients show a better response over serial sessions of treatment, although a dramatic response with a single session has also been noted. However, treatment is usually conducted in the form of six to eight infusions given twice or thrice weekly (acute phase) to prolong the gains. Post this, the sessions may be tapered or stopped based on an individual, case-by-case basis, while continuing the antidepressants. In some cases where this is a nonresponse to other lines of treatment, ketamine therapy may also be given as a continuation and maintenance phase with individualized frequency, although most of the evidence on these lines is anecdotal.

In conclusion, the following points need to be noted:

- Esketamine is not yet available in the Indian market.
- Long-term use of ketamine is not recommended, as there is not enough evidence for its efficacy.

## REFERENCES


1. Rush AJ, Trivedi MH, Wisniewski SR, Nierenberg AA, Stewart JW, Warden D, et al. Acute and longer-term outcomes in depressed outpatients requiring one or several treatment steps: a STAR*D report. Am J Psychiatry. 2006;163(11):1905-17.
2. In: Stahl SM (Ed). Mood Disorders and Antidepressants: Stahl's Essential Psychopharmacology, 4th editon. Cambridge University Press; 2013. pp. 284-369.
3. McIntyre RS, Rosenblat JD, Nemeroff CB, Sanacora G, Murrough JW, Berk M, et al. Synthesizing the Evidence for Ketamine and Esketamine in Treatment-resistant depression: An International Expert Opinion on the Available Evidence and Implementation. Am J Psychiatry. 2021;178(5):383-99.
4. Sanacora G, Katz R. Ketamine: A review for clinicians. Focus. 2018;16(3):243-50.
5. Malhi GS, Bell E, Bassett D, Boyce P, Bryant R, Hazell P, et al. The 2020 Royal Australian and New Zealand College of Psychiatrists clinical practice guidelines for mood disorders. Aust N Z J Psychiatry. 2015;49(12):1087-206.
6. Jagtiani A, Khurana H, Malhotra N. Comparison of efficacy of ketamine versus thiopentone-assisted modified electroconvulsive therapy in major depression. Indian J Psychiatry. 2019;61(3):258-64.
7. Schwenk ES, Viscusi ER, Buvanendran A, Hurley RW, Wasan AD, Narouze S, et al. Consensus guidelines on the use of intravenous ketamine infusions for acute pain management from the American Society of Regional Anesthesia and Pain Medicine, the American Academy of Pain Medicine, and

the American Society of Anesthesiologists. Reg Anesth Pain Med. 2018;43(5):456-66.

8. Swainson J, McGirr A, Blier P, Brietzke E, Richard-Devantoy S, Ravindran N, et al. The Canadian Network for Mood and Anxiety Treatments (CANMAT) Task Force Recommendations for the Use of Racemic Ketamine in Adults with Major Depressive Disorder: Recommandations Du Groupe De Travail Du Réseau Canadien Pour Les Traitements De L'humeur Et De L'anxiété (Canmat) Concernant L'utilisation De La Kétamine Racémique Chez Les Adultes Souffrant De Trouble Dépressif Majeur. Can J Psychiatry Rev Can Psychiatr. 2021;66(2):113-25.
9. In: Stahl SM (Ed). Prescriber's Guide: Stahl's Essential Psychopharmacology, 7th edition. Cambridge University Press; 2020. pp. 321-4.
10. Sarkhel S, Vijayakumar V, Vijayakumar L. Clinical Practice Guidelines for Management of Suicidal Behaviour. Indian J Psychiatry. 2023;65(2):124-30.
11. www.healthquality.va.gov. (2019). VA/DOD Clinical Practice Guideline for the assessment and management of patients at risk for suicide. [Online]. Available from https://www.healthquality.va.gov/guidelines/MH/srb/VADoDSuicideRiskFullCPGFinal5088212019.pdf [Last accessed June, 2025].

CHAPTER 9

# Management of Difficult-to-Treat Generalized Anxiety Disorder

*Sukanto Sarkar, Sukriti Mukherjee*

## INTRODUCTION

Generalized anxiety disorder (GAD) involves persistent anxiety symptoms on most days for several months. Symptoms include general apprehension (i.e., free-floating anxiety) or excessive worry about everyday events such as family, health, finances, school, and work, along with physical symptoms, such as muscle tension, restlessness, and autonomic overactivity. Additional signs are nervousness, difficulty concentrating, irritability, and sleep disturbances. GAD causes significant distress and impairment in life, but the symptoms should not be attributable to another health condition or substance.[1]

Anxiety disorders can occur alone or with other psychiatric conditions, especially depression. They tend to be chronic, and treatment is usually only partially successful.[2] Individuals with GAD are more prone to adverse effects and cannot tolerate high initial doses of selective serotonin reuptake inhibitors (SSRIs).[3]

The "stepped care" approach is recommended to select the most effective intervention. A comprehensive assessment is vital, considering distress, functional impairment, comorbid mental illnesses, substance misuse, medical conditions, and past treatment responses. Psychological therapy, especially cognitive behavioral therapy (CBT), is more effective than pharmacological therapy and should be prioritized when available.[4]

Pharmacological therapy, mainly SSRIs like sertraline, is effective. Patients should be informed about the benefits and disadvantages of each treatment.[4] For GAD, benzodiazepines should be reserved for crises, with SSRIs as the first-line treatment.[2] Serotonin norepinephrine reuptake inhibitors (SNRIs) and pregabalin are alternative first-line options. High-intensity psychological interventions and CBT-based self-help should be encouraged. Antipsychotics, including quetiapine, should be avoided for GAD.[4]

## TREATMENT-REFRACTORY GENERALIZED ANXIETY DISORDER[5] (TABLE 1)

### Assessment

- Check if the person has had an adequate treatment trial. There may be poor medication adherence, inadequate dose, or duration. They may not have had structured CBT with all effective components, enough sessions (weekly for the first 4–6 weeks), completed assigned tasks, or exposure to anxiety triggers. Assess this by checking with the patient's therapist and asking the patient about their therapy experience.
- Review the formulation, noting the social, environmental, and cultural factors that may limit improvement. Assess the social situation, stress levels, loss of function, and quality of life.
- Consider second-line treatments with evidence that have not been tried before, using medications that have been studied less.

### General Principles of Management

- Maintain continuity of care with regular, but not frequent, reviews.
- Encourage the patient to maintain an active life and avoid adopting a sick role.
- Set incremental goals for improving functionality.
- Foster hope for the future, recognizing that the patient's circumstances may change, making previous treatments viable again.
- Seek ongoing peer review and feedback.

### Shifting the Focus of Treatment

- The treatment goal now shifts from achieving symptom remission to managing symptoms and improving functionality while managing a chronic disorder. Enhancing a person's level of function may

**TABLE 1:** Treatment-refractory generalized anxiety disorder.

| | |
|---|---|
| Assessment | • Evaluate adequacy of treatment trial, including medication adherence, adequacy of dosing and duration of trials, and structured CBT<br>• Review social, environmental, and cultural factors that may limit improvement<br>• Review the diagnosis<br>• Rule out comorbid substance use, chronic medical conditions, and other psychiatric conditions |
| General principles of management | • Ensure continuity of care and conduct regular reviews<br>• Encourage an active life and discourage the sick role<br>• Set incremental goals for functional improvement<br>• Foster hope for the future<br>• Consider second-line treatments with evidence before exploring other options<br>• Seek peer review for additional perspectives |
| Shifting the focus of treatment | • Shift the treatment goal to symptom management and functional improvement<br>• Prioritize enhancing quality of life over reducing symptoms<br>• Discuss goals and provide psychoeducation on the recovery model |
| Psychological therapies | • Focus on supporting and adapting to chronic illness<br>• Introduce the recovery model and encourage goal review<br>• Consider supportive psychotherapy and interpretive/exploratory therapy<br>• Use structured treatments such as ACT and mindfulness-based therapies<br>• Ensure experienced clinicians provide these therapies<br>• Conduct an adequate number of sessions before abandoning therapy<br>• Consider continuation or booster sessions for effective modalities |

(ACT: acceptance and commitment therapy; CBT: cognitive behavioral therapy)

significantly enhance their quality of life compared to further symptom reduction efforts. A careful approach is needed, primarily aimed at enhancing quality of life. The clinician should schedule regularly but not overtly frequent appointments.

- Engage in goal-setting discussions with the patient and provide psychoeducation using a recovery-oriented model. Reframe treatment goals to prioritize maximizing functionality over symptom remission.

## Psychological Therapies

- Psychological therapy now focuses on supporting and adapting to chronic illness. Introduce the recovery model and encourage the patient to review their goals.
- Supportive psychotherapy with a dynamic approach and interpretive or exploratory therapy can be beneficial. For maximizing functioning, consider structured treatments including acceptance and commitment therapy or mindfulness-based therapies. These therapies aim to accept the current lived experience and reduce distress.
- Ensure these therapies are provided by experienced clinicians trained in these techniques. Provide an adequate number of sessions before discontinuation of each approach. If a therapy shows some effectiveness, consider continuing or scheduling "booster" sessions.

## Pharmacotherapy[2,5,6]

- If there is no response to the first SSRI, consider switching to another SSRI or an SNRI.
- Sometimes, the response to an SSRI may be delayed. If well tolerated, continue up to 12 weeks.
- If there is no response to SSRI/SNRI, consider switching to pregabalin or agomelatine.
- For resistant cases, benzodiazepines can be considered, but only for a short-term course.
- Combination of medications can be considered in difficult cases.[2]

# MANAGEMENT OF GENERALIZED ANXIETY DISORDER IN PREGNANCY AND LACTATION[7] (TABLE 2)

- *Ability to conceive:* Antidepressants may affect male sperm count and motility.
- *Pregnancy outcomes:* Antidepressant exposure has no significant impact on spontaneous abortion rates, APGAR scores, or birth weight, though there is a slight risk of increased postpartum hemorrhage, but it is not clinically significant.
- *Teratogenicity:* Evidence is conflicting. Some large studies indicate minimal risk, while others find no risk after adjusting for confounders.

**TABLE 2:** Generalized anxiety disorder in pregnancy and lactation.

| | |
|---|---|
| Impact of untreated anxiety disorder during pregnancy | • Significant impact on maternal well-being and potential risks to the child<br>• Treatment should not be avoided if maternal symptoms affect well-being, even if long-term risks are uncertain |
| Individualized treatment decisions | • Decisions on continuing or starting treatment should be tailored to the individual<br>• Options include medication and non-pharmacological methods<br>• Treatment decisions should be made by the patient and her family after receiving detailed information about available treatment options |
| Medication considerations | • Medication may be necessary if the disorder causes severe distress or impairment<br>• Consider the medication with a good response in the past. If treatment-naïve, follow recommendations for non-pregnant patients |
| First-line pharmacological agents | Selective serotonin reuptake inhibitors (SSRIs) (paroxetine to be avoided, sertraline has the best tolerability) |
| Benzodiazepines | Limited data regarding safety. Short-term use only |
| Regular review and the shortest period of treatment | Regularly review the need for treatment<br>Use medication for the shortest period necessary |

- *Neonatal and developmental problems:* Evidence is conflicting. Some studies suggest a link between in utero antidepressant exposure and an increased risk of autism or attention deficit hyperactivity disorder in childhood.
- *Breastfeeding:* SSRIs are generally safer, with sertraline being the safest and paroxetine best avoided.

## MANAGEMENT OF GENERALIZED ANXIETY DISORDER IN THE CHILD AND ADOLESCENT POPULATION[2,8] (TABLE 3)

- Fear and worry are normal in children, but anxiety disorders are common, especially in those with neurodevelopmental disorders.[9] Clinicians must differentiate between normal worries and impairing anxiety disorders, considering developmental variations.
- Anxiety symptoms may improve with age, but anxiety disorders require prompt treatment as they can impact brain development and impair normal experiences. Early and effective treatment can prevent long-term complications.
- Rule out hyperthyroidism, hypoglycemia, pheochromocytoma, migraine, seizure, delirium, brain tumors, cardiac arrhythmia, asthma, and lead poisoning.
- Take a detailed medical history and check for medications such as antiasthma drugs, sympathomimetics, steroids, SSRIs, antipsychotics (akathisia), diet pills, cold medicines, caffeine, and energy drinks, which can precipitate anxiety.
- Rule out depression, bipolar disorder, oppositional-defiant disorder, psychotic disorder, attention deficit hyperactivity disorder (ADHD), Asperger syndrome, and learning disabilities, as anxiety symptoms are common in these conditions.
- Record the baseline severity with rating scales and monitor progress with the same.
- Management should be multimodal, involving psychoeducation, psychotherapy, and pharmacotherapy.
- For mild to moderate anxiety, CBT should be preferred.
- For moderate to severe illness, pharmacotherapy should be added to CBT.
- Discuss treatment options with the child and their parents. Obtain written consent before starting medication.

## MANAGEMENT OF GENERALIZED ANXIETY DISORDER IN THE GERIATRIC POPULATION[10,11] (TABLE 4)

- Proper management of GAD in the geriatric population requires a comprehensive approach integrating medication, therapy, and lifestyle modifications.
- A multidisciplinary team involving physicians, psychiatrists, therapists, and other healthcare professionals ensures comprehensive and coordinated care for geriatric patients with GAD.
- Non-pharmacological treatments should be prioritized, except in severe cases. CBT is effective for GAD in older adults, focusing on identifying and

**TABLE 3:** Management of generalized anxiety disorder (GAD) in the child and adolescent population.

| | |
|---|---|
| Assessment | • Differentiate between normal worries and impairing anxiety disorders, considering developmental variations<br>• Anxiety symptoms may improve with age, but anxiety disorders require prompt treatment<br>• Use rating scales to record baseline severity and monitor progress<br>• Rule out comorbid substance use, chronic medical conditions, and other psychiatric conditions |
| Rule out medical illnesses that mimic symptoms of anxiety disorder | Hyperthyroidism, hypoglycemia, pheochromocytoma, migraine, seizure, delirium, brain tumors, cardiac arrhythmia, asthma, and lead poisoning |
| Check for medications that mimic symptoms of anxiety disorder | Antiasthma medications, sympathomimetics, steroids, SSRIs, antipsychotics (akathisia), cold medicines, and caffeine |
| Rule out psychiatric illnesses that mimic symptoms of anxiety disorder | • Depressive disorder<br>• Bipolar disorder<br>• Oppositional-defiant disorder<br>• Psychotic disorder<br>• ADHD<br>• Asperger syndrome<br>• Learning disabilities |
| General principles of management | • The management plan should involve psychoeducation, psychotherapy, and pharmacotherapy<br>• Discuss the treatment options with the young ones and their parents<br>• Document the written consent before starting the medication<br>• For mild to moderate anxiety, CBT should be preferred<br>• For moderate to severe illness, pharmacotherapy should be added to CBT |
| Pharmacotherapy | • Start at the lowest available dose<br>• Monitor for side effects<br>• Titrate every 7 days for SSRI and 14 days for SNRI<br>• Dosing of medications is similar to adult dosing<br>• SSRIs are the preferred choice<br>• Escitalopram and fluoxetine are better tolerated<br>• After a failed trial of 2 SSRIs, SNRI (venlafaxine) can be tried<br>• Benzodiazepines and TCAs should be avoided except in special cases<br>• Continuation should be for at least 1 year of stable improvement<br>• Taper off slowly and monitor closely during this period |
| Psychological therapies | • Focus on supporting and adapting to chronic illness<br>• Introduce the recovery model and encourage goal review<br>• Consider supportive psychotherapy and interpretive/exploratory therapy<br>• Use structured treatments such as acceptance and commitment therapy (ACT) and mindfulness-based therapies<br>• Ensure experienced clinicians provide these therapies<br>• Conduct an adequate number of sessions before abandoning a particular therapy modality<br>• Consider continuation or booster sessions for effective modalities |

(ADHD: attention deficit hyperactivity disorder; CBT: cognitive behavioral therapy; SNRI: serotonin-norepinephrine reuptake inhibitor; SSRI: selective serotonin reuptake inhibitor; TCA: tricyclic antidepressant)

challenging negative thought patterns, managing worry, and developing coping strategies.

- Educating geriatric patients and their families about GAD, its symptoms, and treatment options can reduce stigma, increase treatment adherence, and enhance outcomes.
- Teaching relaxation techniques such as deep breathing, progressive muscle relaxation, and mindfulness meditation can help manage anxiety and promote calmness.
- Regular physical activity, such as walking and gentle stretching, has been shown to reduce anxiety symptoms in older adults.

**TABLE 4:** Management of GAD in the geriatric population.[10,11]

| | |
|---|---|
| Assessment | • Differentiate between normal worries and impairing anxiety disorders, considering age-related variations<br>• Evaluate the hearing and vision<br>• Use rating scales to record the baseline severity and monitor the progress<br>• Rule out comorbid substance use, chronic medical conditions, and other psychiatric conditions<br>• Degree of cognitive impairment<br>• Limitations in activity<br>• Activities of daily living |
| General principles of management | • The first line of management is a nonpharmacological intervention<br>• If it fails, then opt for pharmacological intervention |
| Nonpharmacological intervention | • Lifestyle modification<br>• Behavioral therapy<br>• CBT<br>• Mindfulness<br>• Yoga, art therapy, music and dance therapy, and social activities |
| Pharmacotherapy | • Start at the lowest available dose<br>• Monitor vigilantly for side effects<br>• SSRI, SNRI, and buspirone are first-line choices<br>• Mirtazapine, pregabalin, TCAs are second-line options<br>• Benzodiazepines should be avoided unless there is no response with first- and second-line drugs<br>• Dosing should be half of the expected adult dose<br>• A trial of at least 4 weeks is essential before rendering it as a failed trial<br>• Continuation should be for at least 1 year of stable improvement<br>• Taper off slowly and monitor closely during this period |

(CBT: cognitive behavioral therapy; GAD: generalized anxiety disorder; SNRI: serotonin-norepinephrine reuptake inhibitor; SSRI: selective serotonin reuptake inhibitor; TCA: tricyclic antidepressant)

- SSRIs and SNRIs are commonly prescribed for GAD in older adults, with careful dosage adjustments due to age-related metabolic changes and potential medication interactions.
- Start medications at the lowest effective dose and titrate slowly to optimize treatment.
- Maintaining social connections and engaging in meaningful activities can provide emotional support and reduce isolation, which are associated with anxiety.
- Promoting a healthy lifestyle, including a balanced diet, adequate sleep, and avoiding excessive caffeine and alcohol, supports mental health in older adults with GAD.
- Regular follow-up with healthcare providers is crucial to monitor treatment progress, adjust medications if necessary, and address emerging concerns or side effects.

**TABLE 5:** Management of GAD in hepatic impairment.[2,12,13]

| | |
|---|---|
| Fluoxetine | • Extensively hepatically metabolized with a long half-life<br>• Reduce dose by at least 50% or administer on alternate days<br>• It takes many weeks to reach steady-state serum levels |
| Other SSRIs | • Reduce dose by 50% and/or reduce dosing frequency<br>• Paroxetine and escitalopram are drugs of choice<br>• Sertraline and paroxetine are used in the management of cholestatic pruritus<br>• Beware of the increased risk of bleeding |
| TCAs | • All are hepatically metabolized, highly protein-bound, and will accumulate<br>• Sedative TCAs are best avoided |
| Venlafaxine/ desvenlafaxine | Reduce dose by 50% in mild and moderate hepatic impairment |
| Vilazodone/ Vortioxetine | No dosage adjustment required |
| Duloxetine/ Agomelatine | Contraindicated in hepatic impairment |

(GAD: generalized anxiety disorder; SSRIs: selective serotonin reuptake inhibitors; TCAs: tricyclic antidepressants)

## MANAGEMENT OF GENERALIZED ANXIETY DISORDER IN PATIENTS WITH MEDICAL COMORBIDITIES

### Hepatic Impairment[2,12,13] (Table 5)

- Limit the number of prescribed drugs.
- Start with lower doses for drugs with high protein binding or extensive first-pass metabolism.
- Be cautious with medications undergoing significant hepatic metabolism.
- Increase intervals between dosages due to prolonged drug half-life in hepatic impairment.

- Avoid medications with long half-lives or those requiring hepatic activation (prodrugs).
- Monitor patients closely for delayed side effects.
- Minimize sedative medications to reduce the risk of hepatic encephalopathy.
- Avoid constipating drugs that may trigger hepatic encephalopathy.
- Avoid hepatotoxic medications, such as MAOIs and chlorpromazine.
- Choose low-risk drugs and regularly monitor liver function tests (LFTs), switching if needed. Cross-hepatotoxicity is possible with structurally related drugs.

## Renal Impairment[2,14,15]

- Start at a low dose and increase slowly. Prescribe as few drugs as possible.
- Be cautious with drugs that are extensively renally cleared, such as pregabalin and gabapentin.
- Monitor patient for adverse effects, as those with renal impairment are more likely to experience and take longer to develop side effects, such as sedation, confusion, and postural hypotension.
- Be vigilant for serotonin syndrome with antidepressants.
- Monitor estimated glomerular filtration rate (eGFR) carefully and frequently.

## Diabetes[2,16,17]

- Nearly one in five diabetes patients has GAD.
- Managing these cases requires collaboration between the endocrinologist and psychiatrist.
- Medication, psychotherapy, and lifestyle modifications can improve the patient's quality of life.
- When pharmacotherapy is considered, SSRIs have a favorable profile.
- Fluoxetine, sertraline, and escitalopram are associated with improved glycemic control.
- TCAs are associated with worsening glycemic control.
- Caution should be taken while prescribing β-blockers to patients on hypoglycemic agents.
- Benzodiazepines should be prescribed for the shortest possible duration.

## REFERENCES

1. World Health Organization. International Statistical Classification of Diseases and Related Health Problems (ICD). [Online] Available from https://www.who.int/standards/classifications/classification-of-diseases [Last accessed June, 2025].
2. Taylor DM, Barnes TRE, Young AH (Eds). The Maudsley Prescribing Guidelines in Psychiatry, 14th edition. Hoboken: John Wiley & Sons; 2021.
3. Nash JR, Nutt DJ. Pharmacotherapy of Anxiety. Handb Exp Pharmacol. 2005;(169):469-501.
4. National Institute for Health and Clinical Excellence. (2011). Generalised anxiety disorder and panic disorder in adults: management. Clinical Guideline [CG113]. [Online] Available from https://www.ncbi.nlm.nih.gov/books/NBK552847/ [Last accessed June, 2025].
5. Andrews G, Bell C, Boyce P, Gale C, Lampe L, Marwat O, et al. Royal Australian and New Zealand College of Psychiatrists clinical practice guidelines for the treatment of panic disorder, social anxiety disorder and generalised anxiety disorder. Aust N Z J Psychiatry. 2018;52(12): 1109-72.
6. Gautam S, Jain A, Gautam M, Vahia V, Gautam A. Clinical Practice Guidelines for the Management of Generalised Anxiety Disorder (GAD) and Panic Disorder (PD). Indian J Psychiatry. 2017;59(Suppl 1):S67-73.
7. McAllister-Williams RH, Baldwin DS, Cantwell R, Easter A, Gilvarry E, Glover V, et al. British Association for Psychopharmacology consensus guidance on the use of psychotropic medication preconception, in pregnancy and postpartum 2017. J Psychopharmacol. 2017;31(5):519-52.
8. Walter HJ, Bukstein OG, Abright AR, Keable H, Ramtekkar U, Ripperger-Suhler J, et al. Clinical Practice Guideline for the Assessment and Treatment of Children and Adolescents With Anxiety Disorders. J Am Acad Child Adolesc Psychiatry. 2020;59(10):1107-24.
9. Simonoff E, Pickles A, Charman T, Chandler S, Loucas T, Baird G. Psychiatric Disorders in Children With Autism Spectrum Disorders: Prevalence, Comorbidity, and Associated Factors in a Population-Derived Sample. J Am Acad Child Adolesc Psychiatry. 2008;47(8):921-9.
10. Wetherell Julie Loebach, Stein Murray B. Anxiety disorders in chapter Geriatric Psychiatry in Kaplan and Sadock's Comprehensive Textbook of Psychiatry. In: Sadock Benjamin, Sadock Virginia, Ruiz Pedro., (Eds). 9th edition. Wolters Kluwer: Lippincott Williams & Wilkins; pp. 4040-47.
11. Subramanyam A, Kedare J, Singh O, Pinto C. Clinical practice guidelines for geriatric anxiety disorders. Indian J Psychiatry. 2018;(Suppl 3):S371-82.
12. Billioti De Gage S, Collin C, Le-Tri T, Pariente A, Bégaud B, Verdoux H, et al. Antidepressants and Hepatotoxicity: A Cohort Study among 5 Million Individuals Registered in the French National Health Insurance Database. CNS Drugs. 2018;32(7):673-84.
13. Telles-Correia D, Barbosa A, Cortez-Pinto H, Campos C, Rocha NBF, Machado S. Psychotropic drugs and liver disease: a critical review of pharmacokinetics and

liver toxicity. World J Gastrointest Pharmacol Ther. 2017;8(1):26-38.
14. Palmer SC, Natale P, Ruospo M, Saglimbene VM, Rabindranath KS, Craig JC, et al. Antidepressants for treating depression in adults with end-stage kidney disease treated with dialysis. Cochrane Database Syst Rev. 2016;2016(5):CD004541.
15. Nagler EV, Webster AC, Vanholder R, Zoccali C. Antidepressants for depression in stage 3-5 chronic kidney disease: a systematic review of pharmacokinetics, efficacy and safety with recommendations by European Renal Best Practice (ERBP)*. Nephrol Dial Transplant. 2012;27(10):3736-45.
16. Hendrieckx C, Halliday JA, Beeney LJ, Speight J (Eds). Diabetes and emotional health: a practical guide for healthcare professionals supporting adults with Type 1 and Type 2 diabetes. London: Diabetes UK, 2019, 2nd edition (UK).
17. Baumeister H, Hutter N, Bengel J. Psychological and pharmacological interventions for depression in patients with diabetes mellitus and depression. Cochrane Database Syst Rev. 2012;12(12):CD008381.

CHAPTER 10

# Management of Difficult-to-Treat Social Anxiety Disorder

*Ravi Philip Rajkumar*

## KEY COMPONENTS OF COGNITIVE-BEHAVIORAL THERAPY FOR SOCIAL ANXIETY DISORDER

- *Social anxiety disorder (SAD),* also known as *social phobia,* is a mental illness characterized by anxiety related to social interactions, performance, or both.[1]
  a. This anxiety involves fears of scrutiny or negative evaluation by others and is often accompanied by somatic manifestations such as blushing, tremors, increased perspiration, or palpitations.
  b. SAD often leads to *avoidance* of feared situations. When avoidance is not possible, patients report significant distress or discomfort.
  c. SAD may be *generalized* or *specific.* In generalized SAD, patients experience significant anxiety in a wide range of social situations. Specific SAD is confined to one or two well-defined situations (e.g., public speaking, eating, or using restrooms in public places).
- Estimates of the prevalence of SAD vary widely between countries. In Western countries, prevalence rates of 8–15% have been reported. The recent National Mental Health Survey in India (2015–16) reported a prevalence of 0.47% for SAD. SAD is about 1.5 times more common in women than in men, with onset typically in late childhood or adolescence.
- SAD is sometimes considered the "*neglected anxiety disorder*" as it is often unrecognized and untreated, despite its chronicity and associated disability.[1,2]
  a. Even with appropriate treatment, around 55–60% of patients remain symptomatic over a period of 5–10 years.
  b. Among patients who respond well to treatment, there is a 30–40% risk of recurrence over the same period.
  c. An earlier age of onset, generalized SAD, and the presence of psychiatric comorbidity are associated with a poorer response to treatment.

## COMORBIDITY IN SOCIAL ANXIETY DISORDER

- Psychiatric *comorbidity* is the rule rather than the exception in SAD. SAD generally precedes the onset of most comorbid disorders. The most common comorbid diagnoses are depression (35–70%), other anxiety disorders (15–45%), and substance use disorders (up to 50%). About 3–15% of patients with SAD have comorbid bipolar disorder. In these cases, symptoms of SAD may be more prominent during depressive episodes and absent or minimal during manic episodes.[2]

## EVIDENCE-BASED TREATMENTS FOR SOCIAL ANXIETY DISORDER

- Evidence-based first-line treatments for SAD include selective serotonin reuptake inhibitors (SSRIs) and cognitive-behavioral therapy (CBT), both of which are equally effective.[3,4]
  a. About 40–60% of patients respond well to their first treatment trial.
  b. If a patient responds well to an initial trial of medication, it should be continued for at least 1 year.
  c. SSRIs with good evidence of efficacy in SAD include *sustained-release paroxetine, escitalopram, sertraline, and fluvoxamine.* Fluoxetine has mixed evidence of efficacy and is not the preferred first-line option.
  d. An adequate medication trial for SAD should last 10–12 weeks.
  e. CBT should be *specifically tailored for SAD* and not delivered in a "generic" form.
     *Key components of CBT for SAD are:*
     - Education
     - Graded exposure to address the harmful effects of avoidance or safety behaviors.
     - Therapist or video feedback for negative self-perceptions.

- Training to focus attention on specific situations rather than the self.
- Behavioral assignments, "homework" between sessions.
- Identifying and "rescripting" past situations of social rejection or trauma.
- Modifying core beliefs about the self, others, and social situations.
- Relapse prevention.[5]

f. *Online CBT* can be a valuable alternative to in-person CBT if access to the latter is difficult.

## DEFINITION AND CLINICAL EVALUATION OF DIFFICULT-TO-TREAT SAD

- There is no widely accepted definition of "treatment-resistant," "treatment-refractory," or "difficult-to-treat" SAD.[1,2,4]
  a. In pharmacotherapy trials, a reduction of 35% or more in symptom severity using a standardized symptom rating scale is used to define a *response*.
  b. In a trial specifically involving patients with difficult-to-treat SAD, *"refractory SAD"* was defined as a Liebowitz Social Anxiety Scale (LSAS) score of >50 even after 10 weeks of adequate treatment with an SSRI. *"Remission"* was defined as LSAS <30 following treatment.
- It is important to differentiate between resistance and "pseudoresistance" in the management of SAD. Pseudoresistance refers to treatment failures caused by errors in diagnosis or inadequate treatment.
  a. The *differential diagnoses of SAD* are listed in **Table 1** and should be considered in any patient who does not respond to treatment. However, it should be borne in mind that many of these conditions can co-occur with SAD.[3]

**TABLE 1:** Differential diagnoses of social anxiety disorder.

| ***Differential diagnosis*** | ***Points of difference with SAD*** |
|---|---|
| Anxious-avoidant personality disorder (AAPD) | AAPD is very similar to SAD and is considered by some experts as a variant of early-onset, generalized SAD. Treatment of both conditions is similar, but AAPD may require long-term cognitive therapy due to associated views of oneself as incompetent or inept |
| Generalized anxiety disorder (GAD) | In GAD, anxiety symptoms are not specifically related to or confined to social or performance situations. GAD also includes symptoms such as irritability, increased muscle tension, and difficulty relaxing, which are not seen in SAD |
| Panic disorder (PD) | • Patients with PD have typical attacks of severe anxiety with a crescendo-decrescendo pattern lasting 5–45 minutes, associated with fear of having another attack (anticipatory anxiety) and secondary agoraphobia<br>• Patients with SAD may experience panic attacks in specific social situations, but these are not spontaneous and are confined to those situations |
| Obsessive-compulsive disorder (OCD) | Patients with OCD may avoid specific social interactions due to their obsessions (e.g., fear of contamination, sexual or aggressive thoughts), but they do not report a fear of social situations, scrutiny, or criticism as in SAD. Compulsions are typical of OCD and are present in SAD |
| Body dysmorphic disorder (BDD) | The core feature of BDD is preoccupation with an exaggerated or imagined defect in one's physical appearance. BDD can lead to secondary social anxiety or avoidance, but body image disturbance is primary. Individuals with BDD may camouflage the perceived "defect" or request cosmetic surgery, which are absent in SAD |
| Post-traumatic stress disorder (PTSD) | Avoidance and anxiety in specific social situations (e.g., interactions with the opposite gender) may occur in some cases of PTSD (e.g., those involving sexual abuse or trauma). PTSD is characterized by emotional numbing, hypervigilance, and "flashbacks" of traumatic incidents, triggered by particular social or interpersonal situations |
| Major depression | Depression can lead to social avoidance and low self-esteem, but is not typically associated with marked anxiety or a fear of scrutiny or negative evaluation, as seen in SAD. Depression typically runs an episodic course, while SAD tends to be continuous |
| Schizotypal disorder | Social anxiety is a diagnostic criterion for schizotypal disorder. However, in this disorder, social anxiety is associated with ideas of reference or persecution rather than fears of negative evaluation. Other symptoms include odd or eccentric beliefs, mannerisms, suspiciousness, and vague or circumstantial speech |

b. Inadequate treatment may be due to inadequate doses of medication, insufficient durations of medication trials, nonadherence to treatment, or failure to use CBT techniques specific to SAD.[5] Nonadherence may be due to adverse effects or psychosocial factors (e.g., difficulties in obtaining medication and nonmedical explanatory models) and should be carefully assessed and managed.

- When undertaking treatment trials in difficult-to-treat SAD, using clinician-rated measures of symptom severity, such as the LSAS at baseline and during follow-ups, is crucial to objectively assess treatment response.

## TREATMENT OPTIONS FOR DIFFICULT-TO-TREAT SAD

- If a patient fails an initial treatment trial in SAD, evidence-based treatment options include **(Flowchart 1)**:
  A. *If the initial treatment was with SSRIs*:
    a. *Switching* to a second SSRI (from the list in c under evidence-based treatment of social anxiety disorder) for 10–12 weeks.

**Flowchart 1:** Algorithm for the management of difficult-to-treat social anxiety disorder.

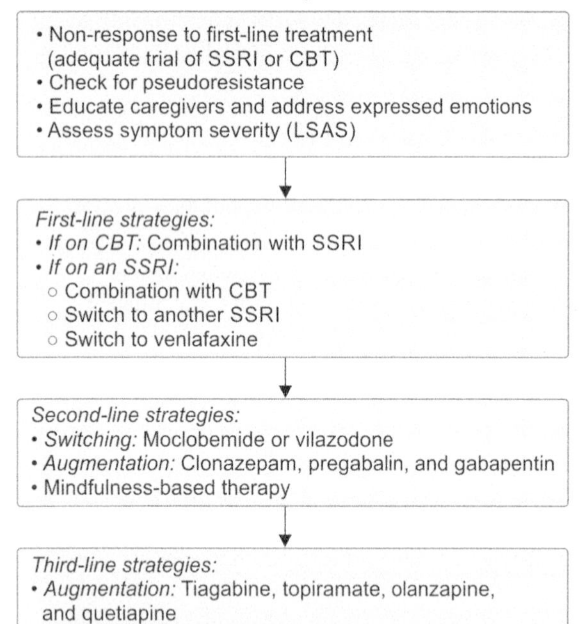


(CBT: cognitive-behavioral therapy; LSAS: Liebowitz Social Anxiety Scale; SSRI: selective serotonin reuptake inhibitor)
Details of doses and trial durations for each medication mentioned in the flowchart are provided in the text.

    b. *Switching* to sustained-release venlafaxine (up to 225 mg/day) for 10–12 weeks.
    c. *Adding* cognitive-behavioral therapy (14–16 sessions, which should be completed within 4 months) to medication.
  B. *If the initial treatment was with CBT:*
    a. Consider *adding* an SSRI for 10–12 weeks.

- If a patient does not respond to treatment options listed above, the following strategies, supported by evidence from randomized controlled trials, may be considered:
  a. *Switching* to the reversible monoamine oxidase inhibitor (MAO-I) moclobemide, 75–600 mg/day for 12 weeks. No significant dietary adjustments are required due to its reversible nature.
  b. *Switching* to the novel antidepressant vilazodone (20–40 mg/day) for 12 weeks.
  c. *Augmentation* with clonazepam (0.5–3 mg/day in 2–3 divided doses) for 10–12 weeks. It is recommended to taper gradually (reduce by one-eighth of the dose weekly) after 3 months due to limited evidence of long-term efficacy and potential for misuse or dependence.
  d. *Augmentation* with pregabalin (450–600 mg/day in two divided doses) for 10 weeks. This drug is effective as maintenance treatment for up to 6 months.
  e. *Augmentation* with gabapentin (minimum effective dose 900 mg/day) for 12 weeks.
  f. *Augmentation* with mindfulness-based psychological interventions (8–12 weekly sessions) delivered by a trained therapist.

- If the above options are not effective, the following strategies can be considered on a case-by-case basis *as augmentation strategies*. They are supported by evidence from open trials:
  a. Anticonvulsants: tiagabine (4–16 mg/day) for 12 weeks or topiramate (25–400 mg/day) for 16 weeks.
  b. *Atypical antipsychotics*: Olanzapine (5–20 mg/day) or quetiapine (50–400 mg/day) for 8 weeks. These drugs may cause sedation or weight gain, and there is no evidence supporting their long-term use.

- In *situational* SAD, there is anecdotal evidence for using propranolol (40–160 mg) "as-needed" for specific anxiety-provoking situations (e.g., public speaking). However, there is no evidence supporting its prolonged use as monotherapy or augmentation in any form of SAD.

- The following drugs have been found ineffective in randomized controlled trials and should not be used as monotherapy or augmentation in SAD: Antipsychotics or anticonvulsants (except the four drugs listed above), atomoxetine, mirtazapine, tricyclic antidepressants, and vortioxetine.
- Though these drugs are not useful in treating SAD, they can be used if necessary to treat comorbid conditions (e.g., atomoxetine for patients with SAD and comorbid attention-deficit/hyperactivity disorder (ADHD), valproate for patients with SAD and bipolar disorder).
- Caregivers should be educated about the nature of SAD. Addressing negative expressed emotions (such as hostility, criticism, or overinvolvement) is important, as high negative expressed emotions may adversely impact treatment response, particularly in adolescents.
- If a patient responds well to pharmacotherapy at any stage, it is recommended to continue treatment for at least 6–12 months before considering tapering or discontinuation of medications.
- Booster sessions (once a month, for up to 12 months) may be required to ensure a sustained response to CBT.

## EMERGING TREATMENT OPTIONS

a. Ketamine (0.25–1 mg/kg subcutaneously or 0.5 mg/kg intravenous infusion) has a rapid anxiolytic effect in SAD that may last up to 2 weeks.
b. Transcranial direct current stimulation (tDCS), involving excitatory stimulation of the left dorsolateral prefrontal cortex given twice a day for 5 days, has an anxiolytic effect in SAD that may be sustained for up to 2 months.
c. Though these treatment approaches show promise, but are still experimental. Their administration requires trained personnel and specialized equipment.

## REFERENCES

1. National Collaborating Centre for Mental Health. Social anxiety disorder: recognition, assessment and treatment. London: National Institute for Health and Care Excellence; 2013.
2. Andrews G, Bell C, Boyce P, Gale C, Lampe L, Marwat O, et al. Royal Australian and New Zealand College of Psychiatrists clinical practice guidelines for the treatment of panic disorder, social anxiety disorder, and generalized anxiety disorder. Aust N Z J Psychiatry. 2018;52(12):1109-72.
3. Tharwani HM, Davidson JRT. Symptomatic and functional assessment of social anxiety disorder in adults. Psychiatr Clin North Am. 2001;24(4):643-59.
4. Williams T, Hattingh CJ, Kariuki CM, Tromp SA, van Balkom AJ, Ipser JC, et al. Pharmacotherapy for social anxiety disorder. Cochrane Database Syst Rev. 2017;10(10):CD001206.
5. Janardhan Reddy YC, Sudhir PM, Manjula M, Arumugham SS, Narayanaswamy JC. Clinical practice guidelines for cognitive-behavioral therapies in anxiety disorders and obsessive-compulsive and related disorders. Indian J Psychiatry. 2020;62(Suppl 2):S230-50.

# CHAPTER 11

# Management of Difficult-to-Treat Somatic Symptom Disorder

*Prerna Kukreti, Saloni Seth*

## INTRODUCTION

- *Somatoform disorders* are a group of psychiatric disorders in which patients present with a myriad of symptoms, which are *often medically unexplained.*[1]
- They can suffer from a *variety of bodily complaints*, such as pain in different locations of the body, from fatigue, or from perceived disturbances of the cardiovascular, gastrointestinal, or other organ functions.
- Many patients complain of multiple symptoms concurrently and over time, but some suffer from only one persisting symptom.
- Apart from bodily complaints, there can also be the *presence of psychological and behavioral features*, including high health anxiety and related checking behavior.
- These bodily complaints are *persistently attributed to organic disease.*
- What makes it even more difficult to diagnose and manage is that *diagnostic and therapeutic approaches to the patients vary* substantially across and within medical specialties, from biomedicine to psychiatry, and these approaches usually are not complementary, but all too often contradictory.[2]
- In psychiatry, different diagnostic categories have been given in different classificatory systems:
  - Somatic symptom disorder (SSD) in DSM-5[1]
  - Somatoform disorders in ICD-10[3]
  - Bodily distress disorder in ICD-11[4]
  - There are also many single functional somatic syndrome diagnoses (like irritable bowel syndrome (IBS) or fibromyalgia syndrome (FMS)[5]
- In somatoform disorders, there is *no well-defined structural organic pathology* that correlates to the symptoms; hence, called functional. *Organic pathology, if present,* it *does not explain the extent of symptoms and distress* due to the same, and successful treatment and remission of the pathology do not relieve the symptoms.[6]
- DSM-5 introduced a new classification category of *SSD*. There are two important changes that are important to consider:
  - The requirement that *somatic symptoms have to be medically unexplained to be dropped.*
  - Certain *psychobehavioral features* are to be present while doing the assessment, which include:
    i. Disproportionate and persistent thoughts about the seriousness of one's symptoms.
    ii. High level of anxiety present persistently about one's health or symptoms.[1]
    iii. Excessive time and energy devoted to these symptoms or to concern about one's health.
  - These symptoms should be present persistently for ≥6 months, although it is not necessary for any symptom to be continuously present.[1]

## ASSESSMENT AND MANAGEMENT OF SSD

- *Assessment and Management of SSD* includes the following:
  - Patients are usually referred with a suspected (differential) diagnosis of SSD in mind to mental health care settings and to psychosomatic and psychiatric consultation liaison services.
  - In such a situation, it is not difficult to ascertain the presence or absence of the relevant diagnostic criteria, and the fact that there is no longer a necessity to ascertain bodily symptoms as being organically unexplained makes it easier to arrive at a diagnosis of somatoform disorder.
  - *Valid self-report questionnaires* are there for screening and for aiding in diagnosis. Some of these include:
    - Patient health questionnaire-15 (PHQ-15) for somatic symptom burden.[7]
    - Whiteley Index for health anxiety **Table 1**.[8]

**TABLE 1 THE PHQ-15 SCREENING INSTRUMENT FOR SOMATIC SYMPTOM DISORDER.**

| *During the past 4 weeks, how much have you been bothered by any of the following problems?* | *Not botherer (0)* | *Bothered a little (1)* | *Bothered a lot (2)* |
|---|---|---|---|
| Stomach pain | O | O | O |
| Back pain | O | O | O |
| Pain in your arms, legs, or joints (knees, hips, etc.) | O | O | O |
| Menstrual cramps or other problems with your periods (women only) | O | O | O |
| Headaches | O | O | O |
| Chest pain | O | O | O |
| Dizziness | O | O | O |
| Fainting spells | O | O | O |
| Feeling your heart pound or race | O | O | O |
| Shortness of breath | O | O | O |
| Pain or problems during sexual intercourse | O | O | O |
| Constipation, loose bowels, or diarrhea | O | O | O |
| Nausea, gas, or indigestion | O | O | O |
| | *Not at all (0)* | *Several days (1)* | *>Half the days (2)* |
| Feeling tired or having low energy | O | O | O |
| Trouble sleeping | O | O | O |
| **Total Score:** | | | |

*Note:* PHQ-15 scores of 5, 10, and 15, represented cutoff points for low, medium, and high somatic symptom severity, respectively.

    - Self-report instruments to assess the psychobehavioral criteria in SSD have also now been published.
- Although diagnostic ascertainment is not a major challenge, the *establishment of a stable doctor-patient relationship as a basis for treatment* very often *remains a difficult initial challenge.*
- Following recommendations for interventions by a Mental Health Professional are advocated:[9]
    - For patients with persistent physical symptoms, *consider the possibility of SSD as early as possible.* Do not equate them with malingering.
    - *Avoid repetitive, especially risky investigations* that serve only to calm the patient.
    - *Screen for other physical symptoms and psychiatric comorbidities* such as anxiety and depression.
    - Assess for *substance use or suicidal ideations.*
    - Assess the patient's experiences, expectations, functioning, beliefs, and illness behavior, especially with regard to catastrophizing, body checking, avoidance, and dysfunctional health care utilization.

## PRACTICE MANAGEMENT STRATEGIES FOR DIFFICULT-TO-TREAT SSD

- *Practice Management Strategies for difficult-to-treat SSDs include:*[10]
    - Accept that patients can have distressing, real physical symptoms and medical conditions with coexisting psychiatric disturbance without malingering or feigning.
    - Consider and discuss the possibility of somatoform disorders with the patient early in the workup, and to make a diagnosis only when all the criteria are met.
    - Once the diagnosis is confirmed, provide patient education on the individual disorder, using empathy and avoiding confrontation.
    - Avoid unnecessary medical tests and referrals.
    - Be cautious when pursuing new symptoms with new tests and referrals.

- Focus on *improving the functioning* of the individual and *not symptoms*, and *on management of the disorder* and *not cure*.
- Advise lifestyle modifications and stress reduction methods.
- Include the patient's family members, if possible.
- Treat psychiatric comorbidities with appropriate interventions.
- Schedule *regular follow-ups* with the patient to provide attention and reassurance, while at the same time *limiting frequent telephone calls and "urgent" visits.*

▪ *Psychotherapy*, especially *cognitive behavioral therapy (CBT)* is an established treatment modality[11] in patients with SSD, but it meets with specific challenges in the initial phases, when patients very often find it difficult to accept that a "talking cure" might help with their primarily bodily symptoms and concerns **(Table 2)**.

▪ The *recommendations for the initial phases of psychotherapy*, which aim at building a sustainable therapeutic relationship,[12] independent of later differentiation as per patient problems and psychotherapy school to be followed (*adapted and translated from Henningsen and Martin)* **(Table 2)**:
- Clarify the motivation of the patient for psychotherapeutic consultation.
- *Acknowledge the patient's symptoms* and the fact that the symptoms have an undetected organic basis.
- Listen attentively to bodily complaints and experiences connected to them (with respect to relationships with doctors and other health professionals, relatives, colleagues, etc.)
- Assess for *emotional aspects of these experiences* (anger, disappointment, fear, etc.)
- In chronic patients, help in supporting and organizing the history of presenting complaints into a coherent narrative.
- Explain to the patient *both psychosocial and biological context factors* (through use of a symptom context diary; not recommended for patients with very high health anxiety).
- Discuss *realistic, i.e., modest treatment goals* and improve coping skills.
- Do not advocate "cure" as a treatment goal.
- *Avoid discussing psychosocial issues too early* and independently of the main somatic complaints. If necessary, "somatize," i.e., enquire about current bodily symptoms.

**TABLE 2:** Key recommendations for practice.[2]

| *Clinical recommendation* | *Evidence rating* | *Comments* |
|---|---|---|
| Fostering a *strong physician-patient relationship* is integral to managing somatoform disorders | C | Recommendations from clinical practice settings |
| *CBT is effective* in treating patients with somatoform disorders | B | Consistent findings from RCT |
| Psychiatric consultation helps improve the effects of somatoform disorders | B | Findings from RCT |

(A: consistent, good-quality patient-oriented evidence; B: inconsistent or limited-quality patient-oriented evidence; C: consensus, disease-oriented evidence, usual practice, expert opinion, or case series)

- *Liaisoning with other departments* is important to obtain relevant information and to assess for further therapeutic interventions. It also sends across the message to the patient that appropriate care for him is being taken and constructive cooperation is possible, and an effective management strategy is being made.

## PHARMACOLOGICAL MANAGEMENT FOR SSD

▪ The following factors are important in planning pharmacological treatment for SSD:
- Take a *pragmatic approach,* i.e., provide symptomatic treatment until a definite etiology and intervention are identified.
- *Prepare patients well before initiation of medication* by explaining the rationale, expected outcome, and common side effects.
- Focus on care rather than cause or cure.
- *Aim at improving the quality of life.*
- Focus on relief, coping, and *return to function.*
- Give *adequate trial for at least 12 weeks* before declaring any drug as ineffective and explain patient to expect improvement over several weeks or months.
- Psychotherapies are not a substitute for pharmacological treatment, as highlighted above, and *different treatments are complementary.*
- *Start low in dosage and titrate gradually* over weeks rather than days, as patients are usually sensitive to side effects because of the nature of the illness.

- *Summary for pharmacological management of SSD:*
  - The evidence indicates that *all classes of antidepressants are superior to placebo* in most subtypes of somatic symptom disorders.
  - *Antidepressants with dual action serotonin and noradrenaline seem more effective than other antidepressants* if pain is the main symptom.[13]
  - *Specific serotonin reuptake inhibitors* seem to *be more effective in hypochondriasis and body dysmorphic disorder.*[14]
  - The *dosages* of antidepressants appear *less than those used in depressive disorder in somatoform and related disorders*, and *higher* than typically used in depression *for hypochondriasis and body dysmorphic disorder.*
  - The *minimum time for improvement is 6 weeks* or more.
  - Limited evidence suggests that the *effect is sustained for up to 24 weeks.*
  - Very limited evidence indicates that *atypical antipsychotics may be effective in somatoform disorder.*
  - There are no systematically conducted trials for antipsychotics in hypochondriasis and body dysmorphic disorder.

## REFERENCES


1. American Psychiatric Association. Diagnostic and statistical manual of mental disorders: DSM-5, 5th edition. Washington, DC: APA; 2013.
2. Henningsen P. Management of functional somatic syndromes and somatoform disorders. Dialogues Clin Neurosci. 2018;20(1):23-31.
3. World Health Organization. The ICD-10 classification of mental and behavioural disorders: clinical descriptions and diagnostic guidelines. Geneva: WHO; 1992.
4. World Health Organization. International Classification of Diseases 11th Revision (ICD-11). Geneva: WHO; 2019.
5. Wessely S, Nimnuan C, Sharpe M. Functional somatic syndromes: one or many? Lancet. 1999;354(9182):936-9.
6. Creed F, Henningsen P, Fink P (Eds). Medically unexplained symptoms, somatisation and bodily distress: developing better clinical services. Cambridge: Cambridge University Press; 2011.
7. Kroenke K, Spitzer RL, Williams JB. The PHQ-15: validity of a new measure for evaluating the severity of somatic symptoms. Psychosom Med. 2002;64(2):258-66.
8. Pilowsky I. Dimensions of hypochondriasis. Br J Psychiatry. 1967;113(494):89-93.
9. National Institute for Health and Care Excellence (NICE). Medically unexplained symptoms: assessment and management [NG75]. London: NICE; 2021.
10. Barsky AJ, Borus JF. Functional somatic syndromes. Ann Intern Med. 1999;130(11):910-21.
11. Allen LA, Woolfolk RL, Escobar JI, Gara MA, Hamer RM. Cognitive-behavioral therapy for somatization disorder: a randomized controlled trial. Arch Intern Med. 2002; 162(7):857-64.
12. Henningsen P, Martin A. Psychotherapy of patients with somatoform disorders. In: Handbook of Psychotherapy for Somatoform Disorders. New Delhi: Springer; 2019.
13. Kroenke K. Efficacy of treatment for somatoform disorders: a review of randomized controlled trials. Psychosom Med. 2007;69(9):881-8.
14. Phillips KA, Albertini RS, Rasmussen SA. A randomized placebo-controlled trial of fluoxetine in body dysmorphic disorder. Arch Gen Psychiatry. 2002;59(4):381-8.

CHAPTER 12

# Differential Diagnosis of Panic Attacks

*Samir Kumar Praharaj*

**Flowchart 1** depicts the diagnostic approach to panic disorder.

**Flowchart 1:** Diagnostic algorithm of panic disorder.

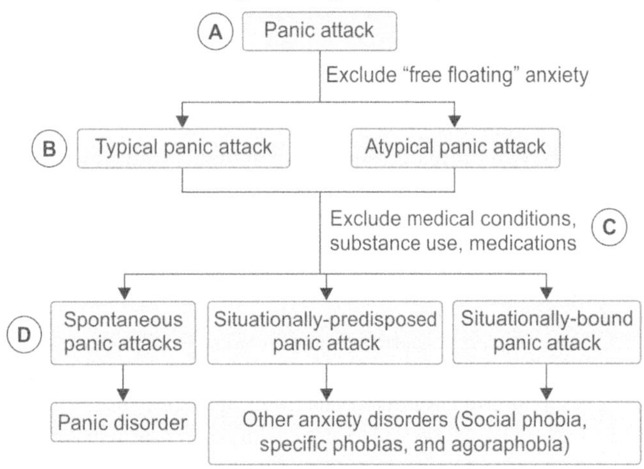


**TABLE 1:** Symptoms during a panic attack.

| *Domain* | *Symptoms* |
|---|---|
| Cardiac | Palpitations, pounding sensation, fast heart rate, chest pain, or discomfort |
| Respiratory | Shortness of breath, smothering feeling, and choking sensation |
| Neurological | Feeling dizzy, fainting sensation, light-headedness, feeling unsteady, chills or heat sensations, numbness or tingling, trembling or shaking, headache[†], and tinnitus[†] |
| Gastrointestinal | Nausea, abdominal distress, and cramps |
| Autonomic | Sweating, mouth dryness |
| Cognitive | derealization, depersonalization, fear of losing control, fear of dying |
| Other | Sore neck[†], Screaming[†], uncontrolled crying[†] |

[†]Seen only in specific cultures

## DESCRIPTION

**A.** *Panic attacks* are characterized by acute episodes of intense fear of an imminent threat in the absence of real danger. It is characterized by (1) *physical* manifestations of autonomic hyperactivity: Palpitations, chest discomfort, choking sensation, shortness of breath, sweating, tremor, dry mouth, abdominal discomfort, dizziness, and paresthesia; (2) *cognitive* manifestations: Thoughts of "losing control," "something bad happening," "dying;" (3) *affective* component: Intense fear or severe anxiety; and (4) *behavioral* manifestations: "Going out for fresh air," "sitting to avoid fall." A list of physical symptoms is provided in **Table 1**. A classical panic attack typically has a *crescendo* and *decrescendo* pattern, with a "steeper crescendo" and a somewhat "flatter decrescendo." The typical duration is 15–30 minutes, though it may last longer. The *postpanic phase* is characterized by fatigue, exertion, and drowsiness. These "episodic" acute anxiety attacks should be differentiated from "free-floating" anxiety, which involves low-grade anxiety symptoms lasting much longer, characteristic of generalized anxiety disorder.

**B.** *Panic subtypes: Typical* panic attacks present with symptoms involving multiple organ systems, such as cardiac, respiratory, gastrointestinal, and vestibular systems. Some patients may exhibit symptoms involving one predominant organ system, which are considered *atypical* panic attacks. The four commonly reported subtypes are: (1) Cardiac subtype, (2) respiratory subtype, (3) gastrointestinal subtype, and (4) vestibular subtype.[1] These presentations may be mistaken for somatic conditions; however, they can be differentiated by: (1) The symptoms are intense, dramatic, and episodic; (2) there are no abnormal laboratory findings; and (3) symptoms recur without any signs of worsening of the medical condition.[1] The differential diagnosis of panic attacks should be based on the predominant phenotype of the anxiety attack. For example, angina or arrhythmia should be considered as a diagnostic possibility with predominant cardiovascular complaints. Specific laboratory investigations will be ordered based on the diagnostic suspicion.

- *Cardiac subtype:* The symptoms in this subtype predominantly include a pounding heart, palpitations, chest pain or discomfort, and a rapid or fluttering heartbeat. These symptoms mimic angina, myocardial infarction, or arrhythmias due to their acute onset and rapid progression. Several patients with atypical chest pain experience panic attacks. Specific characteristics that correlate with panic disorder in persons having chest pain are: (1) No coronary artery disease, (2) atypical chest pain, (3) female gender, (4) young age, and (5) high anxiety level.[2]
- *Respiratory subtype:* These patients present with choking or smothering sensations and shortness of breath and are clinically easily recognized as having hyperventilation. These symptoms are more common in young age, females, and those with comorbid alcohol use.[1] Additionally, carbon dioxide, hyperventilation, and caffeine are common triggers for panic attacks in those with the respiratory subtype.[3] These patients also often have a higher family history of panic disorder.[3]
- *Gastrointestinal subtype:* These patients present with nausea and epigastric discomfort, which can be mistaken for irritable bowel syndrome or functional dyspepsia.
- *Vestibular subtype*: Some patients present with vestibular symptoms such as dizziness, unsteadiness, light-headedness, or faintness, which may be mistaken for vestibular disease.

C. *Panic mimics*: Several medical conditions (listed in **Table 2**) can present with acute anxiety symptoms suggestive of panic attacks and need to be differentiated from classic panic attacks, which are characteristic of primary anxiety disorders. These "panic mimics" have atypical features that help clinicians differentiate them from panic attacks. Examples include *atypical age at onset* (e.g., onset in the elderly in transient ischemic attacks), *shorter duration* (e.g., lasting a few minutes in temporal lobe epilepsy), *associated symptoms of the medical condition* (e.g., vertigo in vestibular disorders), etc. Relevant investigations should be conducted based on the clinical presentation

**TABLE 2:** Medical conditions mimicking anxiety.

| *System* | *Disorder* |
|---|---|
| Cardiovascular | Angina pectoris, myocardial infarction, arrhythmias, congestive cardiac failure, valvular heart disease, hypovolemia, orthostatic and hypotension |
| Respiratory | Bronchial asthma, pulmonary embolism, chronic obstructive pulmonary disease, pneumonia, and acute respiratory distress syndrome |
| Neurological | Complex partial seizure, transient ischemic attack, and myasthenia gravis |
| Endocrine and metabolic | Hyperthyroidism, hypothyroidism, hyperparathyroidism, hypocalcemia, hypercalcemia, hypoglycemia, Cushing's disease, and Addison's disease |
| Otological | Vertigo, Meniere's disease |
| Hematological | Anemia |
| Tumors | Pheochromocytoma, carcinoid tumor, and insulinoma |
| Infections | Brucellosis, neurosyphilis, Lyme borreliosis, and encephalitis |
| Substance use | Caffeine, alcohol, and cannabis |
| Drugs | Stimulants, corticosteroids, β-agonists, decongestants, and antidepressants |

**TABLE 3:** Psychiatric disorders with panic attacks.

| *Disorder* | *Characteristic features* |
|---|---|
| Social anxiety disorder (SAD) | Panic attacks occur only in the context of *social situations*. The primary fear is of *humiliation* or *embarrassment* in social situations |
| Specific phobia | Panic attacks occur only on exposure to the *specific feared stimulus* (e.g., height, insects, snakes, etc.) |
| Post-traumatic stress disorder | Panic attacks occur in situations or thoughts that evoke memories of *trauma* |
| Generalized anxiety disorder (GAD) | *Free-floating anxiety,* which is more persistent, is characteristic of GAD, as opposed to discrete episodes. However, *limited-symptom* panic attacks can occur in GAD |
| Obsessive-compulsive disorder (OCD) | Panic attacks occur on exposure to the *feared situations* (e.g., dirt, contamination, etc.) |
| Depressive disorder | Panic attacks may occur in depression, which may be triggered by *depressive ruminations* |
| Hypochondriasis | Panic attacks occur in the context of fear of having a *life-threatening illness* |
| Separation anxiety disorder | Panic attacks occur only in the context of *separation from key attachment figures* |

to confirm the diagnosis of these medical disorders. It is important to note that panic disorders can be comorbid with these medical conditions.

**D.** *Triggers*: Panic attacks can be further classified based on their triggers, which can include specific situations or thoughts. There are three possibilities: (1) *Spontaneous* panic attacks: These occur without any specific trigger and are characteristic of panic disorder, (2) *Situationally-predisposed* panic attacks: There is a possibility of having a panic attack in specific situations, and (3) *Situationally-bound* panic attacks: Panic attack always occur in those specific situations. The latter two types are seen in other anxiety disorders and are related to specific stimuli (e.g., social situations in social anxiety). Anxiety and other disorders with panic attacks are listed in **Table 3**.

## REFERENCES

1. Sansone RA, Sansone LA. Panic disorder subtypes: deceptive somatic impersonators. Psychiatry (Edgmont). 2009;6:33-7.
2. Huffman JC, Pollack MH. Predicting panic disorders among patients with chest pain: an analysis of the literature. Psychosomatics. 2003;44:222-36.
3. Freire RC, Perna G, Nardi AE. Panic disorder respiratory subtype: psychopathology, laboratory challenge tests, and response to treatment. Harv Rev Psychiatry. 2010;18:220-9.

CHAPTER 13

# Management of Difficult-to-Treat Panic Disorder

*Samir Kumar Praharaj*

## INTRODUCTION

Panic disorder (PD) is common, with a population prevalence varying from 1 to 4%. A diagnosis of panic disorder is based on a history of *recurrent spontaneous panic attacks* and *anticipatory anxiety*, while excluding medical disorders that present with anxiety. Investigations should rule out medical causes of anxiety. An initial work-up should include a full physical examination, urine analysis, urine toxicology, electrolytes, liver function tests, thyroid function tests, complete blood count, and electrocardiogram (ECG). Further investigations depend on the specific presentation (e.g., electroencephalogram and neuroimaging if complex partial seizures are suspected). Additionally, evaluate for comorbid disorders, such as another anxiety disorder, substance use, and depression. Standard treatment of panic disorder includes *pharmacotherapy* and *psychological therapies*. Both are considered first-line options, with medications being essential for rapid symptom control during acute episodes.

## PHARMACOTHERAPY OF PANIC DISORDER

- A key principle of pharmacotherapy of anxiety disorders is to tailor treatment by targeting specific symptoms, such as panic attacks, phobic anxiety, or generalized anxiety, with the goal of suppressing these symptoms. However, not all features of anxiety syndromes are directly responsive to medical interventions (e.g., agoraphobic symptoms in a PD patient). Therefore, it is important to consider *cognitive-behavioral therapy* (CBT) or other psychotherapies for the treatment.[1]
- The first-line treatment option for PD is *specific serotonin reuptake inhibitors* (SSRIs). SSRIs may have superior antipanic efficacy and an earlier onset of action compared to other standard agents. It is important to consider potential drug-drug interactions due to hepatic P450 enzyme inhibition (e.g., paroxetine and fluoxetine substantially inhibit the P450 2D6 isoenzyme at regular clinical doses). *Serotonin norepinephrine reuptake inhibitors* (SNRIs), such as venlafaxine, are also considered alternative first-line agents in PD.[2]
    - Within the SSRI class, there is no available comparative efficacy data that would lead one to select one agent over another. Nevertheless, fluoxetine and paroxetine have stronger evidence for efficacy than sertraline.[2] Pharmacokinetic factors are of some importance in selecting an appropriate SSRI in PD. For example, an agent with a long $t_{1/2}$, such as fluoxetine, should be considered in patients in whom the tapering phase of treatment may be complicated.
    - According to the American Psychiatric Association (APA) treatment guidelines, the recommended daily starting dose for each is as follows: Fluoxetine is 10 mg or less, sertraline 25 mg, paroxetine 10 mg (IR), or 12.5 mg (CR) depending on the formulation used, 10 mg of citalopram, and escitalopram at 5–10 mg. It is further recommended that this lowered starting dose be maintained for approximately 3–7 days and then gradually increased based on tolerability to standard doses. **Table 1** summarizes dosing guidelines for various pharmacological treatments in panic disorder.
    - The SSRIs are generally safe agents for use in special populations such as the elderly, pregnant or lactating women, and children and adolescents. SSRIs have a low teratogenic potential and, although excreted in breast milk, appear, thus far, to have limited effects on the newborn.[3]
    - One caveat to SSRI therapy in elderly patients is the slight risk of a syndrome of inappropriate antidiuretic hormone (ADH) secretion, suggesting the need for electrolyte monitoring in this group.

**TABLE 1:** Dosage guideline for treatment of panic disorder.

| *Drug class* | *Medication* | *Dosage* |
|---|---|---|
| Specific serotonin reuptake inhibitors (SSRIs) | Escitalopram | 10–20 mg |
| | Sertraline | 50–200 mg |
| | Paroxetine | 20–60 mg |
| | Fluvoxamine | 100–300 mg |
| | Fluoxetine | 20–40 mg |
| Serotonin norepinephrine reuptake inhibitors (SNRIs) | Venlafaxine | 75–225 mg |
| Tricyclic antidepressants (TCAs) | Imipramine | |
| | Clomipramine | 75–250 mg |
| | Nortriptyline | |
| | Amitriptyline | |
| Monoamine oxidase inhibitors (MAOIs) | Phenelzine | |
| | Moclobemide | 300–600 mg |
| Benzodiazepines | Clonazepam | 1–4 mg |
| | Alprazolam | 1.5–8 mg |
| | Etizolam | |

- Recent research has shown that the presence of the long allele of the serotonin transporter (*5-HTT*) gene is associated with a favorable response.[4]
- Testing of the functional CYP450 gene variants can be done to avoid over- or underdosing poor or rapid metabolizers. Pharmacogenetic studies are beginning to refine and individualize drug therapy for PD.[5]

- *Treatment resistance* is a relatively uncommon problem and can usually be addressed by careful diagnostic reassessment and then moving through the top four classes of agents in a step-wise manner.[6] Imipramine and other tricyclics should now be considered the second-line agents for panic. Benzodiazepines are third-line anticonvulsants, and the fourth-line, and the classical monoamine oxidase inhibitors (MAOIs) would be considered fifth-line antipanic agents due to their side-effect profile and safety issues. Nevertheless, these medications have similar efficacy as that of SSRIs and SNRIs.[2]
- *Adverse effects:* Panic patients are extremely *side-effect sensitive*, especially to the stimulant properties of agents that modify 5-HT and NE function, and therefore should be commenced on half the usual starting dose used for major depression.[7] Some individuals may experience jitteriness, restlessness, insomnia, and an increase in anxiety symptoms during the initial days of starting treatment, i.e., *jitteriness* or *overstimulation syndrome*. Starting with a lower dose or reducing the dose is sufficient for most patients. Not uncommonly, cotreatment with a benzodiazepine is necessary to minimize the impact of this side-effect. Recent work endorses the benefit of early regular coadministration of the benzodiazepine, clonazepam, with SSRIs for the rapid stabilization of moderate-severe PD.[8] Gradual clonazepam tapering after several weeks of coadministration appears to be well-tolerated and limits the development of physiological dependence associated with long-term benzodiazepine use.
- *Psychoeducation:* PD patients frequently are hypersensitive to medication side effects, and it is recommended to educate patients about the likely course of both primary and side effects of the medications. Careful counseling of the anxious patient concerning the short- and long-term risks and benefits of medications is the key to satisfactory compliance, as these patients are extremely side-effect sensitive.
- *PD with bipolar disorder:* In the bipolar/panic disordered patient, it may be preferable to avoid SSRI use and attempt stabilization of both syndromes with anticonvulsants (e.g., valproate, gabapentin, and lamotrigine), which are now being increasingly used for both syndromes.
- *Duration of treatment:* Guidelines for the duration of SSRI therapy generally depend on the time at which a full response has been obtained. This is usually defined as a remission of both full and limited symptom panic attacks. At this time, a further 6 months of maintenance therapy is considered sufficient,[6] before a trial of SSRI taper is indicated. Some clinicians recommend 12 months of treatment after remission.[9,10] Abrupt discontinuation should be avoided because of the flu-like syndrome that has been observed to occur in this context.[11] Tapering treatment over a week or longer (2–4 weeks) can minimize this risk.
- *Maintenance therapy:* Thus, maintenance pharmacotherapy may be necessary for some patients to protect against relapse. Clinical indications for extended maintenance treatment in a subgroup of patients who might be sensitive to relapse (e.g., patients with multiple previous episodes of panic).
- *Partial response:* Partial responses are relatively common and can often be managed by optimizing the ongoing medication or by adding another therapeutic

agent, such as a benzodiazepine (e.g., clonazepam or tofisopam) or a tricyclic antidepressant (TCA) (e.g., low-dose desipramine).

- *Augmentation strategies:* These strategies may accelerate clinical response to standard medications such as SSRIs. For example, the early co-administration of benzodiazepine clonazepam with SSRIs can facilitate rapid stabilization of acute PD and may also be beneficial for other anxiety disorders.[8] Higher doses of clonazepam (1–3 mg/day) are typically required to achieve acute antipanic efficacy.

## OTHER TREATMENT OF PANIC DISORDER

- *Psychotherapy:* CBT is highly effective for treating PD, with large effect sizes.[1] Two major forms of CBT developed for panic disorder are: (1) *Barlow and Craske's panic control treatment,*[12] and (2) *Clark's cognitive therapy* for panic.[13] The active components for both treatment includes: (1) *Psychoeducation* about panic: Correcting misconceptions about panic symptoms; (2) *Cognitive restructuring:* Identifying and challenging cognitive distortions; (3) *Interoceptive exposure:* Gradual exposure to feared bodily sensations such as palpitations, dyspnea, dizziness; and (4) *In vivo exposure:* Facing feared situations such as unfamiliar areas and driving to gather corrective information, disprove fearful misappraisals, and reduce fear responses. *Applied relaxation* that incorporates exposure to feared stimuli has been demonstrated to be effective.[14]
- *Experimental treatment* approaches for panic disorder include neuromodulation strategies such as transcranial magnetic stimulation,[15] transcranial direct current stimulation,[16] and cannabidiol.[17] However, their efficacy for panic disorder remains uncertain.

## REFERENCES

1. Carpenter JK, Andrews LA, Witcraft SM, Powers MB, Smits JAJ, Hofmann SG. Cognitive behavioral therapy for anxiety and related disorders: a meta-analysis of randomized placebo-controlled trials. Depress Anxiety. 2018;35(6):502-14.
2. Guaiana G, Meader N, Barbui C, Davies SJ, Furukawa TA, Imai H, et al. Pharmacological treatments in panic disorder in adults: a network meta-analysis. Cochrane Database Syst Rev. 2023;11(11):CD012729.
3. Misri S, Burgmann A, Kostaras D. Are SSRIs safe for pregnant and breastfeeding women? Can Fam Physician. 2000;46:631-3.
4. Tiwari AK, Souza RP, Müller DJ. Pharmacogenetics of anxiolytic drugs. J Neural Transm (Vienna). 2009;116(6):667-77.
5. Argueta N, Notari E, Szigeti K. Role of pharmacogenomics in individualizing treatment for Alzheimer's disease. CNS Drugs. 2022;17(4):143-51.
6. Rosenbaum JF, Pollock RA, Jordan SK, Pollack MH. The pharmacotherapy of panic disorder. Bull Menninger Clin. 1996;60(2 Suppl A):A54-75.
7. Louie AK, Lewis TB, Lannon RA. Use of low-dose fluoxetine in major depression and panic disorder. J Clin Psychiatry. 1993;54(11):435-38.
8. Goddard AW, Brouette T, Almai A, Jetty P, Woods SW, Charney D. Early coadministration of clonazepam with sertraline for panic disorder. Arch Gen Psychiatry. 2001;58(7):681-6.
9. Bandelow B, Michaelis S, Wedekind D. Treatment of anxiety disorders. Dialogues Clin Neurosci. 2017;19(2):93-107.
10. Andrews G, Bell C, Boyce P, Gale C, Lampe L, Marwat O, et al. Royal Australian and New Zealand College of Psychiatrists clinical practice guidelines for the treatment of panic disorder, social anxiety disorder and generalised anxiety disorder. Aust N Z J Psychiatry. 2018;52(12):1109-72.
11. Coupland NJ, Bell CJ, Potokar JP. Serotonin reuptake inhibitor withdrawal. J Clin Psychopharmacol. 1996; 16(5):356-62.
12. Hofmann SG, Spiegel DA. Panic control treatment and its applications. J Psychother Pract Res. 1999 Winter; 8(1):3-11.
13. Clark DM, Salkovskis PM, Hackmann A, Wells A, Ludgate J, Gelder M. Brief cognitive therapy for panic disorder: a randomized controlled trial. J Consult Clin Psychol. 1999;67(4):583-9.
14. Ost LG. Applied relaxation: description of a coping technique and review of controlled studies. Behav Res Ther. 1987;25(5):397-409.
15. Zugliani MM, Cabo MC, Nardi AE, Perna G, Freire RC. Pharmacological and neuromodulatory treatments for panic disorder: Clinical trials from 2010 to 2018. Psychiatry Investig. 2019;16(1):50-8.
16. Yosephi MH, Ehsani F, Daghiani M, Zoghi M, Jaberzadeh S. The effects of trans-cranial direct current stimulation intervention on fear: a systematic review of literature. J Clin Neurosci. 2019;62:7-13.
17. Blessing EM, Steenkamp MM, Manzanares J, Marmar CR. Cannabidiol as a potential treatment for anxiety disorders. Neurotherapeutics. 2015;12(4):825-36.

CHAPTER 14

# Differential Diagnoses of Obsessions

*Ravindra Neelakanthappa Munoli*

## INTRODUCTION

An obsession is a repetitive, intrusive, irrational thought, idea, image, or impulse/urge that is ego-dystonic, beyond the person's control, and causes distress. It is a thought phenomenon that borders on other phenomena, including normal worrying, anxiety, depression, and psychosis. Differentiating these conditions aids in differential diagnosis. **Flowchart 1** depicts the possible phenomenology of unwanted thoughts, images, and impulses.

## DIFFERENTIATING OBSESSIONS FROM OTHER PRESENTATIONS (FLOWCHART 1)

- *Obsessions and normal worrying:* People often worry about various aspects of life. Anxious individuals may have intrusive thoughts. The key difference between worry and obsession lies in the context of real-life concerns like work, finances, or relationships in anxiety-related thoughts. Worries typically lack associated compulsions.
- *Obsessions and ruminations in depression:* Ruminations in depression often resemble obsessions but differ in content, focusing on pessimistic self-views, dwelling on the past, or feelings of low self-worth. They typically occur alongside clinical depression symptoms. It is possible for a person to experience both obsessions and depression symptoms as separate phenomena. Obsessive ruminations typically include neutral and mundane thoughts.
- *Obsessions and generalized anxiety:* Recurrent thoughts, ideas, or worries accompanied by avoidant behaviors or seeking reassurance can indicate generalized anxiety disorder. If these concerns encompass multiple aspects of a person's life, they are generally rational, relate to real-life issues, and are more likely part of generalized anxiety rather than obsessions.
- *Obsessions and social anxiety:* In social anxiety, the thoughts or ideas that provoke anxiety are limited to social contexts or interactions. They are often accompanied by social avoidance or reassurance seeking to reduce anxiety or fear, and these reactions are not irrational. These qualities contrast with the features of obsessions.
- *Obsessions and specific phobia:* Contamination obsessions and fear of losing control can be mistaken for phobias. In specific phobias, thoughts or ideas are limited to specific stimuli. Unlike obsessions and compulsions, specific phobias do not involve rituals. Behavioral responses such as avoidance effectively reduce anxiety. Thoughts in specific phobias are confined to the stimulus and are not recurrent, irrational, or intrusive, distinguishing them from obsessions.
- *Obsessions and hypochondriasis:* One common pre-occupation in both obsession and hypochondriasis is the fear of becoming ill or contracting an illness. However, the conviction for this thought is typically less intense in obsessions compared to hypochondriasis. In hypochondriasis, beliefs are ego-syntonic and often

**Flowchart 1:** Establishment of an obsession.

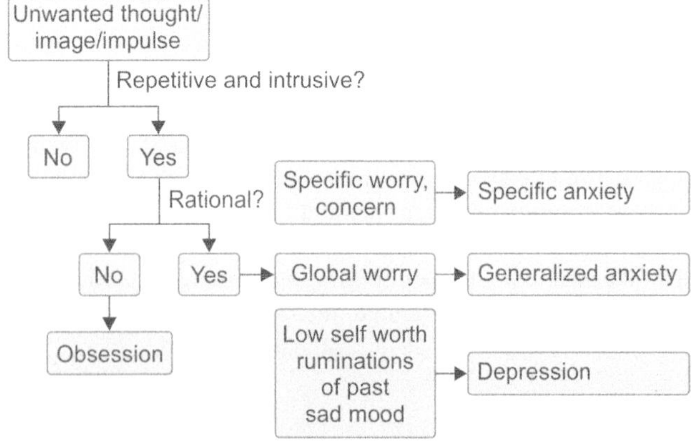

accompanied by somatic sensations or experiences. Conversely, in obsessions, such preoccupations are usually ego-dystonic and may involve other unrelated obsessions and compulsions. It is worth noting that comorbid hypochondriasis is seen in nearly 10% of patients diagnosed with obsessive-compulsive disorder (OCD).[1,2]

- *Obsessions and dysmorphophobia:* In dysmorphophobia, individuals have excessive preoccupation with an imagined defect in their appearance or a specific body part. Insight into this preoccupation is often poorer than in obsessions, and behaviors are driven by concern over the perceived flaw. The repetitive thoughts, ideas, or images typically focus on this single domain. Unlike obsessions, individuals with dysmorphophobia do not necessarily view their concerns as irrational. However, it is noteworthy that one-third of patients with dysmorphophobia also meet criteria for OCD.[3]
- *Obsessions and anorexia nervosa:* In anorexia nervosa, thoughts, ideas, or images primarily revolve around one's body weight and food. The cognitive distortion centers on concerns about body weight or obesity, rather than fear of illness as in hypochondriasis or an imagined defect in appearance as in dysmorphophobia. Unlike obsessions, these thoughts are not typically perceived as irrational or intrusive, and persons with anorexia may not report distress or discomfort due to these thoughts specifically. Furthermore, obsessions generally extend beyond concerns related to food and weight.
- *Obsession, obsessive perfectionism trait, and obsessive-compulsive personality disorder (OCPD):* Here, the person's preoccupation is with perfectionism, and the distress arises from not meeting their own standards of perfection, which they endorse as ideal. They acknowledge the intrusive quality of these thoughts but may find them satisfying, despite the distress they can cause when these standards are not fully achieved. This trait is characteristic of obsessive perfectionism and can be part of OCPD. OCPD involves excessive preoccupation with orderliness, perfectionism, and control over oneself and others. A key difference between obsessions and OCPD is that obsessions are typically experienced as ego-dystonic, whereas in OCPD, the thoughts and preoccupations are ego-syntonic. Furthermore, OCD tends to result in more significant functional impairment compared to OCPD. Additionally, features characteristic of OCPD typically do not respond well to treatment and may not remit easily.
- *Obsessions and pediatric conditions:*
  - *Obsessions and rituals:* During normal development, preschoolers and toddlers often exhibit ritualistic behaviors such as mealtime, bedtime, or play routines. Children may insist on these routines, but if interrupted, delayed, or denied, they typically do not experience severe distress or functional impairment. These behaviors lack the qualities of obsessions and are considered part of normal development.
  - *Obsessions and autism spectrum disorders (ASD):* The core symptoms in ASD include repetitive and stereotypic behaviors, as well as a restricted and narrow range of activities and interests. These symptoms can sometimes be misdiagnosed as OCD, particularly in young children. However, nearly 5% of children with OCD also meet the criteria for ASD.[4] Distinguishing between these conditions can be challenging, especially regarding whether the behaviors are ego-dystonic or result from obsessional fears. A key differentiator is the presence of impairments in reciprocal social communication, which is characteristic of ASD but not OCD. In children with ASD, obsessional concerns are not always apparent. However, when children get upset when their stereotypical and preferred activities are interrupted, it may indicate obsessional concern. Insight in children with OCD usually fluctuates with anxiety and is best assessed when anxiety is at its lowest. Sometimes, obsessional ideas may merge with overvalued ideas or delusional thinking, indicating psychosis; however, insight and nature of the obsession (atypical) may help in differentiating between them.[5]
- *Obsessions and Tourette's disorder/tic disorders:* In OCD, compulsions are driven by an underlying obsessional thought and are usually goal-directed. In contrast, tic disorders are characterized by premonitory experiences that are more sensory in nature or perceived as urges, without the elaborate cognitive distortions seen in obsessions.[6,7] However, tic disorder comorbidity is seen in 30% of OCD patients. About 40% of patients with Tourette's disorder have obsessive-compulsive behaviors, and 20% have OCD.[8]

- *Obsessions and hoarding disorder:* Hoarding can be an obsession within OCD or an independent disorder characterized by persistent difficulty in discarding possessions, regardless of their perceived value. The reluctance to discard these possessions is due to fear of catastrophic consequences. Individuals may engage in complicated rituals before discarding possessions, leading to avoidance of the act. This experience is typically ego-dystonic.[9]
- *Obsession and trichotillomania:* In trichotillomania, individuals feel an urge to pull their hair, often preceded by tension or occurring without any specific trigger, resulting in hair plucking from the scalp and other body parts. This behavior can have an obsessional quality when accompanied by a recurrent urge, resembling a compulsion. However, trichotillomania often presents as a standalone symptom, warranting an independent diagnosis.
- *Obsessions and delusions:* In delusions, there is a lack of insight, rational arguments, or evidence to the contrary are disregarded and are held firmly despite contrary evidence or social pressure.[10] In contrast, individuals with obsessions try to resist their thoughts. Delusions are ego-syntonic, whereas obsessions are ego-dystonic. Oulis et al.[11] listed the phenomenological features distinguishing typical obsessions or compulsions from delusions or repetitive delusional behaviors: (1) Source or origin and sense of ownership of the thought, (2) conviction, (3) consistency with one's belief system, (4) awareness of its inaccuracy, (5) awareness of its symptomatic nature, (6) resistance, and (7) emotional impact. These features help differentiate obsessions from delusions.

## CONCLUSION

Recurrent thoughts, images, and impulses must be thoroughly evaluated to determine their exact nature, aiding in diagnosis. These could be normal thinking patterns or cognitive distortions found in anxiety disorders, depressive disorders, psychosis, or other specified conditions.

## REFERENCES

1. Abramowitz JS, Brigidi BD, Foa EB. Health concerns in patients with obsessive compulsive disorder. J Anxiety Disord. 1999;13:529-39.
2. Bienvenu OJ, Samuels JF, Riddle MA, Hoehn-Saric R, Liang KY, Cullen BA, et al. The relationship of obsessive-compulsive disorder to possible spectrum disorders: results from a family study. Biol Psychiatry. 2000;48(4): 287-93.
3. Pertusa A, Fullana MA, Singh S, Alonso P, Menchón JM, Mataix-Cols D. Compulsive hoarding: OCD symptom, distinct clinical syndrome, or both? Am J Psychiatry. 2008;165(10):1289-98.
4. Geller D, Biederman J, Faraone SV, Bellorde CA, Kim GS, Hagermoser LM. Disentangling chronological age from age of onset in children and adolescents with obsessive compulsive disorder. Int J Neuropsychopharmacol. 2001;4:169-78.
5. Geller D, March J. Practice parameter for the assessment and treatment of children and adolescents with obsessive-compulsive disorder. J Am Acad Child Adolesc Psychiatry. 2012;51(1):98-113.
6. Leckman JF, Walker DE, Cohen DJ. Premonitory urges in Tourette's syndrome. Am J Psychiatry. 1993;150:98-102.
7. Miguel EC, Coffey BJ, Baer L, Savage CR, Rauch SL, Jenike MA. Phenomenology of intentional repetitive behaviors in obsessive-compulsive disorder and Tourette's disorder. J Clin Psychiatry. 1995;56(6):246-55.
8. Leckman JF, Walker DE, Goodman WK, Pauls DL, Cohen DJ. "Just right" perceptions associated with compulsive behavior in Tourette's syndrome. Am J Psychiatry 1994;151:675-80.
9. Pertusa A, Frost RO, Fullana MA, Samuels J, Steketee G, Tolin D, et al. Refining the diagnostic boundaries of compulsive hoarding: a critical review. Clin Psychol Rev. 2010;30(4):371-86.
10. Zink M, Englisch S, Dressing H. Neurobiology confirms psychopathology. On the antagonism of psychosis and obsessive-compulsive syndromes. Psychopathology. 2008;41(5):279-85.
11. Oulis P, Konstantakopoulos G, Lykouras L, Michalopoulou PG. Differential diagnosis of obsessive-compulsive symptoms from delusions in schizophrenia: A phenomenological approach. World J Psychiatry. 2013; 3(3):50-6.

CHAPTER 15

# Management of Difficult-to-treat Obsessive-compulsive Disorder

*Sonia Shenoy*

## A: TREATMENT OF OBSESSIVE-COMPULSIVE DISORDER GENERAL GUIDELINES (FLOWCHART 1)

- Selective serotonin reuptake inhibitors (SSRIs) are the first line of treatment.[1]
- All SSRIs are equally effective.
- Choice of SSRI depends on factors such as previous response, tolerability, and cost.[2]
- Higher doses are recommended **(Table 1)**.
- A minimum of a 12-week trial is recommended (at least 8 weeks at the recommended dose).[3]

**Flowchart 1:** Management of difficult-to-treat obsessive-compulsive disorder (OCD).

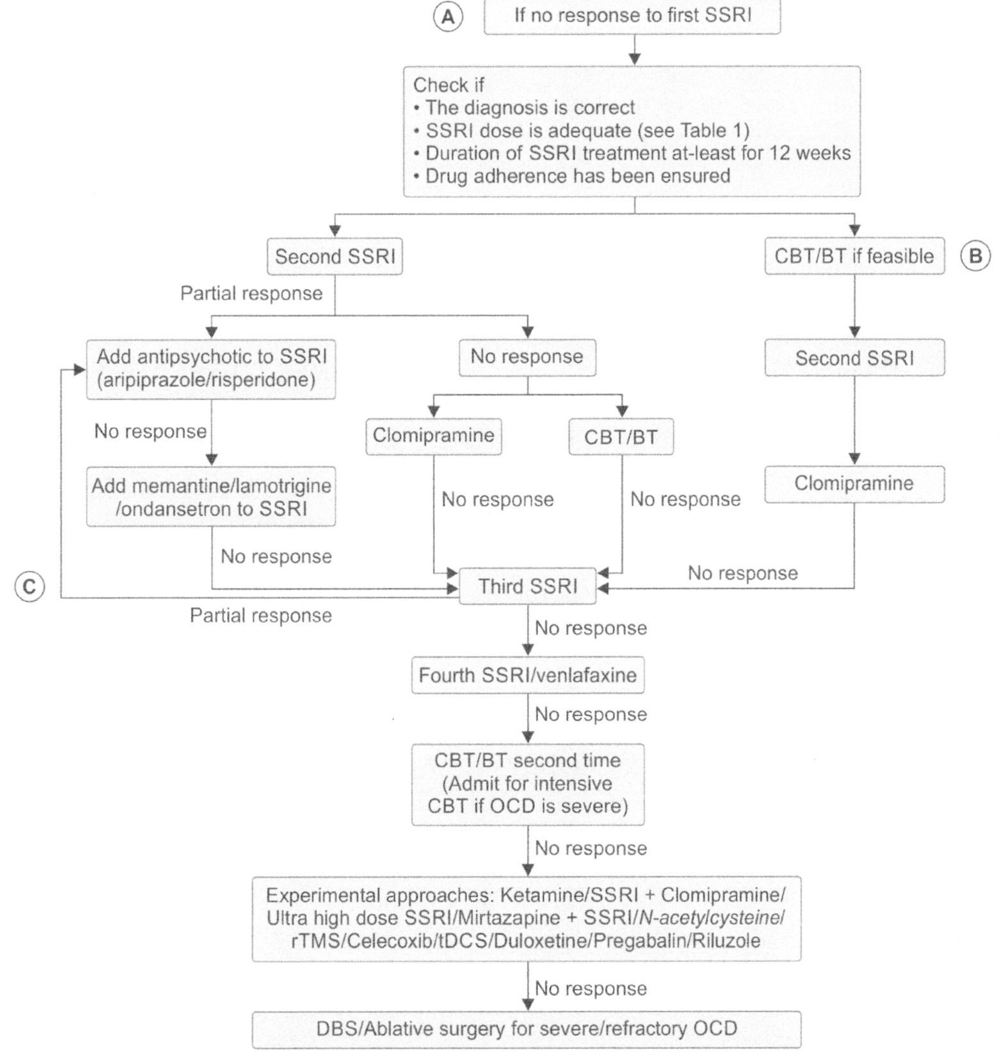


(BT: behavioral therapy; CBT: cognitive behavioral therapy; SSRI: selective serotonin reuptake inhibitor)

**TABLE 1:** Recommended medications for treatment of obsessive-compulsive disorder (OCD).

| *Drugs* | *Recommended dosages* | *Remarks* |
|---|---|---|
| Fluoxetine | 60–80 mg | Can cause loss of appetite and insomnia |
| Sertraline | 150–200 mg | Safer in those with cardiac disorders |
| Escitalopram | 20–30 mg | Most well-tolerated among selective serotonin reuptake inhibitor (SSRI) |
| Paroxetine | 40–60 mg | Has anticholinergic side effects and sedation |
| Fluvoxamine | 200–300 mg | Risk of drug interactions and sedation |
| Citalopram | 40–60 mg | Usually not used; escitalopram is preferred instead |
| Clomipramine | 150–225 mg | Has anticholinergic side effects; better to try an SSRI first |
| Venlafaxine | 225–300 mg | Less evidence compared to SSRIs and clomipramine |

**TABLE 2:** Augmenting agents for treatment of obsessive-compulsive disorder (OCD).

| *Drugs* | *Recommended dosages* | *Remarks* |
|---|---|---|
| Risperidone | 1–3 mg | Low doses beneficial; slight risk of EPS |
| Aripiprazole | 5–10 mg | Can cause akathisia and insomnia |
| Lamotrigine | 100 mg | Low dose uptitration (25 mg once in 2 weeks) |
| Memantine | 10–20 mg | Glutamatergic agent; can cause drowsiness and dizziness |
| Ondansetron | 2–4 mg twice a day | Can cause headache, drowsiness, and GI side effects |
| Granisetron | 1 mg twice a day | Can cause asthenia, constipation, and headache |
| Haloperidol | 2.5–10 mg | Risk of EPS; less evidence compared to risperidone and aripiprazole |

- Clomipramine is as effective as SSRIs but has poorer tolerability due to anticholinergic, neurological, metabolic, and cardiac side effects.
- Augmenting agents may be used if there is a partial response to treatment **(Table 2)**.
- Experimental agents may be considered if there is no response to conventional drugs **(Table 3)**.

## B: COGNITIVE BEHAVIOR THERAPY IN OBSESSIVE-COMPULSIVE DISORDER[4]

- Cognitive behavioral therapy (CBT) and behavioral therapy (BT) are first line of treatments for OCD.
- Exposure and response prevention (ERP), along with belief modification, is recommended.
- CBT/ERP is recommended as monotherapy for mild to moderate OCD if feasible.
- Since 12–20 sessions are needed daily or thrice weekly by qualified therapists, it is often not preferred in low-resource settings.
- Components of CBT/BT include psychoeducation, establishment of a symptom hierarchy, ERP, and cognitive restructuring.
- Other therapies include acceptance and commitment therapy, mindfulness-based therapies alone, or combined with ERP.

## C: RESPONSE TO TREATMENT IN OBSESSIVE-COMPULSIVE DISORDER[5]

- The Yale Brown Obsessive-Compulsive Scale (Y-BOCS) is the gold standard for assessing OCD severity and treatment response.[6]
- Clinically meaningful improvement in OCD symptoms includes reduction in time spent in obsessions and compulsions, distress due to symptoms, interference in daily activities, dysfunction, and avoidance.
- A partial response is determined when there is minimal clinical improvement based on the above criteria.
- An objective measure of partial response is a 25–35% reduction in YBOCS score from baseline, along with a Clinical Global Impression Improvement (CGI-I) score of 3 (minimally improved) for at least 1 week.
- Complete or good response is achieved with ≥35% reduction in Y-BOCS score from baseline, along with a CGI- I score of 1 (very much improved) or 2 (much improved) for at least 1 week.

**TABLE 3:** Experimental agents for the treatment of obsessive-compulsive disorder (OCD).

| *Agents* | *Doses* | *Remarks* |
|---|---|---|
| *N*-acetylcysteine | 600–2,400 mg | Gastrointestinal adverse effects may be problematic |
| Riluzole | 50 mg twice a day | Can cause gastrointestinal side effects and asthenia and rarely hepatotoxicity |
| Pregabalin | 75–225 mg | Can cause sedation and dizziness; also, withdrawal reactions on abrupt cessation |
| Duloxetine | 60 mg | Can cause nausea, dry mouth, and headache |
| Celecoxib | 400 mg | Can cause gastrointestinal side effects; long-term treatment is not preferred |
| Mirtazapine | 30–60 mg | Hastens the response to treatment when added to an SSRI but has no long-term benefits; can cause sedation and weight gain |
| Ketamine | 0.5 mg/kg IV in saline over 40 minutes | Needs monitoring of vitals, can cause dissociation, elevation of blood pressure, and dizziness. It has a rapid and short-lasting benefit |
| rTMS | Stimulation of left DLPFC | Other targets include SMA, OFC, and ACC |
| tDCS | Cathode: Left SMA; anode: left deltoid | 2 mA, 20 minutes, 15 sessions. Other montages include anode over left DLPFC and cathode over right PFC or right DLPFC |

(ACC: anterior cingulate cortex; DLPFC: dorsolateral prefrontal cortex; OFC: orbitofrontal cortex; rTMS: repetitive transcranial magnetic stimulation; SMA: supplementary motor area; tDCS: transcranial direct current stimulation)

- Nonresponse, poor response, or no response is defined as a <25% reduction in Y-BOCS score, along with a CGI-I score of 4 (no change).

## REFERENCES


1. Taylor DM, Barnes TR, Young AH. The Maudsley prescribing guidelines in psychiatry. John Wiley & Sons; 2021.
2. Janardhan Reddy YC, Sundar AS, Narayanaswamy JC, Math SB. Clinical practice guidelines for Obsessive-Compulsive Disorder. Indian J Psychiatry. 2017;59(Suppl 1):S74-90.
3. Koran LM, Hanna GL, Hollander E, Nestadt G, Simpson HB; American Psychiatric Association. Practice guideline for the treatment of patients with obsessive-compulsive disorder. Am J Psychiatry. 2007;164(7 Suppl):5-53.
4. Clark DA. Cognitive-Behavioral Therapy for OCD and Its Subtypes: Second edition: The Guilford Press, New York, 2020.
5. Pallanti S, Quercioli L. Treatment-refractory obsessive-compulsive disorder: methodological issues, operational definitions and therapeutic lines. Prog Neuropsychopharmacol Biol Psychiatry. 2006;30(3):400-12.
6. Goodman WK, Price LH, Rasmussen SA, Mazure C, Fleischmann RL, Hill CL, et al. The Yale-Brown Obsessive Compulsive Scale. I. Development, use, and reliability. Arch Gen Psychiatry. 1989;46(11):1006-11.

CHAPTER 16

# Management of Comorbid Obsessive-Compulsive Disorder and Bipolar Disorder

*Ebin Joseph, Shyam Sundar Arumugham*

## INTRODUCTION

Obsessive-compulsive disorder (OCD) and bipolar disorder (BD) are common psychiatric conditions with a chronic course. Studies show they frequently co-occur beyond chance, with 17% of BD patients also having OCD, and about 18% of OCD patients also having BD.[1] Factors underlying this comorbidity include shared pathophysiology, medication effects (such as antidepressant-induced manic switch or atypical antipsychotic-induced OCD symptoms), mood disorder masquerading as OCD, and atypical variant of a primary condition. However, there is limited research on this, with a poor understanding of the relative contribution of these factors.

There is no overlap in the first-line treatment of these conditions. Mood stabilizers (lithium and valproate) or certain atypical antipsychotics (quetiapine) are indicated for long-term prophylaxis of BD, while selective serotonin reuptake inhibitors (SSRIs) and/or cognitive-behavior therapy (CBT) are the mainstays of treating OCD.[2,3] Aripiprazole and risperidone, which have antimanic properties, may also be helpful for SSRI augmentation in OCD. However, managing this comorbidity can be complicated by the risk of treatment-emergent mania (TEM) with SSRIs. Therefore, effective management requires a nuanced approach that includes an assessment of the patient's clinical profile and formulating an individualized treatment plan.

## CLINICAL PRESENTATION

Although most patients report the onset of OCD before their first mood episode, an earlier onset of mood episode is also not uncommon.[4] There is evidence suggesting a distinct clinical profile of OCD in patients with comorbid BD, including:[5-8]

- Earlier onset of symptoms
- Episodic course of OCD
- Worsening of OCD during depressive episodes and improvement during manic episodes
- Higher suicidality
- Greater severity and functional impairment
- Family loading of mood disorders and obsessive-compulsive related disorders (OCRDs)

Based on these findings, some hypothesize that comorbid BD-OCD is a variant of BD. However, clinical reality is complex, with varied clinical presentations that make it difficult to distinguish the primary condition. Clinicians often encounter one of the following four scenarios:

1. OCD confined to mood episodes
2. Subclinical OCD symptoms during the interepisodic period
3. Clinically significant OCD during the interepisodic period
4. TEM with SSRI

### Obsessive-Compulsive Disorder Confined to Mood Episodes

In this scenario, prioritizing mood stabilization is recommended, and the use of antidepressants should be avoided.[9] Preliminary evidence suggests that mood stabilization with certain atypical antipsychotics, such as aripiprazole, may benefit some patients with this comorbidity.[10] However, there is inadequate evidence to prefer any particular medication. Specific antiobsessive treatments may only be required if OCD symptoms persist without concurrent mood symptoms.

### Subclinical OCD Symptoms during the Inter-Episodic Period of BD

In this scenario, CBT using the principles of exposure and response prevention (ERP) is the first-line treatment. CBT should be recommended whenever possible. SSRIs increase the risk of mood instability and may be avoided.

## Clinically Significant OCD during the Interepisodic Period of BD

Managing this scenario needs a detailed assessment of the evolution of both mood and OCD symptoms and their association with treatment. It is crucial to rule out TEM with SSRI. It may also be helpful to identify a temporal correlation of OCD symptoms with atypical antipsychotic use, although such associations have been reported primarily in patients with schizophrenia. Adjustments to medications may be considered if there is a clear temporal correlation with a specific drug.

If independent manic/hypomanic episodes are identified, it may be necessary to treat both OCD and BD separately. A detailed evaluation of symptoms, primary symptom dimensions, level of distress, and dysfunction caused by OCD will guide treatment decisions.

If symptoms are mild to moderate, consider offering CBT alongside mood stabilizers as the first treatment option to reduce the risk of TEM.

If CBT is not feasible or ineffective, or if symptoms are severe, SSRIs can be considered under the cover of an adequate antimanic treatment. All SSRIs are equally effective in OCD, with the choice guided by empirical considerations. Clomipramine and venlafaxine should be avoided in the early stages due to their increased risk of TEM. Fluoxetine may also be avoided due to its prolonged half-life. Close monitoring is essential due to the potential for TEM and rapid cycling with high doses of SSRIs used for OCD. Augmenting SSRIs with risperidone or aripiprazole may be beneficial if SSRIs alone are inadequate. Other potential augmenting agents for OCD include memantine, N-acetyl cysteine, and ondansetron.

The choice of mood stabilizer is based on the BD profile. Lithium, valproate, and quetiapine are first-line mood stabilizers with good antimanic prophylactic efficacy. The choice is determined by factors such as previous treatment response, clinical profile, drug interactions, comorbidity, tolerability, availability, and affordability. Some patients may require a combination of mood stabilizers or a combination of mood stabilizers and antipsychotics.

## Treatment-Emergent Mania Occurred with Antidepressants

If a patient develops TEM while on SSRIs for OCD, the immediate focus should be on addressing manic symptoms. The SSRI should be discontinued. If the manic symptoms are severe and dysfunctional, antimanic treatment, including atypical antipsychotics or mood stabilizers, may be required. The antimanic agent should be continued until remission of manic symptoms. Further treatment decisions should be based on clinical judgment, as there are no consistent guidelines available.

Cognitive-behavior therapy should be considered for OCD treatment once manic symptoms have improved. If CBT is not available/feasible, trying a different SSRI may be considered. Patients who had a brief, self-limiting hypomanic episode that remitted on discontinuation of the offending agent may be tried on a different SSRI, after discussing the risk with close monitoring for hypomanic or manic symptoms. Family history of BD is another factor that may help in deciding on the need for mood stabilizers. The risks and benefits of antimanic prophylaxis should be discussed. If hypomanic/manic symptoms recur, long-term antimanic treatment in addition to SSRIs may be necessary. Patients with a severe manic episode with poor response to CBT may require continued antimanic prophylaxis in addition to an SSRI. The SSRI and antimanic agent may be chosen as discussed in the previous section.

Although neuromodulatory interventions such as repetitive transcranial magnetic stimulation (rTMS) have shown promise in OCD, their long-term efficacy is unclear. They may be tried judiciously based on the clinical need and availability.

## Treatment of Comorbid Bipolar Disorder–Obsessive-Compulsive Disorder

The treatment of comorbid BD-OCD is mentioned in **Box 1**.

**BOX 1:** The treatment of comorbid BD-OCD.

*A. OCD confined to mood episodes:*
- Mood stabilizer
- *If OCD symptoms are severe:* Mood stabilizer + CBT
- SSRI may be added only if there is persisting OCD resistant to CBT

*B. Subclinical OCD during interepisodic BD:*
- Mood stabilizer + CBT
- SSRI may be added only if the OCD symptoms are dysfunctional and resistant to CBT

*C. Clinically significant OCD during interepisodic BD:*
- *Mild/moderate OCD symptoms:* Mood stabilizer + CBT
- *Severe OCD or CBT resistant OCD:* Mood stabilizer + SSRI

*Contd...*

*Contd...*

| *D. Treatment emergent mania:* |
|---|
| • Stop SSRI and treat mania with antipsychotic or mood stabilizer, if required<br>• CBT can be attempted after remission of manic symptoms<br>• For CBT resistant mania, a combination of a different SSRI with mood stabilizer/atypical antipsychotic can be attempted<br>• Monotherapy with a different SSRI under close monitoring may be attempted in patients with a brief self-remitting hypomanic episode with not family history of BD |
| (BD: bipolar disorder; CBT: cognitive-behavior therapy; OCD: obsessive-compulsive disorder; SSRI: selective serotonin reuptake inhibitor) |

## REFERENCES


1. Amerio A, Stubbs B, Odone A, Tonna M, Marchesi C, Ghaemi SN. The prevalence and predictors of comorbid bipolar disorder and obsessive-compulsive disorder: A systematic review and meta-analysis. J Affect Disord. 2015;186:99-109.
2. Shah N, Grover S, Rao GP. Clinical Practice Guidelines for Management of Bipolar Disorder. Indian J Psychiatry. 2017;59:S51.
3. Reddy YJ, Sundar AS, Narayanaswamy JC, Math SB. Clinical practice guidelines for Obsessive-Compulsive Disorder. Indian J Psychiatry. 2017;59:74.
4. Tonna M, Amerio A, Odone A, Stubbs B, Ghaemi SN. Comorbid bipolar disorder and obsessive-compulsive disorder: Which came first? Aust N Z J Psychiatry. 2016;50:695-8.
5. Saraf G, Paul I, Viswanath B, Narayanaswamy JC, Math SB, Reddy YCJ. Bipolar disorder comorbidity in patients with a primary diagnosis of OCD. Int J Psychiatry Clin Pract. 2017;21:70-4.
6. Jeon S, Baek JH, Yang SY, Choi Y, Ahn SW, Ha K, et al. Exploration of comorbid obsessive-compulsive disorder in patients with bipolar disorder: The clinic-based prevalence rate, symptoms nature and clinical correlates. J Affect Disord. 2018;225:227-33.
7. Mahasuar R, Janardhan Reddy YC, Math SB. Obsessive-compulsive disorder with and without bipolar disorder. Psychiatry Clin Neurosci. 2011;65:423-33.
8. Zutshi A, Kamath P, Reddy YCJ. Bipolar and nonbipolar obsessive-compulsive disorder: a clinical exploration. Comprehensive Psychiatry. 2007;48:245-51.
9. Sharma LP, Reddy YCJ. Obsessive-compulsive disorder comorbid with schizophrenia and bipolar disorder. Indian J Psychiatry. 2019;61:S140-8.
10. Amerio A, Maina G, Ghaemi SN. Updates in treating comorbid bipolar disorder and obsessive-compulsive disorder: A systematic review. J Affect Disord. 2019;256:433-40.

CHAPTER 17

# Management of Difficult-to-Treat Mania

*Varun S Mehta, Surendra Paliwal*

## KEY CONSIDERATIONS

- Approximately 50% of patients will respond to monotherapy with significant improvement in manic symptoms within 3–4 weeks. When symptoms are not controlled, these patients can be classified as having "difficult-to-treat mania".
- Before classifying a patient as "difficult-to-treat mania", the clinician should consider that the symptoms could persist due to:
    a. *Low treatment adherence:* Establish the cause and offer appropriate intervention. For example, if nonadherence is due to an adverse reaction, consider reducing the dose if the adverse effect is dose related. If poor adherence is deliberate and not related to tolerability, long-term lithium may not be indicated due to the risk of "withdrawal" mania and depression. Instead, consider long-acting ("depot") formulations. The choice between first-generation antipsychotic (FGA) and second-generation antipsychotic (SGA) depot formulations should consider patient choice, affordability, and availability, noting that data supporting the use of FGA long-acting injectables (LAIs) is weak. Ensure early and continuing psychoeducation to reduce the risk of relapse due to medication nonadherence.
    b. *Poor tolerability:* Switch to a more tolerable alternative regimen.
    c. *Presence of comorbid disorders:* Identify comorbidities such as anxiety disorders, substance use disorders, and personality disorders, and offer appropriate intervention.
    d. *Secondary to a medical disorder:* Identify medical causes (e.g., hyperthyroidism and head injury) and offer appropriate intervention.
    e. *Ongoing antidepressants:* Taper and discontinue antidepressants.
- Two or more medications from different mechanistic classes are typically considered. For example, consider combining lithium or valproate with a dopamine antagonist/partial agonist.
- The decision to choose a combination agent is typically based on the rapidity of required response, history of partial response to monotherapy, severity of mania, tolerability concerns with combination therapy, and patient willingness.
- Clozapine may be considered for more severe refractory illness.[1]
- Electroconvulsive therapy (ECT) may be considered for patients with severe mania, particularly during pregnancy at any stage of treatment.[2]
- Continue annual physical monitoring to assess the cardiovascular risk factors due to high-premature mortality.

  After addressing points a–e and if symptoms are not controlled with monotherapy, follow the treatment algorithm as shown in **Flowchart 1**.
- *Agents that are not proven to be effective:* N-acetylcysteine, celecoxib, minocycline, Infliximab, allopurinol, eslicarbazepine, gabapentin, lamotrigine, omega-3 fatty acids, topiramate and zonisamide.
- *Agents that have proven to be effective but lack evidence of large RCTs:* Branched chain amino acids, folic acid, l-tryptophan, medroxyprogesterone, memantine, levetiracetam, and phenytoin.

**Flowchart 1:** Treatment algorithm for persistent manic symptoms.

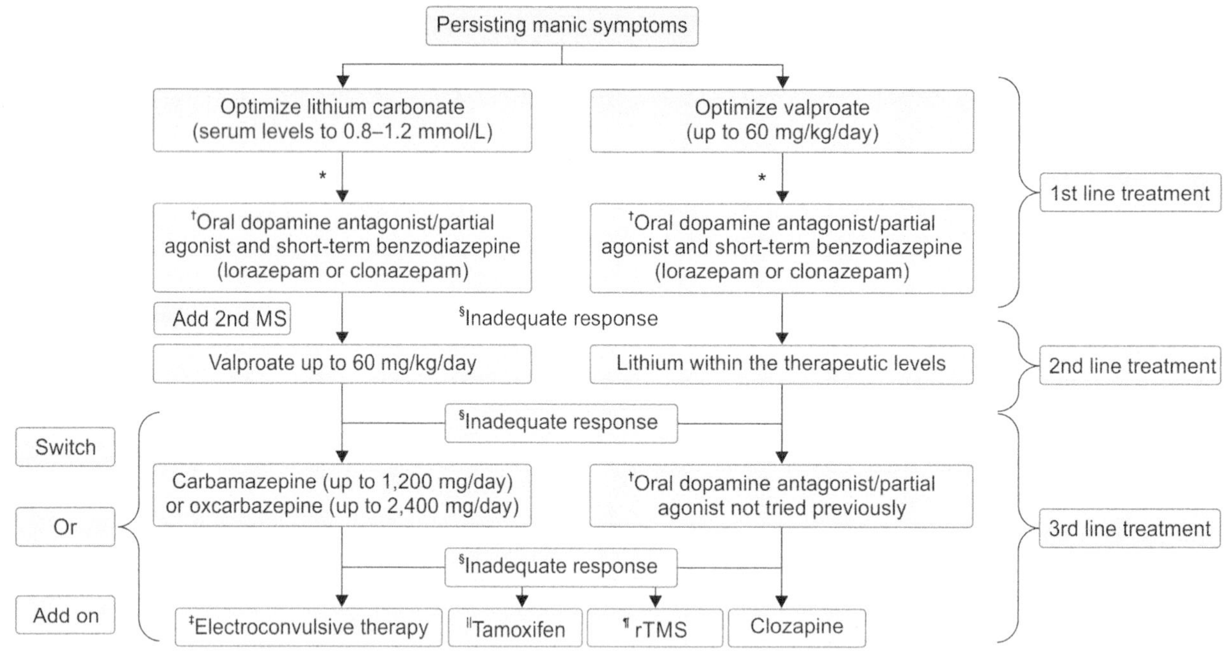


*The combination of mood stabilizer with oral FGA/SGA might be associated with more side effects, especially sedation.

†Not much strong evidence base to support one oral FGA over SGA. Among the oral FGAs, haloperidol has the maximum evidence for effectiveness and rapid onset of actions in the acute phase. However, haloperidol can be considered a second-choice option owing to its propensity to cause extrapyramidal symptoms. Also, the association of depression and tardive dyskinesia with FGAs might preclude their long-term use. Among the oral SGAs, the following can be considered as first-line treatment options: Quetiapine, aripiprazole, risperidone, and asenapine in combination with Li/valproate (CANMAT, 2018).[3] The preferred second-line combination agents can be olanzapine, ziprasidone, and haloperidol (CANMAT, 2018).[3]

‡Keep in mind that all antiepileptic mood stabilizers could affect the seizure threshold and so can be tapered and stopped in case of a poor or inadequate response when electroconvulsive therapy is being considered. Brief pulse therapy with two or three treatments per week is the recommended schedule. Bifrontal electrode placement is preferred over bitemporal as it is associated with faster treatment response and fewer cognitive side effects.

§If no response is observed within 2 weeks with therapeutic doses of antimanic agents, then it can be considered to be an inadequate response.

||Be aware of the risk of uterine cancer and the lack of clinical experience with tamoxifen despite evidence for efficacy.

¶Repetitive transcranial magnetic stimulation (rTMS) in the right prefrontal cortex at 110% motor threshold can also be considered in combination with pharmacotherapy.[4]

## REFERENCES


1. Perugi G, Medda P, Toni C, Mariani MG, Socci C, Mauri M. The Role of Electroconvulsive Therapy (ECT) in Bipolar Disorder: Effectiveness in 522 Patients with Bipolar Depression, Mixed-state, Mania and Catatonic Features. Curr Neuropharmacol. 2017;15:359-71.
2. Li XB, Tang YL, Wang CY, de Leon J. Clozapine for treatment-resistant bipolar disorder: a systematic review. Bipolar Disord. 2015;17:235-47.
3. Yatham LN, Kennedy SH, Parikh SV, Schaffer A, Bond DJ, Frey BN, et al. Canadian Network for Mood and Anxiety Treatments (CANMAT) and International Society for Bipolar Disorders (ISBD) 2018 guidelines for the management of patients with bipolar disorder. Bipolar Disord. 2018;20:97-170.
4. Praharaj SK, Ram D, Arora M. Efficacy of high frequency (rapid) suprathreshold repetitive transcranial magnetic stimulation of right prefrontal cortex in bipolar mania: a randomized sham controlled study. J Affect Disord. 2009; 117:146-50.

CHAPTER 18

# Management of Difficult-to-Treat Bipolar Depression

*Bhawna Yadav, Pooja Sharma, Nishant Goyal*

## INTRODUCTION

Bipolar depression refers to a condition meeting the criteria for a major depressive episode with a history of a manic or hypomanic episode (DSM-5). Bipolar patients, even with treatment, spend more time in a depressed state than in a manic state. The ratio of major depressive to manic/hypomanic episodes is 3:1 for bipolar I and 39:1 for bipolar II disorder, significantly contributing to disability in these illnesses.[1-3] Compared to major depressive disorder (unipolar depression), bipolar depression is more likely to manifest with psychosis, melancholic symptoms, psychomotor retardation (in bipolar I), and "atypical" symptoms.[4] Clear diagnostic criteria help classify the illness, though challenges arise when the initial presentations are depressive episodes before a manic or hypomanic episode is identified. Effective management of bipolar depression is crucial to reduce the burden of illness and the risk of suicide associated with untreated or improperly treated patients.

## CURRENT NOSOLOGICAL STATUS

In DSM-5, bipolar depression is defined as meeting the criteria for a major depressive episode with a history of a manic or hypomanic episode. Similarly, ICD-11 describes it with different codes for varying severity levels and a separate code for the unspecified severity of depressive symptoms.

## APPROACH TO BIPOLAR DEPRESSION

Although there are distinct pathophysiological differences between unipolar and bipolar depression regarding reward processing, emotional regulation, and attentional control, distinguishing between them based solely on clinical symptoms can be difficult. However, accurately identifying bipolar depression from unipolar depression is crucial because treatment strategies differ.[5] Several indicators can guide clinicians in making the correct diagnosis.

## INDICATORS OF BIPOLARITY IN DEPRESSION

Abrupt onset, early onset of the first depressive episode (before age 25), multiple prior episodes (>5), positive family history of bipolar disorder, symptoms such as hypersomnia/increased daytime napping, hyperphagia/weight gain, mood lability, psychomotor retardation, psychotic features, pathological guilt, atypical symptoms such as leaden paralysis, history of treatment resistance, and treatment-emergent mania or activation are indicators of bipolarity.[6,7] Emphasizing accurate diagnosis is crucial due to the already challenging management of bipolar depression.

## CHALLENGES[7-11]

Managing bipolar depression has many challenges, as shown in **Figure 1**. Ensuring adherence to treatment is important before saying a treatment has failed. Some other problems include certain comorbidities that increase the risk of bipolar depression **(Box 1)**, poor response to treatment, and difficulty in achieving remission due to persistent symptoms. Clinicians need to be aware of these factors that can affect clinical response and remission.

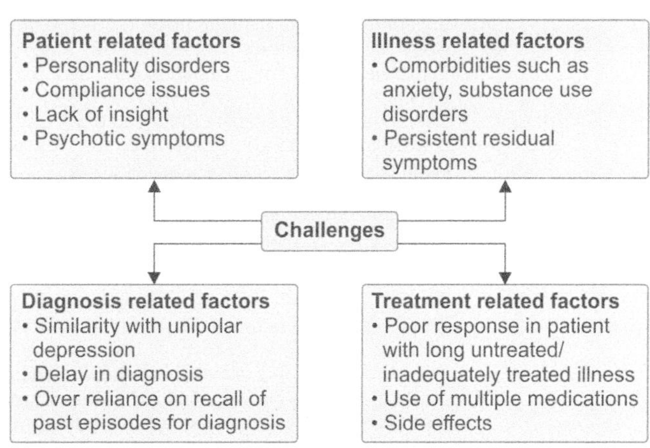


**Fig. 1:** Challenges in the management of bipolar depression.

## DIFFICULT-TO-TREAT DEPRESSION[12,13]

Difficult-to-treat depression (DTD) is defined as "depression that continues to cause significant burden despite usual treatment efforts". Unlike the treatment-resistant depression (TRD) model, DTD views depression as treatable but recognizes it may need special considerations beyond standard treatments.

**BOX 1:** Entities comorbid with bipolar depression.

*Comorbidities*
- Anxiety
- Substance use disorders
- Personality disorders
- Women with mood symptoms during the pregnancy/postpartum period
- Patients with attention-deficit/hyperactivity disorder (ADHD)
- Forensic populations
- Patients presenting for bariatric surgery/obesity treatment

Earlier, a significant reduction in symptoms—typically a 50% reduction on a standard clinician rating scale such as the Hamilton Rating Scale for Depression or Montgomery Åsberg Depression Rating Scale—was the goal. However, recent guidelines have recognized that sustained remission, not simply response, is the preferred goal of treatment. For DTD, treatment focuses on optimal symptom control, daily functioning, and quality of life, using a patient-centered approach with shared

**Flowchart 1:** Decision tree for managing bipolar depression.[17-19]

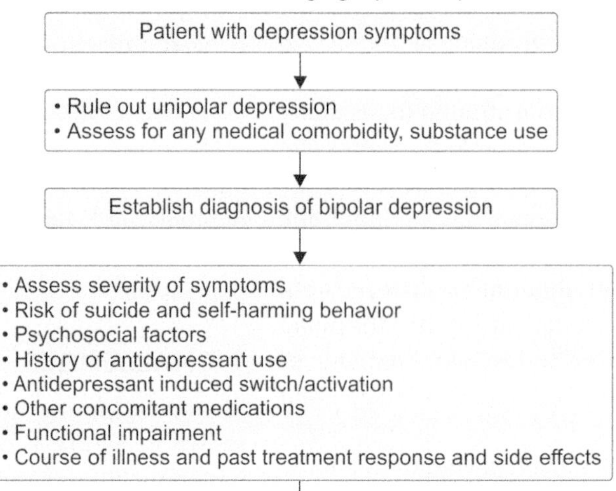


Acute phase

Treatment naive

*First line:* Quetiapine (300–600 mg), lithium (0.8–1.2), lamotrigine †(200 mg), lurasidone (20–120 mg)*, *Combination therapy:* Olanzapine + fluoxetine (5/20–10/40 mg)#, lithium or divalproex + lurasidone

Second line: Monotherapy with divalproex (20–30 mg/kg/day), adjunctive use of antidepressants (SSRI/bupropion (150–450 mg)) with lithium/divalproex, cariprazine (1.5–3 mg)*, sertraline (50–200 mg)*, venlafaxine (75–375 mg)*, ECT

*Third line:* Carbamazepine (600–800 mg)*, olanzapine (5–20 mg)*, tranylcypromine*, fluoxetine*

*Adjunctive agents:* Intravenous ketamine, aripiprazole (5–30 mg), armodafinil, asenapine, eicosapentaenoic acid, pramipexole, levothyroxine, light therapy, *N*-acetylcysteine (2 g/day), SNRI/ MAOI, rTMSc, agomelatine*

On treatment

- Ensure medication compliance
- Optimize the mood stabilizer
- *Not on mood stabilizer:* Lithium, lamotrigine
- *Switch to:* Quetiapine, lurasidone monotherapy
- Poor response to monotherapy with mood stabilizer/antipsychotic: Combination of these with antidepressants
- *ECT to be considered for:* Suicide risk, psychotic depression, catatonia, treatment refractory, rapid response needed
- *Future possible treatments:* Omega-3 fatty acid, modafinil, inositol, and gabapentin

*Psychosocial intervention:* Psychoeducation, interpersonal and social rhythm therapy, cognitive behavior therapy, family-focused interventions

*Novel treatment:* Transcranial direct current stimulation,[17] repetitive transcranial magnetic stimulation,[18] intermittent theta-burst stimulation,[19] Deep transcranial magnetic stimulation[19]

*Not to be used:* Antidepressant monotherapy, aripiprazole, mifepristone (adjunctive), ziprasidone (adjunctive), and levetiracetam (adjunctive)*

decision-making. All treatment options (medications, psychotherapy, neurostimulation, etc.) should be considered timely to optimize outcomes when sustained remission is elusive. Depression is considered significantly resistant if it does not improve after at least two adequate trials of medications from different classes in the current episode. Past treatment failures should also be considered when determining treatment resistance.

## MANAGEMENT

Various guidelines exist for managing bipolar depression, most of which provide similar information with a few differences. Our guidelines, as shown in the decision tree in **Flowchart 1**, are based on the IPS, CANMAT, and NICE guidelines.[14-16]

### Maintenance Phase

- Continue medication started during acute phase of illness.
- Best evidence for lithium, lamotrigine, valproate, and quetiapine
- Carbamazepine is effective but less preferred compared to lithium and valproate.
- Stoppage of antidepressants needs to be considered once bipolar depression remits.
- Maintenance electroconvulsive therapy (ECT) may be considered in patients who have reported to ECT during the acute episode.
- Long-acting injectable risperidone and ziprasidone beneficial to prevent recurrence

### Watch Out For

- *Hypersensitivity:* Carbamazepine and lamotrigine
- *Activation of suicidal ideation/aggression:* During the initial phase with selective serotonin reuptake inhibitors (SSRIs)
- *Delirium:* Due to polypharmacy, excessive anticholinergic side effects, etc.
- *Serotonin syndrome:* With high-dose SSRIs/two or more SSRIs when given together
- Overdose and toxicity, especially with mood stabilizers
- Anticholinergic side effects
- *Elderly:* Start low, go slow.
- *Comorbidities:* Diabetes, hypertension, hyponatremia, thyroid disorders, coronary artery disease (CAD), etc.
- *Interactions:* Drug interactions should be looked out for.

## CONCLUSION

Managing bipolar depression poses many complex challenges for clinicians, making timely and rational decision-making difficult. Reviewing various guidelines for managing difficult-to-treat bipolar depression offers hope that an aggressive yet cautious approach may help these patients achieve a more productive life.

## REFERENCES


1. Post RM. The impact of bipolar depression. J Clin Psychiatry. 2005;66(5):5.
2. Judd LL, Akiskal HS. Depressive episodes and symptoms dominate the longitudinal course of bipolar disorder. Curr Psychiatry Rep. 2003;5(6):417-8.
3. Coryell W, Solomon DA, Fiedorowicz JG, Endicott J, Schettler PJ, Judd LL. Anxiety and outcome in bipolar disorder. Am J Psychiatry. 2009;166(11):1238-43.
4. Mitchell PB, Malhi GS. Bipolar depression: phenomenological overview and clinical characteristics. Bipolar Disord. 2004;6(6):530-9.
5. de Almeida JR, Phillips ML. Distinguishing between unipolar depression and bipolar depression: current and future clinical and neuroimaging perspectives. Biol Psychiatry. 2013;73(2):111-8.
6. Motovsky B, Pecenak J. Psychopathological characteristics of bipolar and unipolar depression-potential indicators of bipolarity. Psychiatr Danub. 2013;25(1):34-9.
7. Suppes T, Kelly DI, Perla JM. Challenges in the management of bipolar depression. J Clin Psychiatry. 2005;66(5):11.
8. Cha B, Kim JH, Ha TH, Chang JS, Ha K. Polarity of the first episode and time to diagnosis of bipolar I disorder. Psychiatry Investig. 2009;6(2):96.
9. Shen YC. Treatment of acute bipolar depression. Tzu-Chi Med J. 2018;30(3):141.
10. Elsayed OH, Ercis M, Pahwa M, Singh B. Treatment-Resistant Bipolar Depression: Therapeutic Trends, Challenges and Future Directions. Neuropsychiatr Dis Treat. 2022;18:2927-43.
11. McIntyre RS, Calabrese JR. Bipolar depression: the clinical characteristics and unmet needs of a complex disorder. Curr Med Res Opin. 2019;35(11):1993-2005.
12. Rush AJ, Thase ME, Dubé S. Research issues in the study of difficult-to-treat depression. Biol Psychiatry. 2003;53(8):743-53.
13. McAllister-Williams RH, Arango C, Blier P, Demyttenaere K, Falkai P, Gorwood P, et al. The identification, assessment and management of difficult-to-treat depression: an international consensus statement. J Affect Disord. 2020;267:264-82.
14. Yatham LN, Kennedy SH, Parikh SV, Schaffer A, Bond DJ, Frey BN, et al. Canadian Network for Mood and Anxiety Treatments (CANMAT) and International Society for Bipolar Disorders (ISBD) 2018 guidelines for the

management of patients with bipolar disorder. Bipolar Disord. 2018;20(2):97-170.

15. Shah N, Grover S, Rao GP. Clinical practice guidelines for management of bipolar disorder. Indian J Psychiatry. 2017;59(Suppl 1):S51.
16. Taylor DM, Barnes TR, Young AH. The Maudsley Prescribing Guidelines in Psychiatry. John Wiley & Sons; 2021.
17. Donde C, Amad A, Nieto I, Brunoni AR, Neufeld NH, Bellivier F, et al. Transcranial direct-current stimulation (tDCS) for bipolar depression: A systematic review and meta-analysis. Prog Neuropsychopharmacol Biol Psychiatry. 2017;78:123-31.
18. Konstantinou G, Hui J, Ortiz A, Kaster TS, Downar J, Blumberger DM, et al. Repetitive transcranial magnetic stimulation (rTMS) in bipolar disorder: A systematic review. Bipolar Disord. 2022;24(1):10-26.
19. Diaz AP, Fernandes BS, Quevedo J, Sanches M, Soares JC. Treatment-resistant bipolar depression: concepts and challenges for novel interventions. Braz J Psychiatry. 2022;44:178-86.

CHAPTER 19

# Management of Difficult-to-Treat Mixed Episode

*Alankrit Jaiswal, Umesh Shreekantiah*

## INTRODUCTION

Mixed mood states have been recognized since Kraepelin's time and were detailed by Weygandt, an assistant of Kraepelin.[1] Mixed affective symptoms in bipolar disorder significantly impact prognosis and complicate management. There is limited research on managing mixed episodes, with most evidence on pharmacological agents extrapolated from studies involving pure manic or bipolar depressive patients.

## DIAGNOSIS

The conceptualization of mixed episode has evolved over the years, but its definition is broadened and unified in the Diagnostic and Statistical Manual's 5th edition (DSM-5). DSM-5 redefined mixed episodes as a specifier applicable to bipolar type I or II, as well as major depressive disorder. It now allows the presence of just three symptoms of opposite mood polarity to qualify for the specifier, marking a significant change in criteria.

## PROBLEMS IN THE MANAGEMENT OF MIXED EPISODES

- A wide range of definitions of mixed episodes in clinical studies
- The FDA employs a narrow definition of mixed episode.[1]
- Mixed episodes can present with wide variations, including predominantly manic, predominantly depressive, or episodes with anxiety, irritability, and agitation.
- Prophylactic management aims to prevent not only future mixed episodes but also manic and depressive episodes.
- Patients with mixed episodes often exhibit varying rates of substance abuse.[2-4]
- Mixed episodes are associated with higher rates of recurrence,[4] psychiatric readmissions,[5] and longer illness duration.[6]
- Higher risk of switch, rapid cycling, and suicide attempts[7]

## DIFFICULT-TO-TREAT MIXED EPISODE (FLOWCHARTS 1 TO 3)

- Mixed features occur in a depressive episode or manic episode and predict poor prognosis.
- Mixed features in depressive episodes increase the likelihood of progression to bipolar disorder.

**Flowchart 1:** Acute treatment of mixed episode.[1,9]

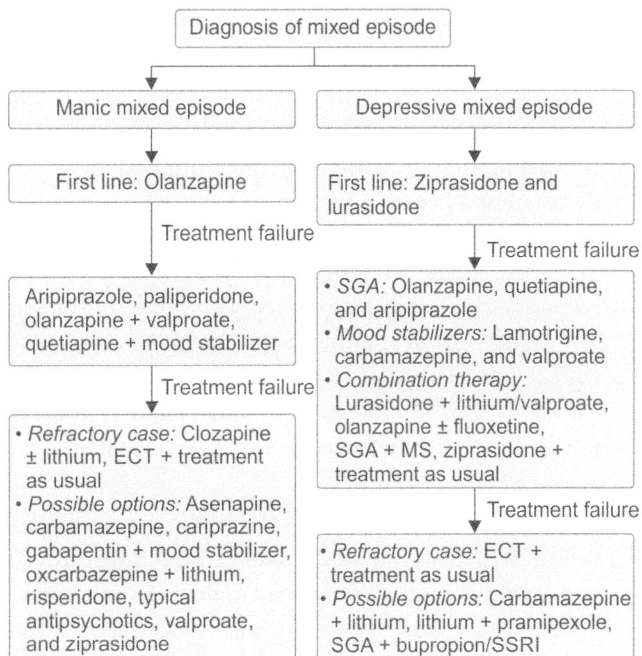


(ECT: electroconvulsive therapy; MS: mood stabilizer; SGA: second generation antipsychotic; SSRI: selective serotonin reuptake inhibitor)

**Flowchart 2:** Prevention of mixed episode.[1,9]

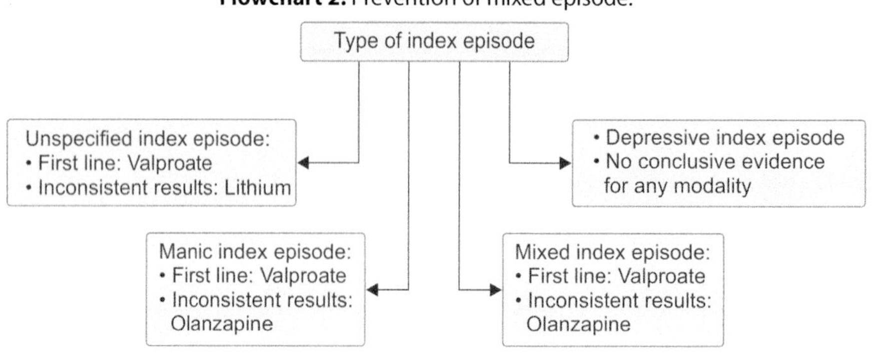


**Flowchart 3:** Maintenance treatment of mixed episode.[1,9]

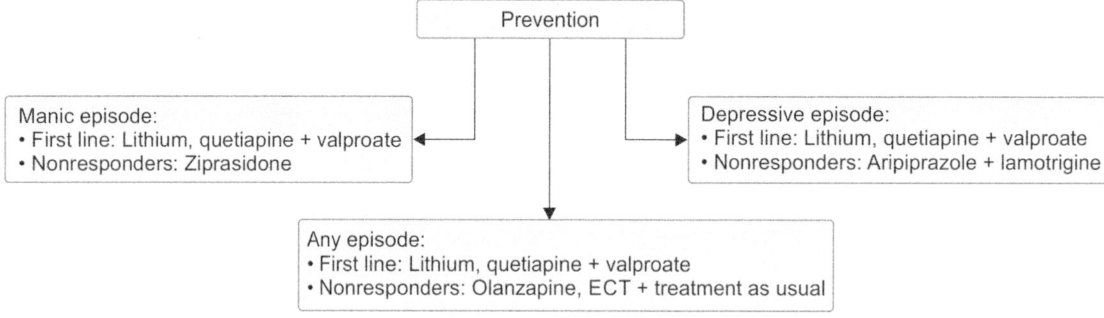


- There is an increased incidence of antidepressant-induced manic/hypomanic switch in mixed depressive episodes.
- Severe and longer episode duration, less interepisodic remission, higher recurrence rate, and a higher incidence of rapid cycling.[8]
- Higher incidence of suicidality[8]
- There are currently no specific guidelines regarding response, remission, and recovery for mixed episodes.
- The definition of treatment resistance or refractory state in mixed episodes is not clearly established.
- Clinically, mixed episodes are more likely to predict poor response to pharmacotherapy in bipolar disorder.[9]

## GENERAL RECOMMENDATIONS

- Using evidence-based interventions tailored to patient's specific needs can lead to positive outcomes.
- Collaborative case formulation, customized to the individual patient, enhances interdisciplinary teamwork and goal sharing.
- Regularly assessing the effectiveness of pharmacological and nonpharmacological interventions at various levels, whenever feasible, is essential.
- Meticulous treatment planning can help prevent relapses and the "revolving door" phenomenon, offering insights for future cost-effectiveness in this patient population.[10]

## REFERENCES

1. Grunze H, Vieta E, Goodwin GM, Bowden C, Licht RW, Azorin JM, et al. The World Federation of Societies of Biological Psychiatry (WFSBP) Guidelines for the Biological Treatment of Bipolar Disorders: Acute and long-term treatment of mixed states in bipolar disorder. World J Biol Psychiatry. 2018;19:2-58.
2. Cassidy F, Ahearn EP, Carroll BJ. Substance abuse in bipolar disorder: Substance abuse in bipolar disorder. Bipolar Disord. 2001;3:181-8.
3. Tohen M, Greenfield SF, Weiss RD, Zarate CA Jr, Vagge LM. The effect of comorbid substance use disorders on the course of bipolar disorder: a review. Harv Rev Psychiatry. 1998;6:133-41.
4. Tundo A, Musetti L, Benedetti A, Berti B, Massimetti G, Dell'Osso L. Onset polarity and illness course in bipolar I and II disorders: The predictive role of broadly defined mixed states. Compr Psychiatry. 2015;63:15-21.
5. Cassidy F, Carroll BJ. The clinical epidemiology of pure and mixed manic episodes. Bipolar Disord. 2001;3:35-40.

6. Perugi G, Micheli C, Akiskal HS, Madaro D, Socci C, Quilici C, et al. Polarity of the first episode, clinical characteristics, and course of manic depressive illness: a systematic retrospective investigation of 320 bipolar I patients. Compr Psychiatry. 2000;41:13-8.
7. Azorin J-M, Aubrun E, Bertsch J, Reed C, Gerard S, Lukasiewicz M. Mixed states vs. pure mania in the French sample of the EMBLEM study: results at baseline and 24 months - European mania in bipolar longitudinal evaluation of medication. BMC Psychiatry. 2009;9:33.
8. Takeshima M. Early recognition and appropriate pharmacotherapy for mixed depression: the key to resolving complex or treatment-refractory clinical cases. Clin Neuropsychopharmacol Therapeut. 2019;10:10-17.
9. Verdolini N, Hidalgo-Mazzei D, Murru A, Pacchiarotti I, Samalin L, Young AH, et al. Mixed states in bipolar and major depressive disorders: systematic review and quality appraisal of guidelines. Acta Psychiatr Scand. 2018;138:196-222.
10. Scherb E, Kerman B. Delivering effective combined treatments in mental health settings with difficult-to-treat patients: A bipolar case study illustrating the role of teamwork and other mediators. J Clin Psychol. 2023;79:1572-92.

CHAPTER 20

# Management of Rapid Cycling Bipolar Disorder

*Sujit Sarkhel*

## INTRODUCTION

The Diagnostic and Statistical Manual of Mental Disorders, Fifth Edition (DSM-5), defines rapid cycling bipolar disorder (RCBD) as the occurrence of at least four distinct episodes of mania, hypomania, or major depression within a 12-month period. These episodes can occur in any order or combination, separated by periods of partial or complete remission lasting at least 2 months, or by a change to an opposite-polarity mood episode.[1]

The estimated 12-month prevalence of RCBD varies, but lifetime prevalence ranges between 26 and 43% among those with bipolar disorder (BD). Those with RCBD experience a significant illness burden, including higher rates of physical health conditions, mixed features, co-occurring substance use disorders, suicidality, lower psychosocial functioning, and more episodes per year.[2]

Prospective studies indicate that RCBD is often a temporary state rather than a fixed trait, though it can persist for years. In one study, the average duration of rapid cycling was 8 years among 109 bipolar patients followed for up to 36 years.[3] Factors such as a depression-(hypo)mania-interval course with partial remission, and quick switches from sadness to (hypo)mania, and presence of agitated/mixed depressions contribute to poorer outcomes.[4]

Remission from individual rapid-cycling mood episodes frequently occurs naturally over the course of the illness rather than solely due to treatment. Therefore, treatment goals often focus on selecting medications suitable for both acute and maintenance phases to prevent new episodes from occurring.

## HISTORY OF PRESENT ILLNESS AND MENTAL STATUS EXAMINATION

It is necessary to evaluate the current episode's nature, severity, and length. Risk factors for RCBD include female gender,[5] younger age of onset, a course with more depressive episodes,[6] and a history of substance use.[7] Common comorbidities such as attention deficit hyperactivity disorder (ADHD) and borderline personality disorder often overlap in symptoms and require accurate diagnosis.[8,9] Given the higher functional impairment and increased risk of suicide attempts in RCBD compared to non-RCBD,[10,11] suicide risk assessment and a comprehensive care strategy are essential. A thorough medical history should include screening for hypothyroidism, as studies have linked autoimmune thyroiditis [thyroid peroxidase (TPO) or thyroglobulin antibodies (TG-abs)] or hypothyroidism with RCBD.[12,13] Antithyroid antibodies may affect mental health even in the absence of thyroid disease.[14]

## INVESTIGATIONS

Laboratory examination of patients with RCBD includes complete blood count, liver and renal function tests, blood biochemistry and metabolic panel, urine screening (both standard and toxicology screen), and thyroid function tests. For elderly patients, a baseline electrocardiogram (ECG) may be helpful. Additional tests such as serum levels of folate, ferritin, vitamin $B_{12}$, or C-reactive protein may be ordered based on clinical necessity.

Patients suspected of having structural brain abnormalities should undergo neuroimaging tests. Biomarker-based methods, including anti-DNA, anti-ENA, anti-NMDA, interleukin 2, 6, and TNF-$\alpha$, can also be considered.[15] Rating scales and diagnostic tools such as the Structured Clinical Interview for DSM Disorders (SCID) and Mini International Neuropsychiatric Interview (MINI) can aid in diagnosis and assessment.

## MANAGEMENT

### Management of Acute Mood Episode

There is limited research on treating mood episodes in patients with RCBD. Current evidence supports the use of olanzapine, aripiprazole, and divalproex for managing RCBD,[16] as well as to treat manic or mixed episodes.[17,18] Quetiapine has shown efficacy in treating depressive episodes according to available evidence.[19] However, antidepressants are generally not recommended for treating depression in RCBD due to concerns about mood destabilization. Citalopram[20] was associated with reports of mood instability, but not fluoxetine (compared to lithium or placebo)[21] or venlafaxine (compared to lithium).[3] In the absence of clear data on treating acute episodes in RCBD, the Canadian Network for Mood and Anxiety Treatments (CANMAT) guideline recommends choosing a treatment for an acute episode in patients with rapid cycling based on their effectiveness in the maintenance phase.[22] The National Institute for Health and Care Excellence (NICE) guideline advises treating RCBD similarly to non-RCBD patients due to the lack of robust evidence for RC-specific therapy.[23] Other medications such as clozapine[24] and risperidone[25] have been mentioned as potentially helpful and warrant further investigation for their role in RCBD treatment.

## Relapse Avoidance/Prophylaxis in Rapid Cycling Bipolar Disorder

Lamotrigine does not offer additional benefit as a preventive therapy as per CANMAT guidelines **Table 1**.[22] However, lamotrigine, aripiprazole, and concomitant levothyroxine have demonstrated superiority over placebo in preventing episodes in individuals with RCBD.[26-29] While there was no clear difference between lithium alone and lithium combined with divalproex in patients with concurrent substance use disorder,[30] combined treatment with carbamazepine and lithium has shown better response rates compared to monotherapy.[31]

**TABLE 1:** Level of evidence for pharmacological rapid cycling bipolar disorder (RCBD) treatment.

| *Grade* | *Medication* | *Discussion* |
|---|---|---|
| A | Levothyroxine | One positive randomized controlled trials (RCT) and multiple positive case reports |
| | Clozapine | One positive RCT, one positive retrospective study, and multiple positive case reports |
| B | Valproate | • One positive open trial and multiple positive case reports<br>• One RCT showing moderate efficacy |
| | Quetiapine | • One positive prospective open-label<br>• One positive open-label, parallel group, and multicentric trial |
| | Aripiprazole | One positive RCT |
| | Olanzapine | One RCT showing similar efficacy to valproate |
| C | Ketamine<br>Pramipexol<br>Topiramate<br>Aripiprazole<br>Bupropion<br>Nimodipine<br>Choline<br>Tryptophan<br>Clonazepam<br>Levetiracetam<br>Chromium | Multiple positive case reports |
| | Carbamazepine | One open trial showing moderate efficacy |
| | Magnesiocard | One pilot study showing moderate efficacy in the acute phase |
| D | Lithium | Two negative RCT, lithium might be effective as an "add-on" treatment |
| | Ethyl-eicosapentaenoate<br>Melatonin<br>Risperidone | One negative RCT |
| | Lamotrigine | • Several positive case reports as an "add-on" treatment<br>• One positive open naturalistic trial, one positive open prospective study<br>• One negative RCT |

(EPA: ethyl-eicosapentanoate; RCT: randomized controlled trials)
*Source*: Bourla A, Ferreri F, Baudry T, Panizzi V, Adrien V, Mouchabac S.[40]

Case reports have highlighted the effectiveness of clozapine, often in combination with lithium or levothyroxine, for treating both psychotic and nonpsychotic RCBD.[32-35] Dosages typically range from 150 to 400 mg daily during acute phases and from 150 to 275 mg/day for relapse prevention. Both retrospective analyses[24] and randomized controlled trials[36] strongly support the use of clozapine in RCBD.

## Alternative Treatments

Levothyroxine has shown significant benefits in the treatment of RCBD. One study on 32 RCBD patients reported that those treated with levothyroxine spent more time in a euthymic state and less time depressed or in a mixed mood compared to pretreatment levels.[29] Levothyroxine, especially at supraphysiological levels, was also associated with remission in RCBD patients resistant to conventional medications in several studies.[12,37,38] Ketamine has also shown positive effects in RCBD based on case reports.[39,40]

**Flowchart 1:** Algorithm of management of rapid cycling bipolar disorder.

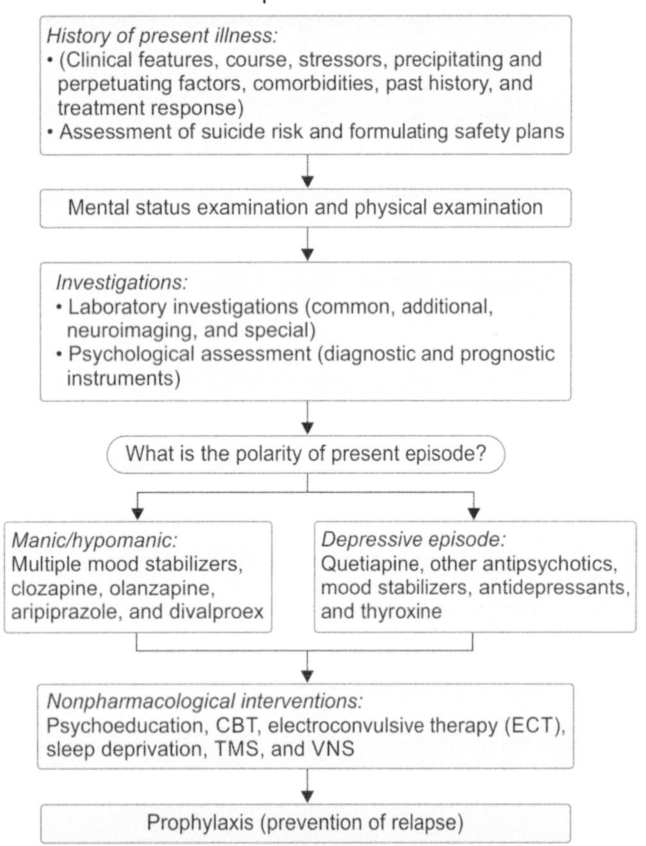


(CBT: cognitive behavioral therapy; TMS: transcranial magnetic stimulation; VNS: vagus nerve stimulation)

Other medications reported to have positive responses in RCBD include Magnesiocard,[41] Nimodipine,[42] Choline,[43] and Tryptophan,[44] levetiracetam,[45] chromium,[46] pramipexole,[47] and clonazepam.[48]

## Nonpharmacological Treatments (Flowchart 1)

Nonpharmacological approaches are considered due to the limited evidence-based pharmacological treatments for both acute and prophylactic management of mood episodes in patients with RCBD. Although not investigated in randomized controlled studies, electroconvulsive therapy (ECT), light therapy, sleep deprivation, transcranial magnetic stimulation (TMS), and vagus nerve stimulation (VNS) have all been used in treating RCBD. Naturalistic studies have shown a significant reduction (13-fold) in sick days per year in RCBD patients receiving maintenance ECT.[49] After an acute ECT treatment, affective episodes were significantly reduced according to an open-label trial in patients with RCBD and ultra-RCBD.[50] Case studies and case series indicate a potential positive effect of sleep restriction, TMS, VNS, and cognitive behavioral therapy in RCBD.[51-55]

## REFERENCES


1. Diagnostic and Statistical Manual of Mental Disorders: DSM-5, 5th edition. American Psychiatric Association; 2013.
2. Carvalho AF, Dimellis D, Gonda X, Vieta E, McIntyre RS, Fountoulakis KN. Rapid cycling in bipolar disorder: a systematic review. J Clin Psychiatry. 2014;75(6):16864.
3. Lorenzo-Luaces L, Amsterdam JD, Soeller I, DeRubeis RJ. Rapid versus non-rapid cycling bipolar II depression: response to venlafaxine and lithium and hypomanic risk. Acta Psychiatr Scand. 2016;133(6):459-69.
4. Roosen L, Sienaert P. Evidence-based treatment strategies for rapid cycling bipolar disorder, a systematic review. J Affect Disord. 2022;311:69-77.
5. Kupka RW, Luckenbaugh DA, Post RM, Leverich GS, Nolen WA. Rapid and non-rapid cycling bipolar disorder: a meta-analysis of clinical studies. J Clin Psychiatry. 2003;64(12):1483-94.
6. Bauer M, Beaulieu S, Dunner DL, Lafer B, Kupka R. Rapid cycling bipolar disorder–diagnostic concepts. Bipolar Disord. 2008;10(1p2):153-62.
7. Schneck CD, Miklowitz DJ, Calabrese JR, Allen MH, Thomas MR, Wisniewski SR, et al. Phenomenology of rapid-cycling bipolar disorder: data from the first 500 participants in the Systematic Treatment Enhancement Program. Am J Psychiatry. 2004;161(10):1902-8.

8. Antonietta Furio M, Popovic D, Vieta E, Stukalin Y, Hagin M, Torrent C, et al. Characterization of rapid cycling bipolar patients presenting with major depressive episode within the BRIDGE-II-MIX study. Bipolar Disor. 2021;23(4):391-9.
9. Coryell W. Rapid cycling bipolar disorder: clinical characteristics and treatment options. CNS Drugs. 2005;19:557-69.
10. Coryell W, Solomon D, Turvey C, Keller M, Leon AC, Endicott J, et al. The long-term course of rapid-cycling bipolar disorder. Arch Gen Psychiatry. 2003;60(9):914-20.
11. Garcia-Amador M, Colom F, Valenti M, Horga G, Vieta E. Suicide risk in rapid cycling bipolar patients. J Affect Disord. 2009;117(1-2):74-8.
12. Bauer MS, Whybrow PC. Rapid cycling bipolar affective disorder: II. Treatment of refractory rapid cycling with high-dose levothyroxine: A preliminary study. Arch Gen Psychiatry. 19901;47(5):435-40.
13. Oomen HA, Schipperijn AJ, Drexhage HA. The prevalence of affective disorder and in particular of a rapid cycling of bipolar disorder in patients with abnormal thyroid function tests. Clin Endocrinol. 1996;45(2):215-23.
14. Müssig K, Künle A, Säuberlich AL, Weinert C, Ethofer T, Saur R, et al. Thyroid peroxidase antibody positivity is associated with symptomatic distress in patients with Hashimoto's thyroiditis. Brain Behav Immun. 2012;26(4):559-63.
15. Sigitova E, Fišar Z, Hroudová J, Cikánková T, Raboch J. Biological hypotheses and biomarkers of bipolar disorder. Psychiatry Clin Neurosci. 2017;71(2):77-103.
16. Suppes T, Brown E, Schuh LM, Baker RW, Tohen M. Rapid versus non-rapid cycling as a predictor of response to olanzapine and divalproex sodium for bipolar mania and maintenance of remission: post hoc analyses of 47-week data. J Affect Disord. 2005;89(1-3):69-77.
17. Sanger TM, Tohen M, Vieta E, Dunner DL, Bowden CL, Calabrese JR, et al. Olanzapine in the acute treatment of bipolar I disorder with a history of rapid cycling. J Affect Disord. 2003;73(1-2):155-61.
18. Suppes T, Eudicone J, McQuade R, Pikalov III A, Carlson B. Efficacy and safety of aripiprazole in subpopulations with acute manic or mixed episodes of bipolar I disorder. J Affect Disord. 2008;107(1-3):145-54.
19. Vieta E, Calabrese JR, Goikolea JM, Raines S, Macfadden W; BOLDER Study Group. Quetiapine monotherapy in the treatment of patients with bipolar I or II depression and a rapid-cycling disease course: a randomized, double-blind, placebo-controlled study. Bipolar Disord. 2007;9(4): 413-25.
20. Ghaemi SN, Whitham EA, Vohringer PA, Barroilhet SA, Amerio A, Sverdlov O, et al. Citalopram for acute and preventive efficacy in bipolar depression (CAPE-BD): a randomized, double-blind, placebo-controlled trial. J Clin Psychiatry. 2021;82(1):6067.
21. Amsterdam JD, Luo L, Shults J. Efficacy and mood conversion rate during long-term fluoxetine v. lithium monotherapy in rapid-and non-rapid-cycling bipolar II disorder. Br J Psychiatry. 2013;202(4):301-6.
22. Yatham LN, Kennedy SH, Parikh SV, Schaffer A, Bond DJ, Frey BN, et al. Canadian Network for Mood and Anxiety Treatments (CANMAT) and International Society for Bipolar Disorders (ISBD) 2018 guidelines for the management of patients with bipolar disorder. Bipolar Disord. 2018;20(2):97-170.
23. National Collaborating Centre for Mental Health (UK). (2023). Bipolar disorder: The NICE guideline on the assessment and management of bipolar disorder in adults, children and young people in primary and secondary care. [online] Available from https://pubmed.ncbi.nlm.nih.gov/29718639/ [Last accessed June, 2025].
24. Kılınçel O, Kılınçel Ş, Gündüz C, Cangür Ş, Akkaya C. The Role of Clozapine as a Mood Regulator in the Treatment of Rapid Cycling Bipolar Affective Disorder. Turk J Psychiatry. 2019;30(4):268-71.
25. Vieta E, Gasto C, Colom F, Martinez A, Otero A, Vallejo J. Treatment of refractory rapid cycling bipolar disorder with risperidone. J Clin Psychopharmacol. 1998;18(2): 172-4.
26. Calabrese JR, Suppes T, Bowden CL, Sachs GS, Swann AC, McElroy SL, et al. A double-blind, placebo-controlled, prophylaxis study of lamotrigine in rapid-cycling bipolar disorder. J Clin Psychiatry. 2000;61(11):841-50.
27. Muzina DJ, Momah C, Eudicone JM, Pikalov A, McQuade RD, Marcus RN, et al. Aripiprazole monotherapy in patients with rapid-cycling bipolar I disorder: an analysis from a long-term, double-blind, placebo-controlled study. Int J Clin Pract. 2008;62(5):679-87.
28. Goldberg JF, Bowden CL, Calabrese JR, Ketter TA, Dann RS, Frye MA, et al. Six-month prospective life charting of mood symptoms with lamotrigine monotherapy versus placebo in rapid cycling bipolar disorder. Biol Psychiatry. 2008;63(1):125-30.
29. Walshaw PD, Gyulai L, Bauer M, Bauer MS, Calimlim B, Sugar CA, et al. Adjunctive thyroid hormone treatment in rapid cycling bipolar disorder: A double-blind placebo-controlled trial of levothyroxine (L-T4) and triiodothyronine (T3). Bipolar Disord. 2018;20(7):594-603.
30. Kemp DE, Gao K, Ganocy SJ, Elhaj O, Bilali SR, Conroy C, et al. A 6-month, double-blind, maintenance trial of lithium monotherapy versus the combination of lithium and divalproex for rapid-cycling bipolar disorder and co-occurring substance abuse or dependence. J Clin Psychiatry. 2009;70 (1):113-21.
31. Denicoff KD, Smith-Jackson EE, Disney ER, Ali SO, Leverich GS, Post RM. Comparative prophylactic efficacy of lithium, carbamazepine, and the combination in bipolar disorder. J Clin Psychiatry. 1997;58(11):470-8.
32. Calabrese JR, Meltzer HY, Markovitz PJ. Clozapine prophylaxis in rapid cycling bipolar disorder. J Clin Psychopharmacol. 1991;11(6):396-7.

33. Frye MA, Altshuler LL, Bitran JA. Clozapine in rapid cycling bipolar disorder. J Clin Psychopharmacol. 1996;16(1):87-90.
34. Lancon C, Llorca PM. Clozapine in the treatment of refractory rapid cycling bipolar disorder. L'encephale. 1996;22(6):468-9.
35. Suppes T, Phillips KA, Judd CR. Clozapine treatment of nonpsychotic rapid cycling bipolar disorder: a report of three cases. Biol Psychiatry. 1994;36(5):38-340.
36. Suppes T, Erkan Ozcan M, Carmody T. Response to clozapine of rapid cycling versus non-cycling patients with a history of mania. Bipolar Disord. 2004;6(4):329-32.
37. Weeston TF, Constantino J. High-dose T4 for rapid-cycling bipolar disorder. J Am Acad Child Adolesc Psychiatry. 1996;35(2):131-2.
38. Afflelou S, Auriacombe M, Cazenave M, Chartres JP, Tignol J. Utilisation de lévothyroxine à haute dose dans le traitement des troubles bipolaires à cycles rapides. Revue de la littérature et premières applications thérapeutiques à propos de 6 cas [Administration of high dose levothyroxine in treatment of rapid cycling bipolar disorders. Review of the literature and initial therapeutic application apropos of 6 cases]. Encephale. 1997;6:209-17.
39. Sampath H, Sharma I, Dutta S. Treatment of suicidal depression with ketamine in rapid cycling bipolar disorder. Asia-Pacific Psychiatry. 2016;8(1):98-101.
40. Bourla A, Ferreri F, Baudry T, Panizzi V, Adrien V, Mouchabac S. Rapid cycling bipolar disorder: Literature review on pharmacological treatment illustrated by a case report on ketamine. Brain Behav. 2022;12(2):e2483.
41. Chouinard G, Beauclair L, Geiser R, Etienne P. A pilot study of magnesium aspartate hydrochloride (Magnesiocard®) as a mood stabilizer for rapid cycling bipolar affective disorder patients. Prog Neuropsychopharmacol Biol Psychiatry. 1990;14(2):171-80.
42. Goodnick PJ. Nimodipine treatment of rapid cycling bipolar disorder. J Clin Psychiatry. 1995;56(7):330.
43. Stoll AL, Sachs GS, Cohen BM, Lafer B, Christensen JD, Renshaw PF. Choline in the treatment of rapid-cycling bipolar disorder: clinical and neurochemical findings in lithium-treated patients. Biol Psychiatry. 1996;40(5):382-8.
44. Sharma V, Barrett C. Tryptophan for treatment of rapid-cycling bipolar disorder comorbid with fibromyalgia. Can J Psychiatry. 2001;46(5):452-3.
45. Bräunig P, Krüger S. Levetiracetam in the treatment of rapid cycling bipolar disorder. J Psychopharmacol. 2003;17(2):239-41.
46. Amann BL, Mergl R, Vieta E, Born C, Hermisson I, Seemueller F, et al. A 2-year, open-label pilot study of adjunctive chromium in patients with treatment-resistant rapid-cycling bipolar disorder. J Clin Psychopharmacol. 2007;27(1):104-6.
47. Hegde A, Singh A, Ravi M, Narayanaswamy JC, Math SB. Pramipexole in the treatment of refractory depression in a patient with rapid cycling bipolar disorder. Indian J Psychol Med. 2015;37(4):473-4.
48. Sugimoto T, Murata T, Omori M, Wada Y. Clonazepam augmentation therapy in a male at early adolescence with rapid cycling bipolar disorder. General Hospital Psychiatry. 2003;1(25):57-9.
49. Minnai GP, Salis PG, Oppo R, Loche AP, Scano F, Tondo L. Effectiveness of maintenance electroconvulsive therapy in rapid-cycling bipolar disorder. J ECT. 2011;27(2):123-6.
50. Mosolov S, Born C, Grunze H. Electroconvulsive therapy (ECT) in bipolar disorder patients with ultra-rapid cycling and unstable mixed states. Medicina. 2021;57(6):624.
51. Marangell LB, Suppes T, Zboyan HA, Prashad SJ, Fischer G, Snow D, et al. A 1-year pilot study of vagus nerve stimulation in treatment-resistant rapid-cycling bipolar disorder. J Clin Psychiatry. 2008;69(2):183-9.
52. Dell'Osso B, Altamura AC. Augmentative transcranial magnetic stimulation (TMS) combined with brain navigation in drug-resistant rapid cycling bipolar depression: a case report of acute and maintenance efficacy. World J Biol Psychiatry. 2009;10(4-2):673-6.
53. Leibenluft E, Turner EH, Feldman-Naim S, Schwartz PJ, Wehr TA, Rosenthal NE. Light therapy in patients with rapid cycling bipolar disorder: preliminary results. Psychopharmacol Bull. 1995;31(4):705-10.
54. Reilly-Harrington NA, Deckersbach T, Knauz R, Wu Y, Tran T, Eidelman P, et al. Cognitive behavioral therapy for rapid-cycling bipolar disorder: a pilot study. J Psychiatr Pract. 2007;13(5):291-7.
55. Papadimitriou GN, Christodoulou GN, Katsouyanni K, Stefanis CN. Therapy and prevention of affective illness by total sleep deprivation. J Affect Disord. 1993;27(2):107-16.

CHAPTER 21

# Antidepressant-induced Affective Switch

*Arvind Nongpiur, Subhash Das*

## INTRODUCTION

Antidepressants were introduced post-World War II, with early reports of antidepressant-induced switches initially refuted. Tricyclic antidepressants (TCAs) were implicated,[1] and Bunney[2] suggested the switch might be due to drugs altering monoamines. Peet[3] found higher switch rates in unipolar depressed patients using TCAs compared to selective serotonin reuptake inhibitors (SSRIs) or placebos. Debates continued on whether switching to mania was part of bipolar disorder's natural course.[4] Akiskal and Mallya[5] described bipolar III patients as prone to switching when treated with TCAs. Due to these ambiguities, DSM-IV-TR[6] classified antidepressant-induced switches as substance-induced mood disorders. However, DSM-5[7] now diagnoses a manic or hypomanic episode during antidepressant treatment as bipolar.

## DEFINITION OF MANIC SWITCH

Switching between mania and depression is normal in bipolar illness. With the advent of psychopharmacology, many agents, especially antidepressants, are believed to cause a switch from depression to mania/hypomania, and typical antipsychotics from mania to depression. However, there is no clear consensus on what constitutes a switch, and most meta-analyses have not reached a definitive conclusion on using antidepressants in bipolar disorders.[3,8,9] To bring uniformity to research, the International Society for Bipolar Disorders (ISBD) Task Force[10] defined a *treatment emergent affective switch* (TEAS) as at least 2 consecutive days of full syndromic hypomanic, manic, or mixed state, lasting more than 50% of time each day, occurring within 8 weeks after the last treatment change. This definition aims to standardize research.

## WHO ARE AT RISK OF SWITCHING?

Clinicians need to know the risk factors or predictors to avoid using antidepressants in susceptible patients. Gitlin[11] reviewed the controversies surrounding antidepressant use in bipolar disorders, and Ghaemi et al.[12] found no benefit in combining a mood stabilizer with an antidepressant over using mood stabilizer alone. The ISBD Task Force[13] could not fully endorse antidepressants for bipolar patients but noted some individuals might benefit. Salvadore et al.[14] highlighted inconsistent study findings, indicating no specific predictors for a switch. The ISBD Task Force[13] outlined situations where antidepressants should be avoided in acute bipolar depression treatment, such as:

- Monotherapy in bipolar I
- Patients with two or more core manic symptoms
- Psychomotor agitation
- Patients with a history of rapid cycling
- Patients presenting in mixed states
- Those with a past history of mania, hypomania, or mixed states with antidepressant.

Further, Valenti et al. [15] found that an earlier age at onset is also a risk factor for a switch.

Another clinical challenge is treating patients presenting with depression who may actually be bipolar and are at risk of iatrogenic switching to mania. The CANMAT and ISBD guidelines for managing bipolar disorder[16] have enumerated features that may predict bipolarity, adapting observations from Mitchell et al.[17] and Schaffer et al.[18] as those with:

- Earlier age of illness onset (before 25 years)
- Brief, highly recurrent depressive episodes
- Family history of BD
- Depression with psychotic features

- Atypical features such as reverse vegetative symptoms of hypersomnia and hyperphagia, leaden paralysis, or psychomotor agitation
- Postpartum depression or psychosis
- Antidepressant-induced irritability, manic symptoms, or rapid cycling.

## GUIDING PRINCIPLES IN ANTIDEPRESSANT INDUCED AFFECTIVE SWITCH

The use of antidepressants in treating bipolar disorders is not fully endorsed by most guidelines due to the risk of switching to mania, worsening illness, or causing rapid cycling. Antidepressants seem to take longer or may not work as effectively in bipolar depression compared to unipolar depression,[19] yet some studies have reported small but significant symptom improvement with adjunctive antidepressant.[20] There is no conclusive guideline, but the following considerations are important when using antidepressants for bipolar depression. **Table 1** lists antidepressants and their propensity to cause switches **(Flowchart 1)**.

- Antidepressants increase the risk of a switch to mania. Tricyclics, tetracyclics, and SNRIs have a higher risk, while SSRIs and bupropion are less prone to causing switches, especially when used with a mood stabilizer. Bipolar I patients have higher switch rates

**TABLE 1:** Antidepressants' propensity to cause treat emergent effective switch (TEAS).

| *Class of drug* | *Drug type* | *Literature/evidence regarding the switch present* | *Remark* |
|---|---|---|---|
| TCA | Amitriptyline | Yes[19] | Being dual-action monoamine, it is more likely to cause switch compared to single-action drugs like serotonin. Also, antidepressants are less likely to induce switch if they are used along with antimanic drugs.[19] Antidepressants without the cover of mood stabilizers are avoided in bipolar I disorder[22] |
| | Amoxapine | – | |
| | Desipramine | Very limited evidence is present[14] | |
| | Doxepin | – | |
| | Imipramine | Yes[19] | Being dual-action monoamine, it is more likely to cause switch compared to single-action drugs like serotonin. Also, antidepressants are less likely to induce switch if they are used along with antimanic drugs.[19] Antidepressants without the cover of mood stabilizers are avoided in bipolar I disorder[22] |
| | Nortriptyline | – | |
| | Protriptyline | Yes[23] | Rare induction of mania |
| | Trimipramine | – | |
| SSRI | Citalopram | Yes[24,25] | |
| | Dapoxetine | – | |
| | Escitalopram | Yes[25] | |
| | Fluoxetine | Yes[24,25] | Olanzapine and fluoxetine combination has been recommended for use in bipolar depression (as first-line treatment [26] and second-line treatment[16]) |
| | Paroxetine | Yes[24,25] | |
| | Sertraline | Yes[25,27] | Do not increase switch rate in bipolar II depression.[22] Risk for switch is comparatively less than venlafaxine but more than bupropion[23] |
| | Vilazodone | – | |
| | Vortioxetine | Very limited evidence is present[28-30] | |

*Contd...*

*Contd...*

| *Class of drug* | *Drug type* | *Literature/evidence regarding the switch present* | *Remark* |
|---|---|---|---|
| SNRI | Duloxetine | Yes[14] | Being dual-action monoamine, it is more likely to cause switch compared to single-action drugs like serotonin. Also, antidepressants are less likely to induce switch if they are used along with antimanic drugs.[19] Antidepressants without the cover of mood stabilizers are avoided in bipolar I disorder[22] |
| | Desvenlafaxine | Very limited evidence is present[31] | Being almost similar to venlafaxine, its propensity to induce mania, especially in those who are vulnerable, is likely to be the same as venlafaxine |
| | Levomilnacipran | Very limited literature present.[32] | Individuals with bipolar disorders are vulnerable[31] |
| | Venlafaxine | Yes[19,22] | Being dual-action monoamine, it is more likely to cause switch compared to single-action drugs like serotonin. Also, antidepressants are less likely to induce switch if they are used along with antimanic drugs.[19] Antidepressants without the cover of mood stabilizers are avoided in bipolar I disorder[22] |
| MAOI | Selegiline, isocarboxazid, phenelzine, tranylcypromine | Very limited literature available for MAOIs as a class possibly because it is used less frequently nowadays[33] | MAOIs and bupropion likely to cause milder manic switch in comparison to the TCAs or fluoxetine[34] |
| Others | Mirtazapine | Yes[26] | Low doses may be used for treating insomnia; low doses may cause manic switch in the vulnerable ones[26] |
| | Trazodone | Yes[26,35] | Low doses may be used for treating insomnia; low doses may cause manic switch in the vulnerable ones[26] |
| | Nefazodone | Very limited evidence is present[36] | |
| | Tianeptine | Very limited literature[37] | |
| | Agomelatine | Yes[26] | |
| | Bupropion | Limited evidence is present[38-40] | May be dose related; risk for manic switch increases with increase in dosage[40] |

and more severe symptoms compared to bipolar II.[13] Antidepressant monotherapy should be monitored for a switch in bipolar II patients.[19]

- Depressive episodes are shorter in bipolar compared to unipolar depression. Antidepressants should be tapered by 12 weeks if remission is achieved, and only those who relapse after discontinuation should be offered longer treatment.[19]
- In those who switch while on an antidepressant, consider stopping the antidepressant and offering an antipsychotic. Antipsychotics (e.g., haloperidol, olanzapine, quetiapine, or risperidone) should be offered even if the antidepressant is not stopped.[21]
- As second-line treatment in bipolar I, SSRIs or bupropion may be added to lithium or divalproex, but antidepressants should not be used as monotherapy.[16]
- For bipolar II patients, CANMAT and ISBD recommend bupropion, sertraline, and venlafaxine as second-line monotherapy treatments, and fluoxetine as a third-line option.[16]

In **Table 1**, all drugs except tianeptine, agomelatine, and bupropion are US FDA approved for the treatment of depression[41,42]

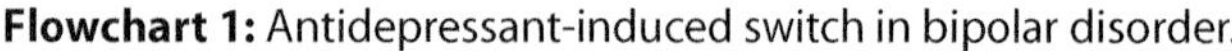

**Flowchart 1:** Antidepressant-induced switch in bipolar disorder.

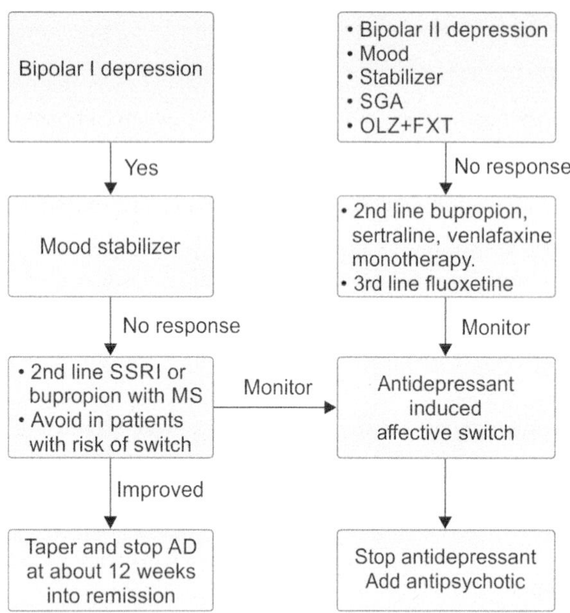


(FXT: fluoxetine; OLZ: olanzapine; SGA: second-generation antipsychotics; SSRI: selective serotonin reuptake inhibitor)

## REFERENCES


1. Lewis JL, Winokur G. The Induction of Mania: A Natural History Study with Controls. Arch Gen Psychiatry. 1982;39(3):303-6.
2. Bunney W, Murphy D, Goodwin F, Borge G. The switch process from depression to mania: relationship to drugs which alter brain amines. Lancet. 1970;295(7655):1022-7.
3. Peet M. Induction of mania with selective serotonin re-uptake inhibitors and tricyclic antidepressants. Br J Psychiatry. 1994;164:549-50.
4. Angst J, Sellaro R. Historical perspectives and natural history of bipolar disorder. Biol Psychiatry. 2000;48(6):445-57.
5. Akiskal HS, Mallya G. Criteria for the "soft" bipolar spectrum: treatment implications. Psychopharmacol Bull. 1987;23:68-73.
6. American Psychiatric Association. Diagnostic and Statistical Manual of Mental Disorders, Fourth Edition Text Rev. IV TR. Arlington, VA: American Psychiatric Association; 2000.
7. American Psychiatric Association. Diagnostic and Statistical Manual of Mental Disorders, fifth edition (DSM-5). Arlington, VA: American Psychiatric Association; 2013.
8. Grunze HCR. Switching, Induction of Rapid Cycling, and Increased Suicidality with Antidepressants in Bipolar Patients: Fact or Overinterpretation? CNS Spectr. 2008;13(9):790-5.
9. Salvi V, Fagiolini A, Swartz HA, Maina G, Frank E. The use of antidepressants in bipolar disorder. J Clin Psychiatry. 2008;69(8):1307-18.
10. Tohen M, Frank E, Bowden CL, Colom F, Ghaemi SN, Yatham LN, et al. The International Society for Bipolar Disorders (ISBD) Task Force report on the nomenclature of course and outcome in bipolar disorders. Bipolar Disord. 2009;11(5):453-73.
11. Gitlin MJ. Antidepressants in bipolar depression: an enduring controversy. Int J Bipolar Disord. 2018;6(1):25.
12. Ghaemi SN, Wingo AP, Filkowski MA, Baldessarini RJ. Long-term antidepressant treatment in bipolar disorder: meta-analyses of benefits and risks. Acta Psychiatr Scand. 2008;118(5):347-56.
13. Pacchiarotti I, Bond DJ, Baldessarini RJ, Nolen WA, Grunze H, Licht RW, et al. The International Society for Bipolar Disorders (ISBD) task force report on antidepressant use in bipolar disorders. Am J Psychiatry. 2013;170(11):1249-62.
14. Salvadore G, Quiroz JA, Machado-Vieira R, Henter ID, Manji HK, Zarate CA Jr. The neurobiology of the switch process in bipolar disorder: a review. J Clin Psychiatry. 2010;71(11):1488-501.
15. Valentí M, Pacchiarotti I, Bonnín CM, Rosa AR, Popovic D, Nivoli AM, et al. Risk factors for antidepressant-related switch to mania. J Clin Psychiatry. 2012;73(2):e271-6.
16. Yatham LN, Kennedy SH, Parikh SV, Schaffer A, Bond DJ, Frey BN, et al. Canadian Network for Mood and Anxiety Treatments (CANMAT) and International Society for Bipolar Disorders (ISBD) 2018 guidelines for the management of patients with bipolar disorder. Bipolar Disord. 2018;20(2):97-170.
17. Mitchell PB, Goodwin GM, Johnson GF, Hirschfeld RMA. Diagnostic guidelines for bipolar depression: a probabilistic approach. Bipolar Disord. 2008;10:144-52.
18. Schaffer A, Cairney J, Veldhuizen S, Kurdyak P, Cheung A, Levitt A. A population-based analysis of distinguishers of bipolar disorder from major depressive disorder. J Affect Disord. 2010;125:103-10.
19. Goodwin G, Haddad P, Ferrier I, Aronson J, Barnes T, Cipriani A, et al. Evidence-based guidelines for treating bipolar disorder: Revised third edition recommendations from the British Association for Psychopharmacology. J Psychopharmacol. 2016;30(6):495-553.
20. McGirr A, Vöhringer PA, Ghaemi SN, Lam RW, Yatham LN. Safety and efficacy of adjunctive second-generation antidepressant therapy with a mood stabiliser or an atypical antipsychotic in acute bipolar depression: a systematic review and meta-analysis of randomised placebo-controlled trials. Lancet Psychiatry. 2016;3(12): 1138-46.
21. NICE. (2014). Bipolar Disorder: Assessment and Management (NICE2014). [online] Available from https://www.nice.org.uk/guidance/cg185. [Last accessed June, 2025].
22. Taylor DM, Barnes TRE, Young AH. The Maudsley Prescribing Guidelines in Psychiatry, 14th ed. West Sussex (UK): Wiley Blackwell; 2021.

23. Saef MA, Yilanli M, Saadabadi A. Protriptyline. StatPearls. Treasure Island (FL): StatPearls Publishing; 2023.
24. Bryois C, Ferrero F. Mania Induced by Citalopram. Arch Gen Psychiatry. 1994;51(8):664-5.
25. Çiray RO, Halaç E, Turan S, Tunçtürk M, Özbek M, Ermiş Ç. Selective serotonin reuptake inhibitors and manic switch: A pharmacovigilance and pharmacodynamical study. Asian J Psychiatr. 2021;66:102891.
26. Wichniak A, Jarkiewicz M, Okruszek Ł, Wierzbicka A, Holka-Pokorska J, Rybakowski JK. Low Risk for Switch to Mania during Treatment with Sleep Promoting Antidepressants. Pharmacopsychiatry. 2015;48(3):83-8.
27. Leverich GS, Altshuler LL, Frye MA, Suppes T, McElroy SL, Keck PE Jr, et al. Risk of switch in mood polarity to hypomania or mania in patients with bipolar depression during acute and continuation trials of venlafaxine, sertraline, and bupropion as adjuncts to mood stabilizers. Am J Psychiatry. 2006;163(2):232-9.
28. Aydin EP, Dalkiran M, Özer OA, Karamustafalioğlu KO. Hypomanic switch during vortioxetine treatment: a case report. Psychiatry Clin Psychopharmacol. 2019;29(1):114-6.
29. Songur E. Vortioxetine-Induced Hypomania: A Case Report. Psychiatr Danub. 2021;33(2):198-9.
30. Tunc EB, Tunc S. Vortioxetine Induced Hypomania: A Case Presentation and Review of the Literature. Clin Psychopharmacol Neurosci. 2022;20(2):394-7.
31. Kalia R, Magsalin RM, Khan AY, Kahn DA. Mania possibly induced by desvenlafaxine. J Psychiatr Pract. 2010;16(1):58-62.
32. National Alliance on Mental Illness. (2023). Levomilnacipran. [online] Available from https://nami.org/About-Mental-Illness/Treatments/Mental-Health-Medications/Types-of-Medication/Levomilnacipran-(Fetzima) [Last accessed June, 2025].
33. Mayorga L, Ilzarbe L, Gracia H, Lufi S, Viladegut O, Pablo B. Role of MAOI drugs as triggers of manic episodes in bipolar disorders: A case report and a narrative review. Eur Psychiatry. 2022;65:S407.
34. Stoll AL, Mayer PV, Kolbrener M, Goldstein E, Suplit B, Lucier J, et al. Antidepressant-associated mania: a controlled comparison with spontaneous mania. Am J Psychiatry. 1994;151(11):1642-5.
35. İzci F, Ülger E, Yolcu S. Manic Episode as a Result of Adding Trazodone to a Patient under Escitalopram Treatment. Alpha Psychiatry. 2021;22(1):67-9.
36. Zaphiris HA, Blaisdell GD, Jermain DM. Probable nefazodone-induced mania in a patient with unreported bipolar disorder. Ann Clin Psychiatry. 1996;8(4):207-10.
37. Yıldırım SG, Başterzi AD, Göka E. Tianeptine Induced Mania: A Case Report. J Clin Psychiatry. 2004;7(3):177-80.
38. Aggarwal A, Sharma RC. Bupropion-induced mania and hypomania: a report of two cases. J Neuropsychiatry Clin Neurosci. 2011;23(2):E51-2.
39. Masand P, Stern TA. Bupropion and secondary mania. Is there a relationship? Ann Clin Psychiatry. 1993;5(4):271-4.
40. Goren JL, Levin GM. Mania with bupropion: a dose-related phenomenon? Ann Pharmacother. 2000;34(5):619-21.
41. US Food and Drug Administration. (2019). Depression Medicines. [online] Available from https://www.fda.gov/consumers/free-publications-women/depression-medicines [Last accessed June, 2025].
42. Jilani TN, Gibbons JR, Faizy RM, Saadabadi A. Mirtazapine. StatPearls. Treasure Island (FL): StatPearls Publishing; 2023.

# How to Manage Premenstrual Mood Syndromes?

*Alka Subramanyam, Prerna Khar, Vinyas Nisarga*

## PREMENSTRUAL SYNDROME

### INTRODUCTION

Premenstrual syndrome (PMS) refers to a condition denoted by the presence of at least one somatic, emotional, or behavioral symptom in women of reproductive age. The symptoms of PMS typically appear during the luteal phase of the menstrual cycle and dissipate after the periods begin. They must be present consecutively for at least two consecutive cycles and interfere with the individual's ability to meet personal and occupational demands. Mood symptoms include irritability, sadness, anger, fatigue, restlessness, mood swings, crying, and anxiety.[1]

### PREMENSTRUAL DYSPHORIC DISORDER

It is considered the most severe form of PMS.[2] According to DSM-5, it involves five symptoms present in the final week before menstruation (luteal phase), improving within a few days after menstruation, and minimal, or absent post-menses (follicular phase). Symptoms include a minimum of one mood symptom (marked mood lability, irritability or anger, sad mood, anxiety, or feelings of tension) and at least one additional symptom (decreased interest, difficulty concentrating, fatigue, changes in appetite like overeating, and sleep disturbances such as insomnia or hypersomnia, emotionally distressed, or physical symptoms such as breast tenderness or swelling, joint or muscle pain, bloating, or weight gain). These mood symptoms must be present daily for at least two consecutive menstrual cycles. They cause significant distress or interference in social, occupational, or relationship settings and are not attributable to other psychiatric disorders, medical conditions, or substance effects.[2]

#### Etiology

- The key mechanism of premenstrual dysphoric disorder (PMDD) is increased sensitivity of serotonin receptors in the brain to fluctuations in progesterone levels.
- Progesterone crosses the blood-brain barrier and interacts with brain neurochemistry.
- Progesterone receptors (PRs) are present in the hypothalamus, hippocampus, amygdala, and frontal cortex.
- Research suggests that the brain effects of progesterone on mood are due to its metabolite, allopregnanolone, which is a positive modulator of the gamma-aminobutyric acid (GABA) receptor. The luteal phase surge of allopregnanolone is responsible for PMS symptoms such as irritability, anxiety, low mood, food cravings, and abdominal bloating.
- The expression of genes in the epigenetic ESC/E(Z) complex, which is estrogen-sensitive, differs in women with PMDD versus healthy control women. This increases neuronal excitability, making it resistant to GABA-A receptor modulators and causing emotional symptoms.
- The role of inflammation in PMS is under investigation, with various studies showing inconclusive and contradictory findings.[3]

### TREATMENT

Treatment mainly targets brain neurotransmitters and the hypothalamus-pituitary-ovarian axis.[1]

- *First line: Selective serotonin reuptake inhibitors (SSRIs):* Women with PMS/PMDD have fewer serotonin transporters and atypical serotonergic transmission. They also have a heightened serotonin response in the follicular phase compared to the secretory phase. Additionally, its availability in the brain is influenced by ovarian sex steroids, which act on the monoamine oxidase (MAO), the enzyme primarily responsible for amine neurotransmitter degradation, including serotonin. Hence, SSRIs are the first choice.

**Flowchart 1:** Management of premenstrual mood syndromes.[3,4]

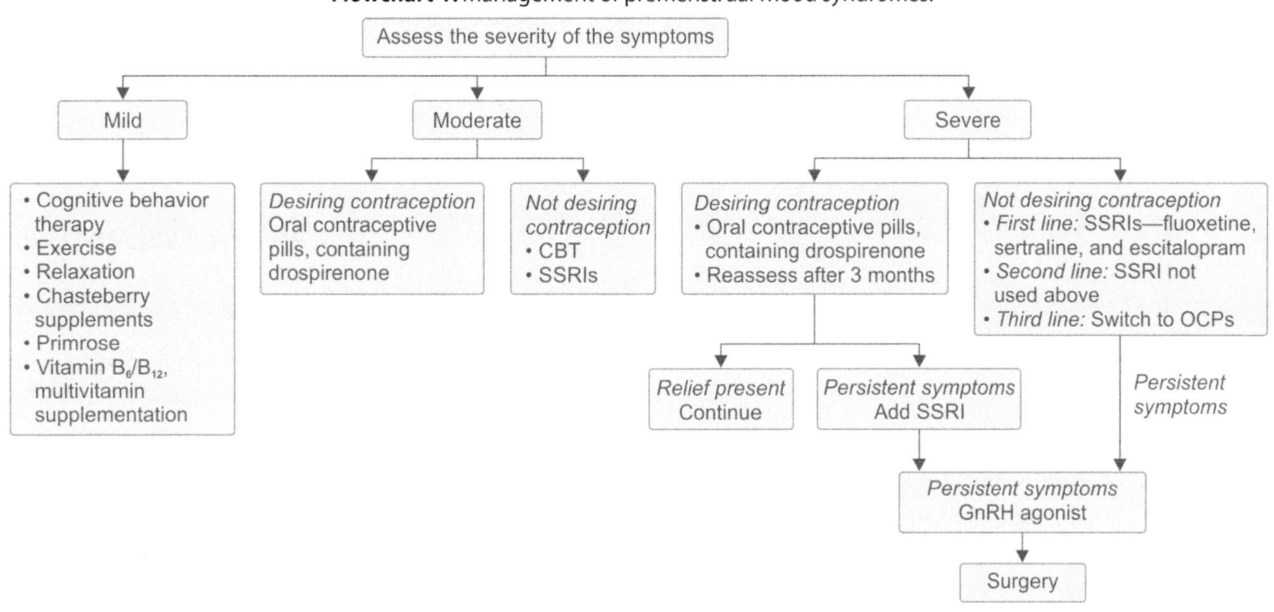


(CBT: cognitive behavioral therapy; GnRH: gonadotropin-releasing hormone; SSRI: selective serotonin reuptake inhibitor; OCP: oral contraceptive pill)

- *Dosing regimens:*
  - *Continuous:* Prescribed at antidepressant doses without breaks, usually for severe PMDD.
  - *Intermittent:* SSRIs can show effects within a few days for PMS/PMDD, allowing for dosing to start 14 days before expected menses (luteal phase dosing) or at the onset of symptoms (symptom-onset dosing).
  - *Semi-intermittent:* Low dose in the proliferative phase and a higher dose in the secretory (luteal) phase.

A 2013 Cochrane review found SSRIs effective for PMS/PMDD symptoms irrespective of the dosing regimen.[3]

- *Second line: Combined hormonal contraception (CHC)/combined oral contraceptive pills (COCPs):* These block the ovulatory surge of sex hormones, thus inhibiting PMS symptoms. The most widely used COCP is a combination of drospirenone (progesterone) and ethinyl estradiol.
- *Third line: Progesterone and selective progesterone receptor modulator (SPRMs):* These have an antagonistic action on PRs. Ulipristal acetate (UPA) has shown promising results in emotional and behavioral symptoms of PMDD in an randomized controlled trial (RCT) at a low dose of 5 mg/day. It may be considered when SSRIs are ineffective or poorly tolerated and is available in India.
- *Newer drugs:* Currently under evaluation and trial.
  - *Sepranolone (isoallopregnanolone):* A GABA-A receptor modulating steroid antagonist (GAMSA) that antagonizes the effects of allopregnanolone.
  - *Zuranolone and ganaxolone:* Positive allosteric modulators of the GABA-A receptor, these neuroactive steroids are being studied for PMS/PMDD.[3,4]

Management of PMS has been summarized in **Flowchart 1**.

## REFERENCES

1. Tiranini L, Nappi RE. Recent advances in understanding/management of premenstrual dysphoric disorder/premenstrual syndrome. Fac Rev. 2022;11:11.
2. American Psychiatric Association. Diagnostic and Statistical Manual of Mental Disorders, 5th edition . Washington, D.C.: American Psychiatric Publishing; 2013.
3. Marjoribanks J, Brown J, O'Brien PMS, Wyatt K. Selective serotonin reuptake inhibitors for premenstrual syndrome. Cochrane Database Syst Rev. 2013;2013(6):CD001396.
4. Casper RF, Yonkers KA. (2019). Treatment of premenstrual syndrome and premenstrual dysphoric disorder. [online] Available from https://www.uptodate.com/contents/treatment-of-premenstrual-syndrome-and-premenstrual-dysphoric-disorder [Last accessed June, 2025].

CHAPTER 23

# Approach to Diagnosis and Management of Insomnia

*Anindya Das, Ravi Gupta*

## DEFINITION

Insomnia is the inability to initiate or maintain sleep despite adequate opportunities for the sleep resulting in a number of symptoms during wakefulness. The International Classification of Sleep Disorders, 3rd edition (ICSD-3), defines insomnia as the presence of nighttime symptoms accompanied by daytime symptoms, such as fatigue, headache, poor concentration, irritability, and concerns about sleep. These symptoms are considered clinically salient as a disorder when they occur at least three times per week. Short-term and chronic insomnia are distinguished by a threshold criterion of 3 months for the persistence of symptoms.[1] The previous concept of primary and secondary insomnia has been revised to comorbid insomnia. It is a common clinical condition, with a prevalence of 10% in the general adult population.[2]

## CLINICAL DIAGNOSIS

The clinical work-up of sleep complaints includes obtaining a detailed history from the patient (including the chronology of complaints, symptom analysis, sleep schedule, bedtime routine, medication history, and nonprescribed drug/alcohol use), as well as from the bed partner to gather additional information. Sleep diary/log, actigraphy, and occasionally polysomnography help narrow the diagnosis. Physical examination may reveal other contributing or comorbid conditions.

*The 3P model* (predisposing, precipitating, and perpetuating factors) helps explore contributing factors that are useful for intervention.[3] Identifying predisposing factors such as anxious predispositions, general hyperarousal, or circular thinking; precipitating events, such as stressors, and medical disorders; or perpetuating conditions, such as learned negative sleep behavior and cognitive distortions, can be especially useful.

Objectively rating of the severity of complaints with a standardized instrument (e.g., Insomnia Severity Index[4]) helps in monitoring across time and/or response to treatment. Similarly, scales such as Dysfunctional Beliefs and Attitudes about Sleep,[5] help provide additional information to guide treatment **(Flowchart 1)**.

## MANAGEMENT

Once the diagnosis of insomnia is made, management depends on the chronicity, profile, and preferences of the patient, as well as the available resources. Cognitive behavior therapy for insomnia (CBT-I) is considered as the first-line treatment, particularly for chronic insomnia.[6] While drug therapy is preferred for short-term insomnia, there is also sufficient evidence supporting its use for chronic insomnia.[7]

The CBT-I can be delivered face-to-face, either individually or in groups, as well as digitally. It is efficacious in physical and psychiatric comorbidities. It is a multimodal approach, consisting of the following components[8] **(Flowchart 2)**:

- Education on sleep hygiene and mechanisms of sleep. It includes, among others, establishing a conducive sleep environment, winding down routine at bedtime, and avoiding arousing activities such as reading or viewing screens, and vigorous exercise within 4 hours of bedtime. Additionally, educating patients about the regulation of sleep and wakefulness (e.g., the two-process model) helps allay their anxiety.
- Behavioral component includes *stimulus control, sleep restriction, relaxation training, and paradoxical intention.*
    - *Stimulus control* addresses the conditioned association of the bed and bedroom with arousal. It involves avoiding the bedroom when not sleepy and going to bed only when feeling sleepy. Additionally, the bed should be used exclusively for

**Flowchart 1:** Diagnostic algorithm for insomnia.

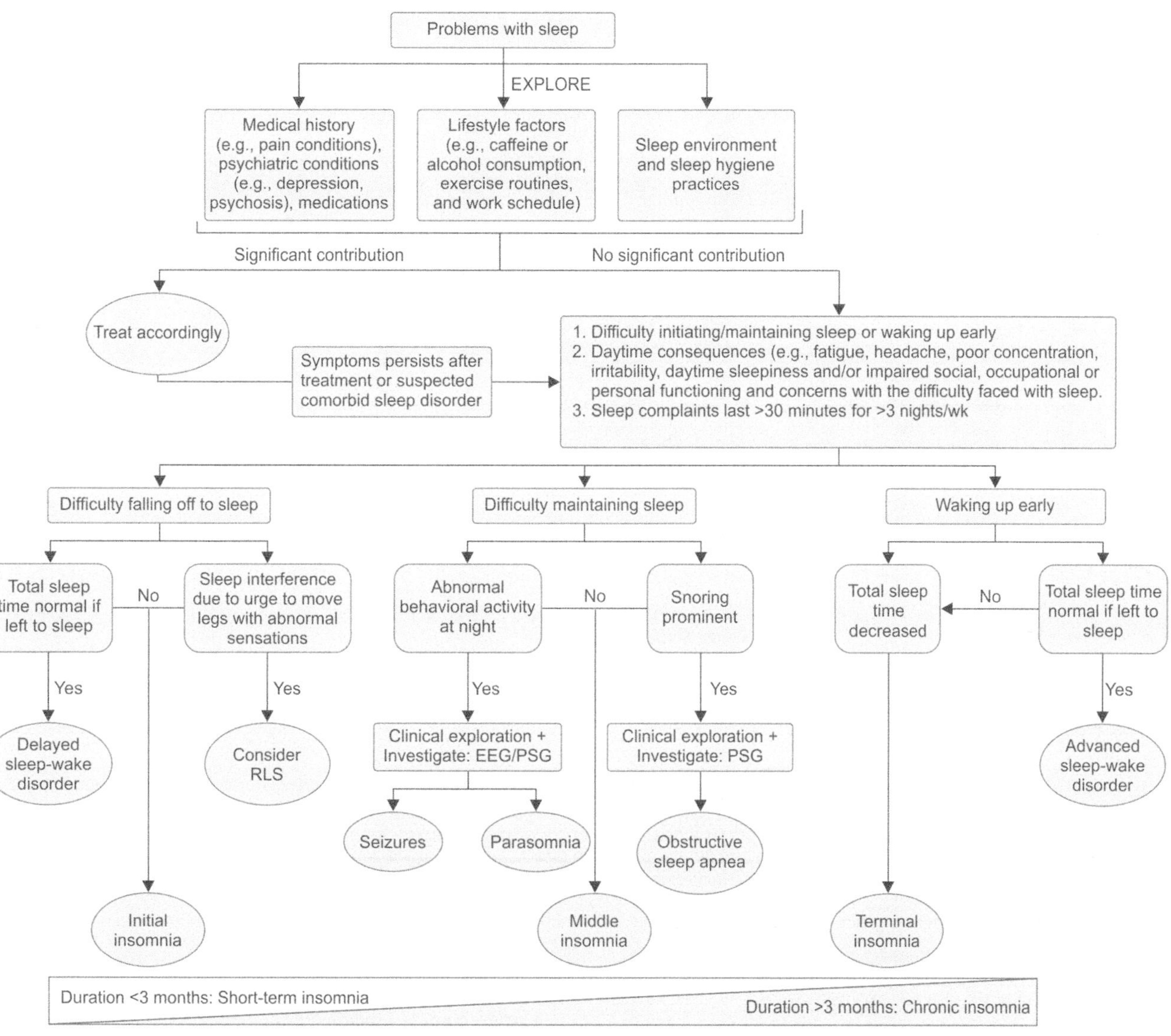


*Note:* Supplement clinical history from bed partner, sleep log/diary, actigraphy if available, occasionally PSG
(RLS: restless leg syndrome; PSG: polysomnography)

sleep and sex. Similarly, one should get out of bed once awake, within 10–15 minutes.

- *Sleep restriction* aims to reduce time in bed to match the reported total sleep time. This requires a prerequisite of maintaining a sleep log for 1-week. Based on the log, a sleep schedule is prescribed (with a minimum of five hours) to restrict time in bed. Once sleep efficiency (the percentage of time asleep relative to time in bed) exceeds 85%, bedtime can be incrementally extended by 15 minutes. Sleep restriction is contraindicated in patients with mood and psychotic disorders, epilepsy, or those operating heavy machinery, driving, and in pilots.
- *Relaxation* includes various techniques of diaphragmatic breathing, alternate tensing and relaxing of muscle groups, etc.
- *Paradoxical intention* addresses the anxiety of being unable to fall asleep. Patients are encouraged to stay awake for as long as possible. However, its efficacy remains uncertain.

- The cognitive component addresses maladaptive thoughts, including sleep-related worries, unrealistic expectations, and catastrophic thinking of the

**Flowchart 2:** Treatment algorithm.

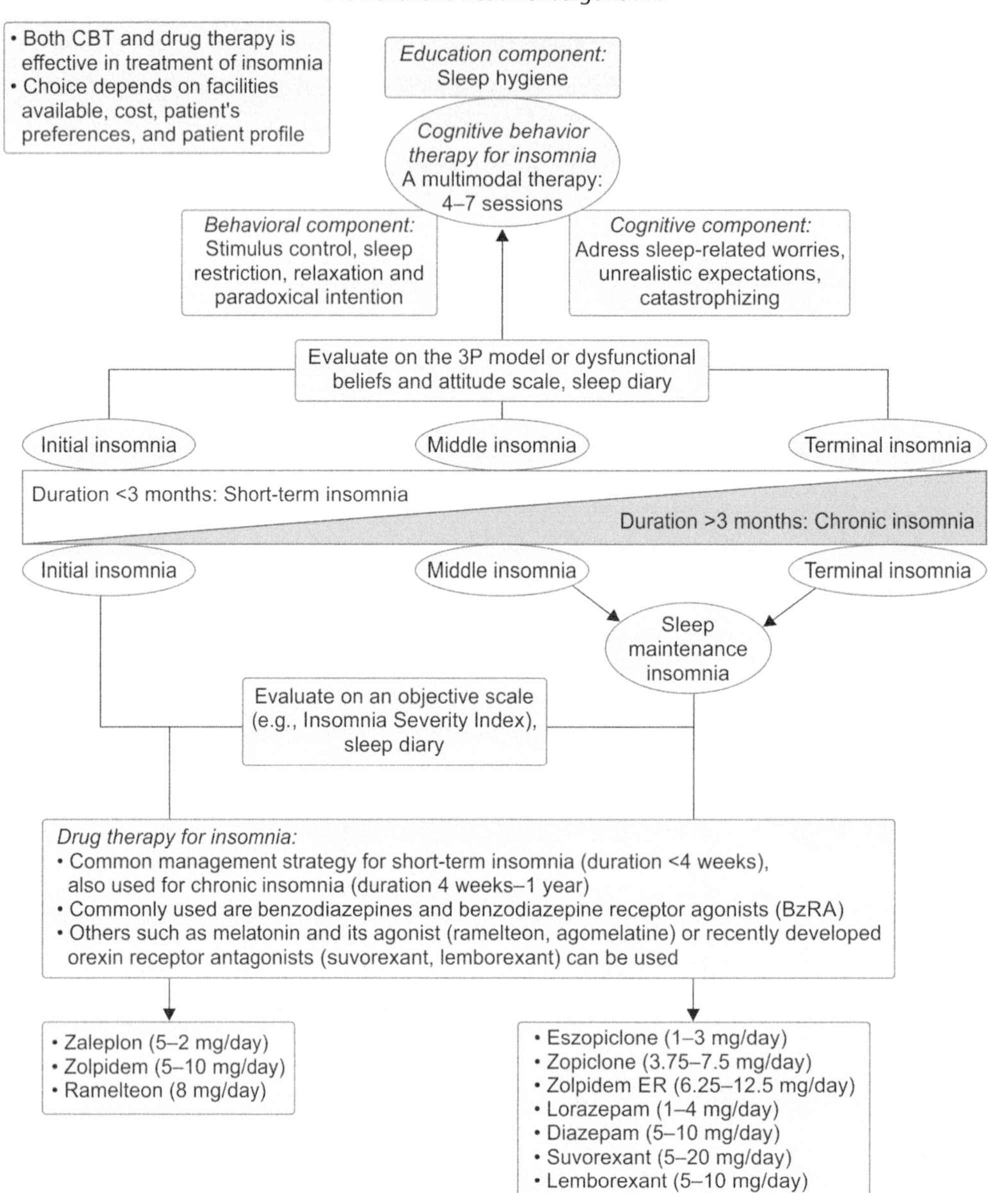


(CBT: cognitive behavioral therapy)

consequences of insomnia. General principles of CBT are used to modify thoughts.

Other components of CBT-I include problem solving technique, time-management, priority-determination, and activity scheduling, which are used as per requirement.

Drug therapy is often preferred due to its greater accessibility, though it is associated with significant adverse effects. Various medications have hypnotic properties (e.g., antihistaminic doxylamine, antidepressant doxepin and trazodone, and antipsychotic quetiapine). Meta-analysis of various double-blind randomized controlled trials suggests the efficacy of benzodiazepines (BZDs), BZD receptor agonists (z-drugs), and orexin receptor antagonists. Melatonin and its analogs do not show any benefit,[9] except ramelteon that is useful in sleep initiation. Overall, irrespective of acute and long-term treatment, lemborexant and eszopiclone have the best profile, considering efficacy, acceptability, and tolerability.[9] However, the choice of drugs for individual patients depends on cost, side effects, tolerability, and the potential for abuse.

**TABLE 1:** Drugs used for insomnia and its profile.

| Drug | Indication | | Special note |
|---|---|---|---|
| | **Initial insomnia, dose** | **Sleep maintenance insomnia, dose** | |
| *Benzodiazepines* | | | |
| Lorazepam | Yes, 1–4 mg/day | Yes, 1–4 mg/day | Intermediate half-life |
| Flurazepam | Yes, 10–30 mg/day | Yes, 10–30 mg/day | |
| Diazepam | Yes, 5 mg/day | Yes, 5–10 mg/day | Long half-life |
| Nitrazepam | Yes, 2.5–5 mg/day | Yes, 5–10 mg/day | |
| *Z-drugs* | | | |
| Zaleplon | Yes, 5–10 mg/day | – | Ultrashort half-life |
| Zolpidem | Yes, 5–10 mg/day | – | Short half-life |
| Zolpidem ER | Yes, 6.25 mg/day | Yes, 12.5 mg/day | |
| Zopiclone | Yes, 3.75–7.5 mg/day | Yes, 3.75–7.5 mg/day | Intermediate half-life |
| Eszopiclone | Yes, 1–3 mg/day | Yes, 1–3 mg/day | Intermediate half-life |
| *Melatonin receptor agonist* | | | |
| Ramelteon | Yes, 8 mg/day | – | Absence of withdrawal insomnia |
| *Orexin receptor antagonist* | | | |
| Suvorexant | Yes, 5–20 mg/day | Yes, 5–20 mg/day | Effective for last third of the night insomnia without daytime sedation |
| Lemborexant | Yes, 5–10 mg/day | Yes, 5–10 mg/day | |
| Daridorexant | Yes, 25–50 mg/day | Yes, 25–50 mg/day | |

Prescribing hypnotics requires caution due to potential risks, including daytime drowsiness, cognitive and psychomotor impairment, an increased risk of falls in the elderly, and the potential for abuse in a small subset of insomnia patients. The common concern regarding tolerance and dependence with long-term use of BZDs and benzodiazepines receptor agonists (BzRA) is largely unfounded. However, caution is advisable for their long-term use. Generally, shorter-acting BZDs (e.g., alprazolam) have a higher potential for abuse, while those with longer half-lives carry a greater risk of daytime adverse effects **(Table 1)**.

## REFERENCES


1. American Academy of Sleep Medicine. International Classification of Sleep Disorders. 3rd ed. Darian, IL: American Academy of Sleep Medicine; 2014.
2. Grewal RG, Doghramji K. Epidemiology of Insomnia. In: Attarian HP (Ed). Clinical Handbook of Insomnia. Current Clinical Neurology. Cham: Springer; 2017. pp. 13-25.
3. Ebben MR, Spielman AJ. Non-pharmacological treatments for insomnia. J Behav Med. 2009;32:244-54.
4. Bastien CH, Vallières A, Morin CM. Validation of the Insomnia Severity Index as an outcome measure for insomnia research. Sleep Med. 2001;2:297-307.
5. Morin CM, Vallières A, Ivers H. Dysfunctional beliefs and attitudes about sleep (DBAS): Validation of a brief version (DBAS-16). Sleep. 2007;30:1547-54.
6. Brasure M, Fuchs E, MacDonald R, Nelson VA, Koffel E, Olson CM, et al. Psychological and behavioral interventions for managing insomnia disorder: an evidence report for a clinical practice guideline by the American College of Physicians. Ann Intern Med. 2016;165:113.
7. Sateia MJ, Buysse DJ, Krystal AD, Neubauer DN, Heald JL. Clinical practice guideline for the pharmacologic treatment of chronic insomnia in adults: an American Academy of Sleep Medicine clinical practice guideline. J Clin Sleep Med. 2017;13:307-49.
8. Krystal AD, Prather AA, Ashbrook LH. The assessment and management of insomnia: an update. World Psychiatry. 2019;18(3):337-352.
9. De Crescenzo F, D'Alò GL, Ostinelli EG, Ciabattini M, Di Franco V, Watanabe N, et al. Comparative effects of pharmacological interventions for the acute and long-term management of insomnia disorder in adults: a systematic review and network meta-analysis. Lancet. 2022;400:170-84.

# Assessment and Treatment of Sleep Disturbance in Mood and Anxiety Disorders

*Ravi Gupta, Lokesh Kumar Saini, Kaustav Kundu*

## BACKGROUND

Sleep disorders are common among patients with mood and anxiety disorders. This chapter adheres to the International Classification of Diseases 11th Revision (ICD-11) classification for mood and anxiety disorders. According to the available literature, nearly all types of sleep disorders are common among patients with mood and anxiety disorders, with obstructive sleep apnea (OSA), insomnia, and restless legs syndrome (RLS) being most prevalent.

### Mood Disorders

Many sleep disorders have a bidirectional relationship with depression. Several factors contribute to this relationship, including shared neurobiology, particularly common neural substrates and chronobiological mechanisms; psychiatric symptoms arising as an epiphenomenon of poor sleep caused by sleep disorders; and physiological changes caused by psychotropic medications that increase the risk for sleep disorders.

#### *Depression*

- Depression has bidirectional association with insomnia. While some studies suggest that insomnia serves as a transdiagnostic marker for various psychiatric disorders, others indicate that optimal management of insomnia can prevent and improve depressive symptoms.[1]
- Studies have reported that RLS increases the risk for depressive symptoms by impairing sleep quality due to associated periodic limb movements during sleep (PLMS). On the other hand, antidepressants, particularly mirtazapine, increase the risk of having RLS.[2]
- While hypersomnia is a characteristic feature of atypical depression, depressive symptoms are common in patients with narcolepsy, Kleine–Levin Syndrome, and idiopathic hypersomnia.[3,4]
- Depression is associated with prolonged sleep-onset latency, recurrent awakenings, and terminal insomnia. Delayed circadian rhythm, manifesting as delayed sleep wake phase disorder, increases the future risk of depression.[5,6]
- OSA and depression share overlapping symptoms, leading to many patients with OSA being misdiagnosed as having depression.[7,8] Moreover, untreated OSA has been found to increase the risk of incidental depression.[8] Another possibility is that both disorders are comorbid, as positive airway pressure therapy (PAP) has not been consistently found to improve depressive symptoms.[7]
- Nonrapid eye movement (NREM) parasomnias such as sleep-walking, sleep-related eating disorder (SRED), as well as REM sleep parasomnias, such as REM sleep behavior disorder (RBD) and nightmare disorder, are common among patients with depression.[9] While nightmare appears to be independent of antidepressants, RBD has been linked to the use of selective serotonin reuptake inhibitors, and sedating antidepressants and Z-drugs are associated with SRED and sleep-walking.[9]

#### *Bipolar Disorder*

- Patients having bipolar disorder are at a greater risk for OSA. It could be related to medication induced weight gain or effect of antipsychotics on the basal tone of upper airway muscles.[6,10]
- Delayed sleep-wake phase disorder has been reported among patients having bipolar disorder.[11] It could either be a consequence of bipolar disorder or results from shared genetic mechanisms.[11] Moreover, prolonged sleep-onset latency, prolonged awakenings, and variability of sleep-wake schedule are observed not only during active phase of bipolar disorder, but also during remission.[6]

- RLS is also relatively common among patients with bipolar disorder and is often associated with the use of psychotropic medications, particularly antipsychotics.[2,6]
- Both REM parasomnias, such as REM sleep behavior disorder, nightmares, and sleep paralysis, as well as NREM parasomnias, including selective estrogen receptor degraders (SERDs), are common among patients with patients taking sedating antidepressants and Z drugs.[9]

### *Anxiety Disorders*

- Anxiety disorders are associated with hyperactive HPA axis activity, as well as emotional and cognitive hyperarousal; hence, comorbid insomnia is relatively common among these patients.[12]
- Nearly one in ten patients with panic disorder experience nocturnal panic attacks, which can be difficult to distinguish from sleep-terrors.[9] Contrary to sleep-terror, patients with nocturnal panic attacks are fully awake and can vividly recall the dream upon awakening. They may also have difficulty going back to sleep.[9] Similarly, sleep paralysis is not uncommon among patients with panic attack.[9]
- REM parasomnias, such as nightmare disorder and sleep paralysis, have also been reported in patients with social anxiety disorder and generalized anxiety disorder.[9]

## MAJOR GROUPS OF SLEEP DISORDERS OBSERVED AMONG PATIENTS WITH MOOD AND ANXIETY DISORDERS

**Table 1** outlines the common presentations of sleep disorders observed in patients with mood and anxiety disorders, along with their assessment and treatment strategies.

**TABLE 1:** Sleep disorders among patients with mood and anxiety disorders.

| S.N. | *Sleep-related breathing disorder* | *Hypersomnia* | *Circadian rhythm sleep disorders* | *Sleep-related movement disorders* | *Parasomnia* |
|---|---|---|---|---|---|
| Major complaints by patients | • Snoring<br>• Witnessed pauses in breath<br>• Poor quality sleep<br>• Dreamy sleep<br>• Multiple voiding at night<br>• Daytime tiredness or sleepiness<br>• Cognitive impairment<br>• Irritabilty | *Idiopathic hypersomnia:*<br>• Sleepiness during daytime, mostly despite optimal sleep at night<br>• Usually, starts during adolescence<br>*Narcolepsy:*<br>• Poor sleep quality at night<br>• Sleep attacks during daytime<br>• Sleep paralysis<br>• Hypnogogic hallucinations<br>• Hypnopompic hallucinations<br>• Cataplexy may be present<br>*Kleine–Levin Syndrome:* Periodic hypersomnia lasting at least 2 days and at least two episodes | *Delayed sleep wake phase disorder* is characterized by going to bed late at night and waking up late in morning with preserved total sleep time. Dysfunction occurs when patients are to wake up early in morning to match with environmental timing | *Restless legs Syndrome:*<br>• Urge to move legs with or without dysesthesias; Symptoms occur at rest and improve with movement or counterirritant; Symptoms start in the evening or at night<br>• Symptoms are not explained by leg edema, venous stasis, arthralgia, myalgia, leg cramps, etc. | *Sleep terror:* Waking up from sleep screaming, inconsolable, appears disoriented for some time<br>*Sleep walking:* Gets up from bed and walks around, engaged in complex behaviors with amnesia for the event<br>*SRED:* Similar to sleep-walking along with eating at night<br>*Sleep paralysis:* Waking up from sleep with inability to move for some time. Patients often report difficulty breathing/ someone sitting on chest at that time<br>*Nightmare:* Waking up from sleep with bad dream and tachycardia<br>*REM sleep behavior disorder:* Acting on a dream with complex body movements |

*Contd...*

*Contd...*

| S.N. | Sleep-related breathing disorder | Hypersomnia | Circadian rhythm sleep disorders | Sleep-related movement disorders | Parasomnia |
|---|---|---|---|---|---|
| Screening instruments | • Berlin questionnaire[13]<br>• NoSAS[14]<br>• STOP-Bang[15] | • Swiss Narcolepsy Scale[16]<br>• Ullanlinna Narcolepsy Scale[17] | | • Cambridge Hopkins for ascertainment of RLS[18]<br>• Modified RLS Diagnostic Questionnaire[19] | • Munich parasomnia screening [20]<br>• Arousal disorder questionnaire[21]<br>• REM sleep behavior disorder screening questionnaire[22] |
| Diagnostic modality to be used | Home sleep apnea testing<br>Attended polysomnography | • Sleep diary<br>• Actigraphy<br>• Attended polysomnography with multiple sleep latency test | • Sleep diary<br>• Actigraphy | Serum iron profile<br>Serum $B_{12}$<br>Serum creatinine<br>Liver function test<br>Multiple suggested immobilization test | Attended video-synchronized polysomnography with extended EEG montage |
| Differential diagnosis | • Central sleep apnea<br>• Obesity hypoventilation syndrome | • From one another insufficient sleep syndrome<br>• Drug induced hypersomnia<br>• Sleep apnea | • Insomnia<br>• Hypersomnia | • From RLS mimics as mentioned above<br>• Drug induced akathisia | • SRED must be differentiated from night eating syndrome<br>• Nightmare and sleep terror must be differentiated from nocturnal panic attack<br>• RBD must be differentiated from sleep-walking<br>• Sleep-related hypermotor epilepsy |
| Approach to the treatment | • Avoidance of offending agents weight management<br>• Sleep hygiene<br>• Regular exercise<br>• PAP therapy<br>• Maxillofacial surgery in cases of anatomical issues | • Sleep hygiene<br>• Scheduled napping<br>• Avoid the sedating medications<br>• Pemoline, armodafinil and other stimulants<br>• SSRI for cataplexy | • Chronotherapy<br>• Time melatonin<br>• Bright light therapy | • Avoidance of offending agents dopaminergic medications like l-dopa, pramipexole, ropinirole<br>• Alpha 2 delta ligands, e.g., gabapentin and pregabalin | • Avoidance of offending agents<br>• Clonazepam at night |

(RBD: REM sleep behavior disorder; REM: rapid eye movement; SRED: sleep-related eating disorder)

## DIAGNOSIS OF SLEEP DISORDERS IN PATIENTS WITH MOOD AND ANXIETY DISORDERS

**Flowcharts 1 to 5** depict diagnostic algorithm for RLS, OSA, hypersomnia, parasomnias, and diagnosis of circadian rhythm sleep disorders (CRSD).

**Flowchart 1:** Diagnosis of restless legs syndrome (RLS).

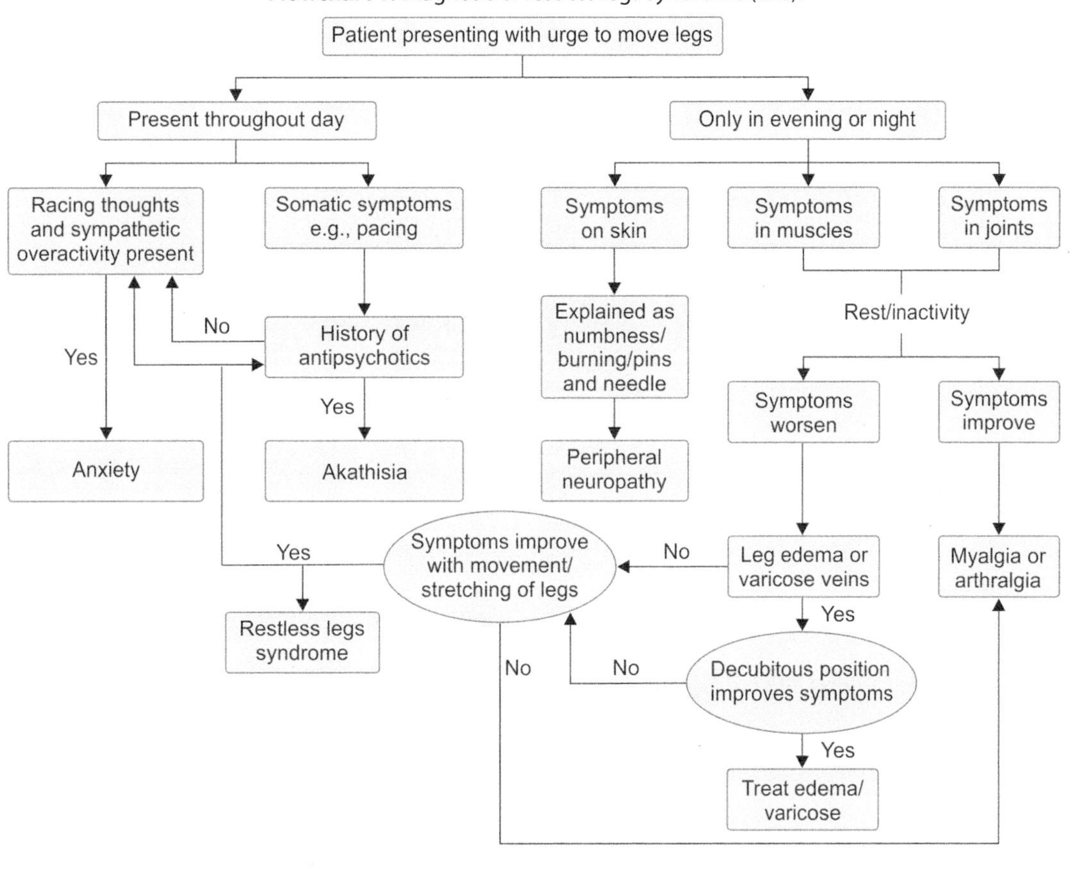


**Flowchart 2:** Diagnosis of obstructive sleep apnea (OSA).

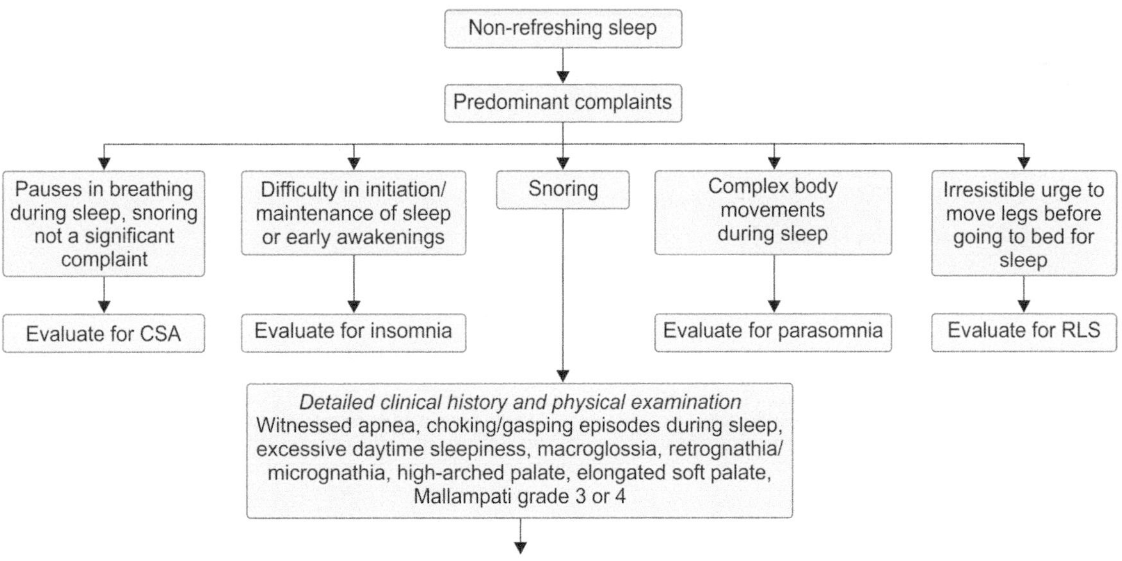


*Contd...*

*Contd...*

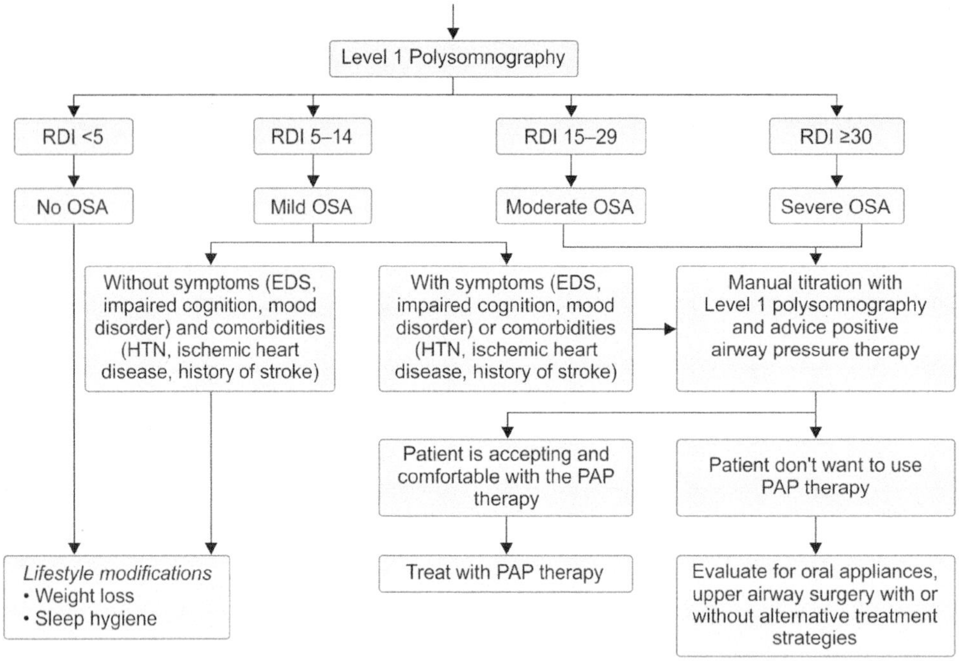

Level 1 Polysomnography

- RDI <5 → No OSA → *Lifestyle modifications* • Weight loss • Sleep hygiene
- RDI 5–14 → Mild OSA
  - Without symptoms (EDS, impaired cognition, mood disorder) and comorbidities (HTN, ischemic heart disease, history of stroke) → *Lifestyle modifications* • Weight loss • Sleep hygiene
  - With symptoms (EDS, impaired cognition, mood disorder) or comorbidities (HTN, ischemic heart disease, history of stroke) → Manual titration with Level 1 polysomnography and advice positive airway pressure therapy
- RDI 15–29 → Moderate OSA → Manual titration with Level 1 polysomnography and advice positive airway pressure therapy
- RDI ≥30 → Severe OSA → Manual titration with Level 1 polysomnography and advice positive airway pressure therapy

Manual titration with Level 1 polysomnography and advice positive airway pressure therapy:
- Patient is accepting and comfortable with the PAP therapy → Treat with PAP therapy
- Patient don't want to use PAP therapy → Evaluate for oral appliances, upper airway surgery with or without alternative treatment strategies

(EDS: Ehlers-Danlos syndrome; PAP: positive airway pressure; RDI: respiratory disturbance index)

**Flowchart 3:** Diagnosis of hypersomnia.

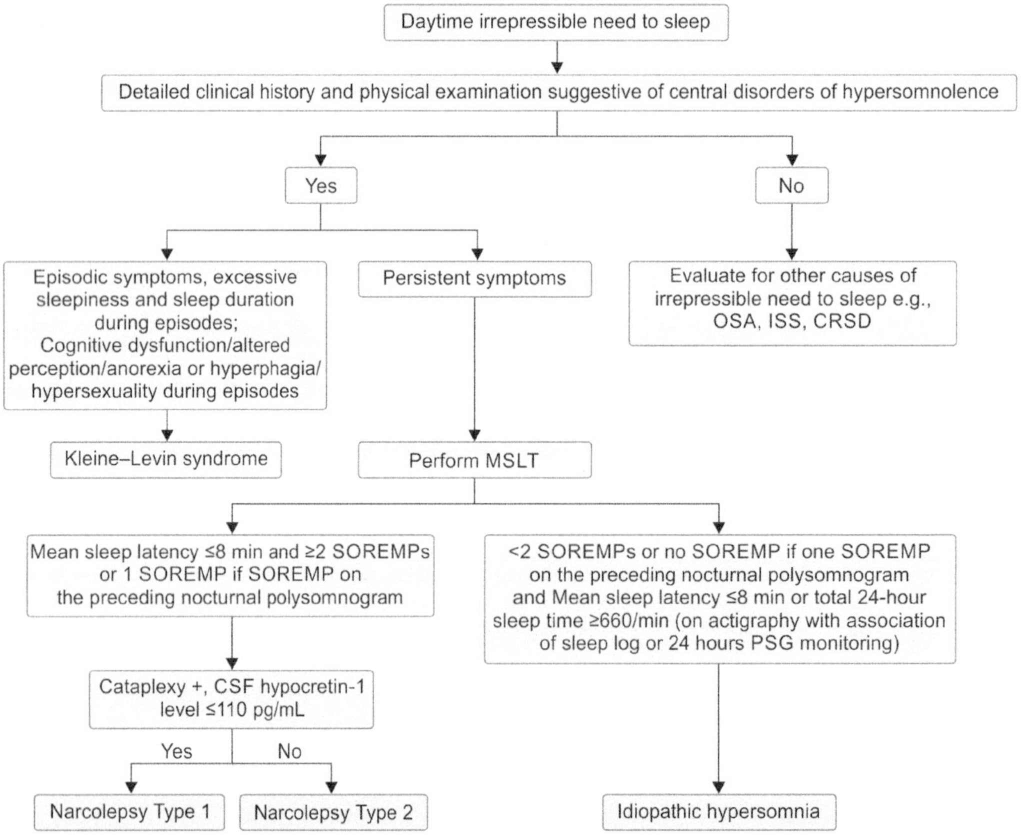

Daytime irrepressible need to sleep → Detailed clinical history and physical examination suggestive of central disorders of hypersomnolence

- Yes
  - Episodic symptoms, excessive sleepiness and sleep duration during episodes; Cognitive dysfunction/altered perception/anorexia or hyperphagia/hypersexuality during episodes → Kleine–Levin syndrome
  - Persistent symptoms → Perform MSLT
    - Mean sleep latency ≤8 min and ≥2 SOREMPs or 1 SOREMP if SOREMP on the preceding nocturnal polysomnogram → Cataplexy +, CSF hypocretin-1 level ≤110 pg/mL
      - Yes → Narcolepsy Type 1
      - No → Narcolepsy Type 2
    - <2 SOREMPs or no SOREMP if one SOREMP on the preceding nocturnal polysomnogram and Mean sleep latency ≤8 min or total 24-hour sleep time ≥660/min (on actigraphy with association of sleep log or 24 hours PSG monitoring) → Idiopathic hypersomnia
- No → Evaluate for other causes of irrepressible need to sleep e.g., OSA, ISS, CRSD

(CRSD: circadian rhythm sleep disorders; CSF: cerebrospinal fluid; ISS: insufficient sleep syndrome; MSLT: multiple sleep latency test; OSA: obstructive sleep apnea; PSG: polysomnography; SOREM: sleep-onset REM)

**Flowchart 4:** Diagnosis of parasomnia.

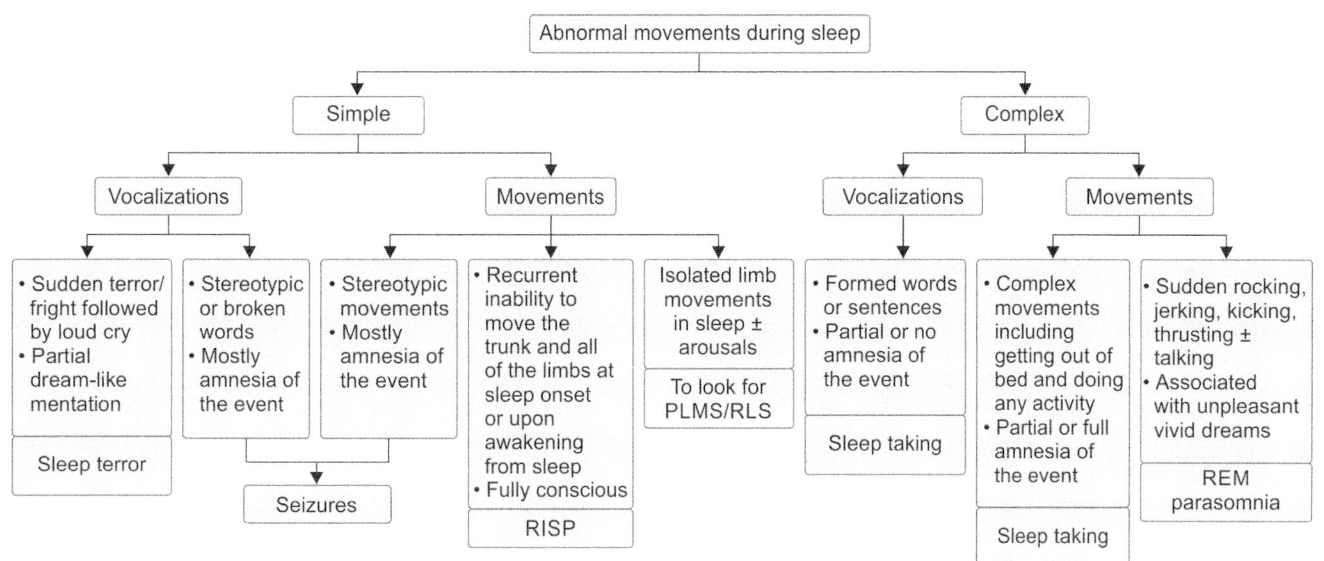


(PLMS: periodic limb movements of sleep; REM: rapid eye movement; RISP: recurrent isolated sleep paralysis; RLS: restless leg syndrome)

**Flowchart 5:** Diagnosis of Circadian Rhythm Sleep Disorders (CRSD).

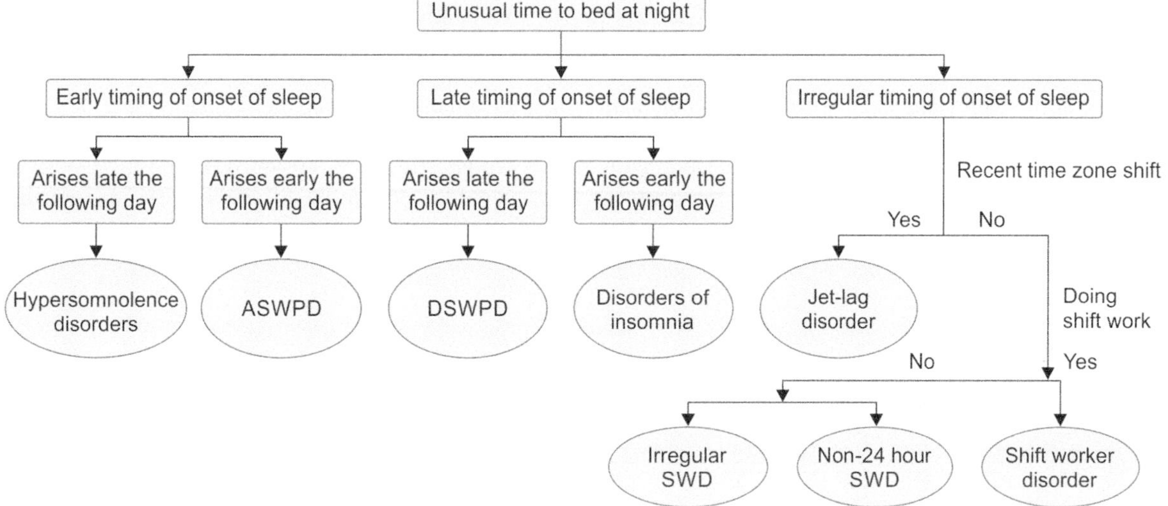


(ASWPD: advanced sleep-wake phase disorder; DSWPD: delayed sleep-wake phase disorder; SWD: sleep wake disorder)

## REFERENCES


1. Nutt DJ, Wilson S, Paterson L. Sleep disorders as core symptoms of depression. Dialogues Clin Neurosci. 2008;10(3):329-36.
2. Patatanian E, Claborn MK. Drug-induced restless legs syndrome. Ann Pharmacother. 2018;52(7):662-72.
3. Barateau L, Lopez R, Franchi JAM, Dauvilliers Y. Hypersomnolence, hypersomnia, and mood disorders. Curr Psychiatry Rep. 2017;19(2):1-11.
4. Dauvilliers Y, Lopez R, Ohayon M, Bayard S. Hypersomnia and depressive symptoms: methodological and clinical aspects. BMC Med. 2013;11(1):78.
5. Crouse JJ, Carpenter JS, Song YJC, Hockey SJ, Naismith SL, Grunstein RR, et al. Circadian rhythm sleep-wake disturbances and depression in young people: implications for prevention and early intervention. Lancet Psychiatry. 2021;8(9):813-23.
6. Geoffroy PA, Micoulaud Franchi JA, Lopez R, Poirot I, Brion A, Royant-Parola S, et al. How to characterize and

treat sleep complaints in bipolar disorders? Encephale. 2016;43(4):363-73.

7. BaHammam AS, Kendzerska T, Gupta R, Ramasubramanian C, Neubauer DN, Narasimhan M, et al. Comorbid depression in obstructive sleep apnea: an under-recognized association. Sleep Breath. 2016;20(2):447-56.
8. Edwards C, Almeida OP, Ford AH. Obstructive sleep apnea and depression: a systematic review and meta-analysis. Maturitas. 2020;142:45-54.
9. Waters F, Moretto U, Dang-Vu TT. Psychiatric illness and parasomnias: a systematic review. Curr Psychiatry Rep. 2017;19(7):1-11.
10. Stubbs B, Vancampfort D, Veronese N, Solmi M, Gaughran F, Manu P, et al. The prevalence and predictors of obstructive sleep apnea in major depressive disorder, bipolar disorder and schizophrenia: a systematic review and meta-analysis. J Affect Disord. 2016;197:259-67.
11. Talih F, Gebara NY, Andary FS, Mondello S, Kobeissy F, Ferri R. Delayed sleep phase syndrome and bipolar disorder: Pathogenesis and available common biomarkers. Sleep Med Rev. 2018;41:133-40.
12. Khurshid KA. Comorbid insomnia and psychiatric disorders: an update. Innov Clin Neurosci. 2018;15(3-4):28.
13. Netzer NC, Stoohs RA, Netzer CM, Clark K, Strohl KP. Using the Berlin Questionnaire to identify patients at risk for the sleep apnea syndrome. Ann Intern Med. 1999;131(7):485-91.
14. Marti-Soler H, Hirotsu C, Marques-Vidal P, Vollenweider P, Waeber G, Preisig M, et al. The NoSAS score for screening of sleep-disordered breathing: a derivation and validation study. Lancet Respir Med. 2016;4(9):742-8.
15. Chung F, Abdullah HR, Liao P. STOP-Bang questionnaire: a practical approach to screen for obstructive sleep apnea. Chest. 2016;149(3):631-8.
16. Sturzenegger C, Baumann CR, Lammers GJ, Kallweit U, Lm Van Der Zande W, Bassetti CL. Swiss Narcolepsy Scale: a simple screening tool for hypocretin-deficient narcolepsy with cataplexy. Clin Transl Neurosci. 2018; 2(2):34.
17. Hublin C, Kaprio J, Partinen M, Koskenvuo M, Heikkilä K. The Ullanlinna Narcolepsy Scale: Validation of a measure of symptoms in the narcoleptic syndrome. J Sleep Res. 1994;3(1):52-9.
18. Allen RP, Burchell BJ, MacDonald B, Hening WA, Earley CJ. Validation of the self-completed Cambridge-Hopkins questionnaire (CH-RLSq) for ascertainment of restless legs syndrome (RLS) in a population survey. Sleep Med. 2009;10(10):1097-100.
19. Kumar R, Krishnan V, Das A, Kumar N, Gupta R. Modification and Validation of a Diagnostic Questionnaire for Restless Legs Syndrome: Modified-Restless Legs Syndrome Diagnostic Questionnaire (m-RLS-DQ). Ann Indian Acad Neurol. 2023;26(4):475-83.
20. Fulda S, Hornyak M, Müller K, Cerny L, Beitinger PA, Wetter TC. Development and validation of the Munich Parasomnia Screening (MUPS): a questionnaire for parasomnias and nocturnal behaviors. Somnologie [Internet]. 2008;12(1):56-65.
21. Loddo G, La Fauci G, Vignatelli L, Zenesini C, Cilea R, Mignani F, et al. The Arousal Disorders Questionnaire: a new and effective screening tool for confusional arousals, Sleepwalking and Sleep Terrors in epilepsy and sleep disorders units. Sleep Med [Internet]. 2021;80:279-85.
22. Stiasny-Kolster K, Mayer G, Schäfer S, Möller JC, Heinzel-Gutenbrunner M, Oertel WH. The REM sleep behavior disorder screening questionnaire—a new diagnostic instrument. Mov Disord. 2007;22(16):2386-93.

CHAPTER 25

# Management of Schizophrenia—Positive Symptoms

*Harsh Pathak, Vanteemar S Sreeraj, Ganesan Venkatasubramanian*

## INTRODUCTION

Schizophrenia is a severe and debilitating disorder with a lifetime prevalence of 0.7%.[1] Being a heterogeneous disorder, it presents with various symptoms, including positive, negative, and cognitive symptoms. Since the time of Kraepelin, positive symptoms have been a prominent feature of schizophrenia[2] and are sometimes considered synonymous with the disorder.

Positive symptoms, such as delusions and hallucinations, are predominant in the initial presentation of schizophrenia. Since the advent of chlorpromazine, antipsychotics have been the primary treatment for these symptoms.[1] Recently, adjunctive treatments such as psychosocial intervention and neuromodulation have also been proposed for managing positive symptoms in schizophrenia.

Management of positive symptoms of schizophrenia includes the following steps **(Flowchart 1)**:

**Flowchart 1:** Overview of management of positive symptoms in schizophrenia.

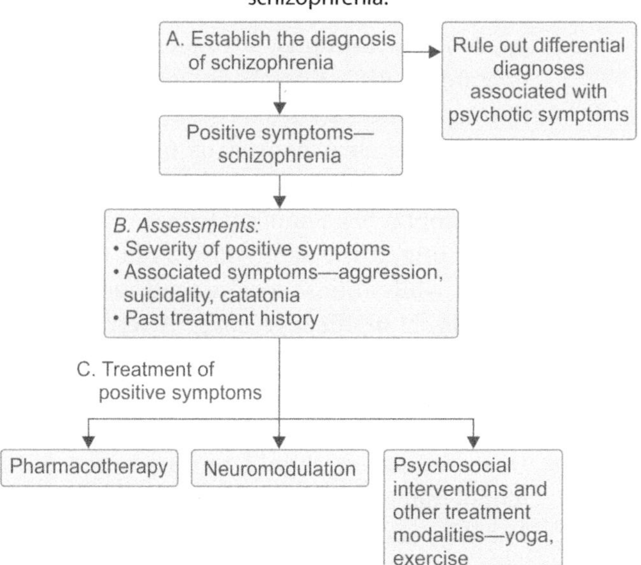


A. *Establish the diagnosis:* To diagnose schizophrenia, a comprehensive evaluation is needed, including detailed interviews with patients and caregivers. The diagnosis is confirmed using the current nosological system [Diagnostic and Statistical Manual of Mental Disorders (DSM) or International Classification of Diseases (ICD)] after ruling out other disorders with psychotic symptoms, such as severe depression with psychotic symptoms or substance-induced psychosis.

B. *Assessment:* A detailed evaluation includes assessing the severity of positive symptoms and any associated symptoms that may increase the risk of harm to self or others, such as aggression or suicidality. Also, reviewing the past treatment history (including pharmacological treatment, adherence, and response), detailed medical history, and substance use history is necessary. Based on this assessment, the appropriate treatment setting and options are chosen.

C. *Treatment of positive symptoms:*
   - *Pharmacotherapy* ***(Flowchart 2)****:*
     - The first-line treatment for positive symptoms is antipsychotics. The choice of antipsychotic depends on various factors, including patient preference and side effect profile.
     - All antipsychotics have similar efficacy for positive symptoms, except for amisulpride, olanzapine, and risperidone, which can be considered among the first agents for treating positive symptoms.[3]
     - Antipsychotics should be initiated at the minimum therapeutic dose. For first-episode schizophrenia, the required dose is generally lower than for multiepisode schizophrenia.[4] Most guidelines recommend at least a 6-week antipsychotic trial to consider it adequate.[5] However, if there is no response by 2–3 weeks, consider changing the antipsychotic.[6,7]

**Flowchart 2:** Pharmacotherapy in the treatment of positive symptoms in schizophrenia.

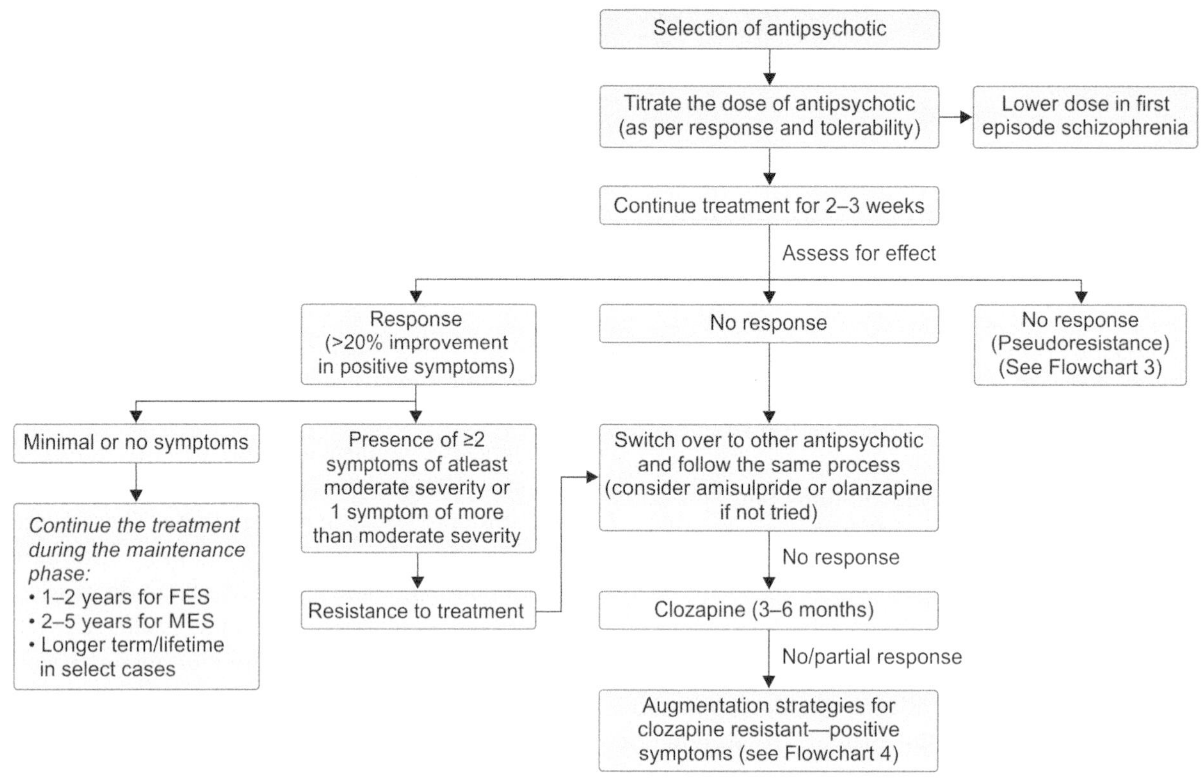


(FES: first episode schizophrenia, MES: multiepisode schizophrenia)

The second antipsychotic trial should also last for a minimum of 6 weeks.

- If patients have a partial response (i.e., <20% reduction in symptoms on a structured scale), optimize the antipsychotic dose and monitor for a delayed response for up to 10 weeks.[7]
- If no improvement is observed, or if the patient continues to experience two or more symptoms of moderate severity, or a single positive symptom of more than moderate severity, switching the antipsychotic can be considered.
- Long-acting injectable (LAI) antipsychotics can be considered in the first episode if the patient prefers them, or poor adherence is suspected.
- Following symptom improvement in the acute phase, during the maintenance phase of treatment, antipsychotics should be continued for 1-2 years in first-episode schizophrenia and 2-5 years in multiepisode schizophrenia.[4] Most guidelines recommend long-term maintenance treatment to prevent relapses. Nevertheless, gradual tapering down and discontinuation can be planned for those who show good recovery.[8]
- In certain situations, such as a history of multiple relapses on/off treatment, suicidal attempts, more severe illness, and the presence of residual psychotic symptoms, a longer duration of treatment with antipsychotics, potentially even lifelong, may be needed.[9]
- There is no clear consensus on the dose of antipsychotics during the maintenance phase of schizophrenia. Some guidelines recommend continuing at the same dose as in the acute phase, while others recommend reducing to the minimum effective dose.[4] A retrospective study indicated that a 30% reduction in the antipsychotic dose during the maintenance phase was adequate for sustained remission.[10]
- Dose reduction should be attempted 6-12 months after initiating the maintenance phase.[11] The dose should be reduced by no >25% of the previous dose every 6 months.[12]

- In case of acute exacerbation or relapse after the initial response, assess for nonadherence. Consider a trial of LAI antipsychotics if the nonadherence is due to poor insight or lack of support **(Flowchart 3)**. LAI antipsychotics may reduce the risk of relapse and rehospitalizations.[13] However, if nonadherence is due to poor tolerability, consider switching to an antipsychotic with fewer side effects **(Flowchart 3)**.
- Assess for psychosocial factors that may have led to worsening of symptoms. If a relapse of positive symptoms occurs while on treatment, consider the possibility of antipsychotic failure and change the antipsychotic.
- If there is no improvement or if improvement plateaus, consider factors that may influence the response to treatment, including substance use, rapid metabolism of medication, poor absorption, drug interactions, and other effects on drug metabolism (such as smoking), as well as psychosocial factors, to rule out pseudoresistance to treatment **(Flowchart 3)**.
- If there is no response, the presence of two or more positive symptoms of moderate severity, or one severe positive symptom after adequate trials of two antipsychotics, treatment resistance is considered. For treatment-resistant positive symptoms, clozapine is the treatment of choice.[14]
- Additionally, emerging evidence supports the role of clozapine as a second-line agent following a failed trial of amisulpride.[15,16]
- In certain scenarios, such as suicidality, aggression, substance use, and psychogenic polydipsia, clozapine is effective alongside treatment-resistance.[17]
- In the Indian population, a dose of 120–250 mg/day is typically sufficient to reach a serum clozapine level >350 μg/L.[18] It is recommended to give clozapine a minimum trial of 3–6 months at the maximum tolerable dose to assess its effectiveness.
- In case of partial or no response to clozapine, various augmentation and add-on strategies can be employed, including electroconvulsive therapy (ECT), antipsychotics (aripiprazole, amisulpride, and risperidone), antidepressants (fluoxetine and mirtazapine), and antiepileptics/mood stabilizers (valproate, lamotrigine, lithium, and topiramate) **(Flowchart 4)**.[19] The adequate trial duration for these augmentation strategies is 3–6 months, though the evidence base for this stage is limited.
- Treatment resistance is defined as the presence of two or more positive symptom domains of at least moderate severity after an adequate trial of

**Flowchart 3:** Management of pseudoresistance.

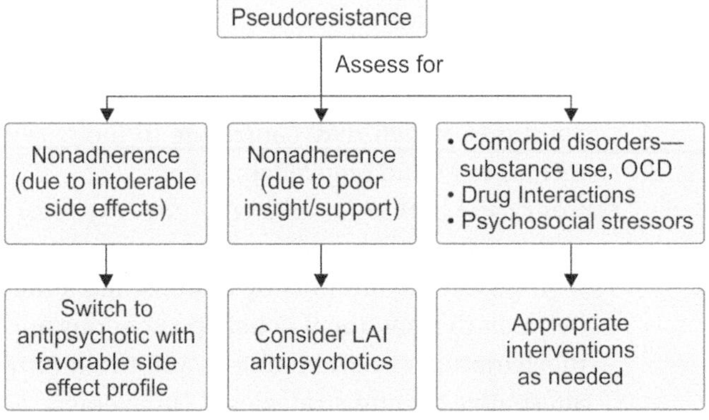


(LAI: Long-acting injectable, OCD: Obsessive compulsive disorder)

**Flowchart 4:** Augmentation strategies for clozapine-resistant positive symptoms in schizophrenia.

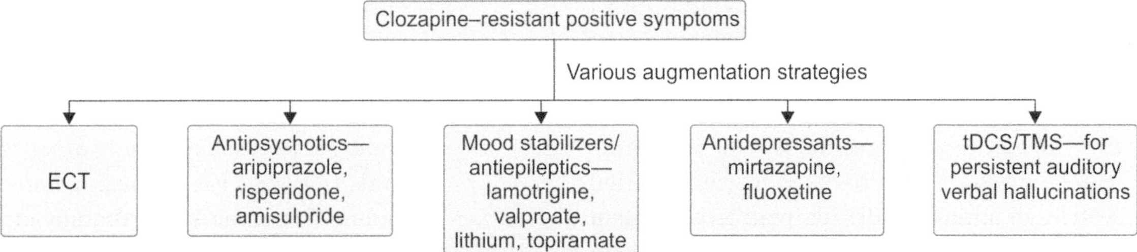


(ECT: electroconvulsive therapy, tDCS: transcranial direct current stimulation, TMS: transcranial magnetic stimulation)

two antipsychotics, or a single positive symptom domain be of more than moderate severity persisting after such trials.[5] In case of resistant symptoms, consider changing to another antipsychotic, switching to clozapine, or using augmentation strategies. It is important to note that some positive symptoms, such as persistent auditory verbal hallucinations, may persist at moderate severity despite overall improvement. Handling such symptoms generally follows the same algorithm as for treatment resistance, but somatic modalities such as transcranial magnetic stimulation or transcranial direct current stimulation may also be considered.

- Antipsychotic polypharmacy should generally be avoided. However, it may be considered in certain situations, such as poor response to clozapine. Another exception is the use of partial dopamine agonists such as aripiprazole as an add-on for antipsychotic-induced hyperprolactinemia.[20] A recent nationwide cohort study of schizophrenia noted that higher dose polypharmacy is associated with a reduced risk of hospitalization for medical comorbidities or psychiatric causes. Also, across all doses combined, no significant differences were noted between polypharmacy or monotherapy for the risk of hospitalization for nonpsychiatric causes.[21]
- Antipsychotic discontinuation or deprescription can be considered in patients who have shown good recovery. This should follow the exponential 6-monthly 25% dose reduction in the maintenance phase, as mentioned earlier.[7]

- *Neuromodulation:*
  - Neuromodulation techniques are mainly used as adjunctive treatment strategies for positive symptoms.
  - These techniques involve ECT, transcranial electric stimulation [including transcranial direct current stimulation (tDCS)], and transcranial magnetic current stimulation (TMS).
  - ECT has been employed since the 20th century for various psychiatric disorders, including schizophrenia. It can be used in combination with other antipsychotics for treatment-resistant schizophrenia and as an augmenting agent with clozapine.[19,22,23] ECT can also be considered in situations requiring rapid response, such as aggression, suicidality, and catatonia. Modified bilateral ECTs are generally administered for 6–12 sessions, with three sessions per week on alternate days. Maintenance ECTs can be considered in some cases, especially for individuals with clozapine-resistant schizophrenia who show a good response to ECT.[24]
  - TMS[25] and tDCS[26] have been used as add-on treatments primarily for persistent auditory verbal hallucinations.
- *Psychosocial interventions:* Psychosocial intervention play an important role in schizophrenia treatment, addressing both psychological and social factors contributing to the symptoms. They are:
  - *Psychoeducation:* It involves providing information about schizophrenia and its treatment, focusing on relapse prevention. It enhances treatment adherence and reduces relapse rates,[27] and may positively impact overall functioning.
  - *Family intervention:* It includes psychoeducation of the family members regarding the illness and its treatment and facilitates better communication and conflict resolution. It helps identify and reduce negative expressed emotions, which may contribute to increased relapse rates and rehospitalization.[27]
  - *Cognitive behavior therapy for psychosis (CBTp):* It aims to reduce distress associated with positive symptoms by establishing a link between dysfunctional beliefs/perceptions and the symptoms, reevaluating it, and promoting alternative coping strategies.[28] On average, 20 sessions are administered.
  - Other cognitive approaches,[28] such as metacognitive therapy, metacognitive training, metacognitive insight, and reflection therapy, can also be administered.
  - Assertive community treatment (ACT), an intensive community-based treatment may reduce frequent relapses due to nonadherence secondary to poor social support or supervision.[29]
  - Virtual reality (VR)-based psychological treatments[30] such as avatar therapy or VR-CBT, have shown promising results in reducing positive symptoms.

- *Other treatment modalities*: These include yoga, mind-body exercises, and other physical exercises. The current findings are preliminary and need to be substantiated with future studies.
  - *Yoga and other mind-body exercises:* Yoga and other mind-body exercises have been shown add-on benefits in the symptoms of schizophrenia, including positive symptoms.[31]
  - *Other exercises:* Resistance exercises appears to be beneficial with regard to positive symptoms.[32]

## REFERENCES


1. Jauhar S, Johnstone M, McKenna PJ. Schizophrenia. Lancet. 2022;399(10323):473-86.
2. Kendler KS. Phenomenology of Schizophrenia and the Representativeness of Modern Diagnostic Criteria. JAMA Psychiatry. 2016;73(10):1082-92.
3. Huhn M, Nikolakopoulou A, Schneider-Thoma J, Krause M, Samara M, Peter N, et al. Comparative efficacy and tolerability of 32 oral antipsychotics for the acute treatment of adults with multi-episode schizophrenia: a systematic review and network meta-analysis. Lancet. 2019;394(10202):939-51.
4. Correll CU, Martin A, Patel C, Benson C, Goulding R, Kern-Sliwa J, et al. Systematic literature review of schizophrenia clinical practice guidelines on acute and maintenance management with antipsychotics. Schizophrenia (Heidelb). 2022;8(1):5.
5. Howes OD, McCutcheon R, Agid O, de Bartolomeis A, van Beveren NJM, Birnbaum ML, et al. Treatment-Resistant Schizophrenia: Treatment Response and Resistance in Psychosis (TRRIP) Working Group Consensus Guidelines on Diagnosis and Terminology. Am J Psychiatry. 2017;174(3): 216-29.
6. Leucht S, Busch R, Hamann J, Kissling W, Kane JM. Early-onset hypothesis of antipsychotic drug action: a hypothesis tested, confirmed and extended. Biol Psychiatry. 2005;57(12):1543-9.
7. Taylor DM, Barnes TRE, Young AH. The Maudsley Prescribing Guidelines in Psychiatry, 14th edition. United States: Wiley; 2021.
8. Asian Network of Early Psychosis Writing Group. Guidelines for Discontinuation of Antipsychotics in Patients Who Recover From First-Episode Schizophrenia Spectrum Disorders: Derived From the Aggregated Opinions of Asian Network of Early Psychosis Experts and Literature Review. Int J Neuropsychopharmacol. 2022;25(9): 737-58.
9. Grover S, Chakrabarti S, Kulhara P, Avasthi A. Clinical Practice Guidelines for Management of Schizophrenia. Indian J Psychiatry. 2017;59(Suppl 1):S19-33.
10. Kumar V, Rao NP, Narasimha V, Sathyanarayanan G, Muralidharan K, Varambally S, et al. Antipsychotic dose in maintenance treatment of schizophrenia: A retrospective study. Psychiatry Res. 2016;245:311-6.
11. Shimomura Y, Kikuchi Y, Suzuki T, Uchida H, Mimura M, Takeuchi H. Antipsychotic treatment in the maintenance phase of schizophrenia: An updated systematic review of the guidelines and algorithms. Schizophr Res. 2020; 215:8-16.
12. Liu CC, Takeuchi H. Achieving the Lowest effective antipsychotic dose for patients with remitted psychosis: a proposed guided dose-reduction algorithm. CNS Drugs. 2020;34(2):117-26.
13. Leucht C, Heres S, Kane JM, Kissling W, Davis JM, Leucht S. Oral versus depot antipsychotic drugs for schizophrenia: A critical systematic review and meta-analysis of randomised long-term trials. Schizophr Res. 2011;127(1):83-92.
14. Siskind D, McCartney L, Goldschlager R, Kisely S. Clozapine v. first- and second-generation antipsychotics in treatment-refractory schizophrenia: systematic review and meta-analysis. Br J Psychiatry. 2016;209(5):385-92.
15. Kahn RS, Winter van Rossum I, Leucht S, McGuire P, Lewis SW, Leboyer M, et al. Amisulpride and olanzapine followed by open-label treatment with clozapine in first-episode schizophrenia and schizophreniform disorder (OPTiMiSE): a three-phase switching study. Lancet Psychiatry 2018;5(10):797-807.
16. Okhuijsen-Pfeifer C, Huijsman EAH, Hasan A, Sommer IEC, Leucht S, Kahn RS, et al. Clozapine as a first- or second-line treatment in schizophrenia: a systematic review and meta-analysis. Acta Psychiatr Scand. 2018;138(4):281-8.
17. Meyer JM, Stahl SM. The Clozapine Handbook: Stahl's Handbooks. Cambridge: Cambridge University Press; 2019
18. Suhas S, Kumar V, Damodharan D, Sharma P, Rao NP, Varambally S, et al. Do Indian patients with schizophrenia need half the recommended clozapine dose to achieve therapeutic serum level? An exploratory study. Schizophr Res. 2020;222:195-201.
19. Siskind DJ, Lee M, Ravindran A, Zhang Q, Ma E, Motamarri B, et al. Augmentation strategies for clozapine refractory schizophrenia: A systematic review and meta-analysis. Aust NZJ Psychiatry. 2018;52(8):751-67.
20. Lähteenvuo M, Tiihonen J. Antipsychotic polypharmacy for the management of schizophrenia: evidence and recommendations. Drugs. 2021;81(11):1273-84.
21. Taipale H, Tanskanen A, Tiihonen J. Safety of antipsychotic polypharmacy versus monotherapy in a nationwide cohort of 61,889 patients with schizophrenia. Am J Psychiatry. 2023;180(5):377-85.
22. Sinclair DJ, Zhao S, Qi F, Nyakyoma K, Kwong JS, Adams CE. Electroconvulsive therapy for treatment-resistant schizophrenia. Cochrane Database Syst Rev. 2019;(3):CD011847.

23. Ali SA, Mathur N, Malhotra AK, Braga RJ. Electroconvulsive therapy and schizophrenia: a systematic review. Mol Neuropsychiatry. 2019;5(2):75-83.
24. Keepers GA, Fochtmann LJ, Anzia JM, Benjamin S, Lyness JM, Mojtabai R, et al. The American Psychiatric Association Practice Guideline for the Treatment of Patients With Schizophrenia. AJP. 2020;177(9):868-72.
25. Marzouk T, Winkelbeiner S, Azizi H, Malhotra AK, Homan P. Transcranial magnetic stimulation for positive symptoms in schizophrenia: a systematic review. Neuropsychobiology. 2019;79(6):384-96.
26. Cheng PWC, Louie LLC, Wong YL, Wong SMC, Leung WY, Nitsche MA, et al. The effects of transcranial direct current stimulation (tDCS) on clinical symptoms in schizophrenia: A systematic review and meta-analysis. Asian J Psychiatry. 2020;53:102392.
27. McDonagh MS, Dana T, Kopelovich SL, Monroe-DeVita M, Blazina I, Bougatsos C, et al. Psychosocial interventions for adults with schizophrenia: an overview and update of systematic reviews. Psychiatr Serv. 2022;73(3): 299-312.
28. Moritz S, Klein JP, Lysaker PH, Mehl S. Metacognitive and cognitive-behavioral interventions for psychosis: new developments. Dialogues Clin Neurosci. 2019;21(3):309-17.
29. Arahanthabailu P, Purohith AN, Kanakode R, Praharaj SK, Bhandary RP, Venkata Narasimha Sharma PS. Modified assertive community treatment program for patients with schizophrenia: Effectiveness and perspectives of service consumers from a South Indian setting. Asian J Psychiatry 2022;73:103102.
30. Chan KCS, Hui CLM, Suen YN, Lee EHM, Chang WC, Chan SKW, et al. Application of immersive virtual reality for assessment and intervention in psychosis: A Systematic Review. Brain Sci. 2023;13(3):471.
31. Wei GX, Yang L, Imm K, Loprinzi PD, Smith L, Zhang X, et al. Effects of mind-body exercises on schizophrenia: a systematic review with meta-analysis. Fro Front Psychiatry. 2020;11:819
32. Yu Q, Wong KK, Lei OK, Nie J, Shi Q, Zou L, et al. Comparative effectiveness of multiple exercise interventions in the treatment of mental health disorders: a systematic review and network meta-analysis. Sports Med Open. 2022;8(1):135.

# Treatment of Difficult-to-Treat Auditory Hallucination

*Swarna Buddha Nayok, Vanteemar S Sreeraj, Ganesan Venkatasubramanian*

## INTRODUCTION

Auditory hallucinations (AH) are present in about 60% of patients with schizophrenia.[1-3]

Among them, about 30% may continue to experience AH even after receiving treatment with antipsychotic medications. This chapter offers various treatment options for managing difficult-to-treat AH. A combination of strategies may be required for successful treatment outcomes.

It is important to note that "difficult-to-treat" AH consists of "treatment-resistant schizophrenia" as well as "persistent AH". The term "treatment resistance" is preferred when moderate or more severe symptoms persist across multiple domains of schizophrenia, despite adequate trials with two antipsychotics. Persistent AH, on the other hand, it refers to predominantly persistent moderate or more severe hallucinations even when other symptoms have responded to treatment. For example, "persistent AH" may occur during the initial trial of an antipsychotic, where all other schizophrenia symptoms have responded to treatment. Psychological/psychosocial interventions and brain stimulation approaches may be considered in such cases, regardless of whether the patient is resistant to pharmacotherapy. Treatment duration and adherence must be considered in "difficult-to-treat" AH at any stage in the illness course.[4] In this chapter, we consider difficult-to-treat AH within the context of schizophrenia. The step-by-step approach to managing difficult-to-treat AH is represented in **Flowchart 1**, with additional details provided in **Table 1** outlining various management strategies.

**Flowchart 1:** Difficult-to-treat auditory hallucinations in schizophrenia.

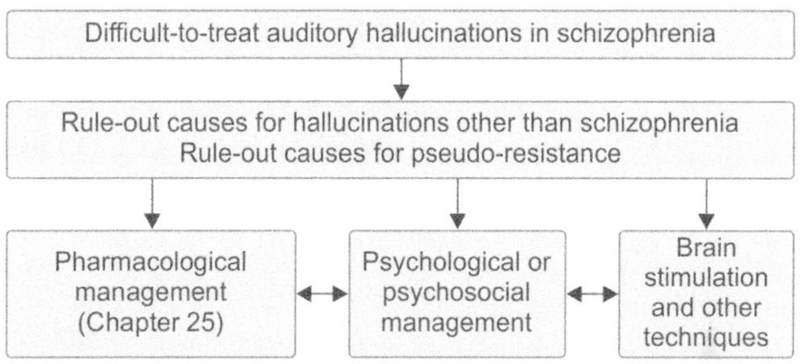


## RULING OUT OTHER REASONS FOR DIFFICULT-TO-TREAT AUDITORY HALLUCINATIONS [2,5,6]

- Although not always possible, effort must be made to differentiate AH from other overlapping psychopathological phenomena such as imagery, obsessive thoughts, musical hallucinations/involuntary musical imagery/"ear-worms", elementary hallucinations, akoasms, pseudohallucinations, hypnogogic/hypnopompic hallucinations, and hallucination-like experiences during derealization/depersonalization.
- AH can be present in any other psychotic disorders, such as mania/depression with psychotic symptoms. Often, when faced with such hallucinations, it is prudent to revisit the diagnosis and treat the underlying cause.
- AH is also found in other nonpsychotic psychiatric disorders, such as borderline personality disorder and dissociative identity disorder, unipolar and bipolar disorder, anxiety spectrum disorders, autism, substance use disorders (chronic use, intoxication, and withdrawal), and posttraumatic stress disorder.
- AH is often associated with other neurological, medical, or surgical disorders/conditions, such as Parkinson's disease, dementia, Lewy-body, Alzheimer's, Parkinson's, vascular, frontotemporal, dementia, stroke, migraine, delirium, epilepsy, Huntington's disease, lesions of the thalamus, temporal lobe, and

**TABLE 1:** Management types, targets, and methods for difficult-to-treat auditory hallucinations (AH).

| *Type of management* | *Target* | *Method/protocol* |
|---|---|---|
| Brain stimulation—ECT[2] | Resistant schizophrenia | • Bitemporal/bifrontal ECT for 8–16 sessions<br>• ECT may be the first choice of treatment when commanding AH is associated with significant suicidality/homicidal |
| Brain stimulation—TMS[13,14] | AH | • rTMS (till 40 sessions in 8 weeks), low-frequency rTMS at left temporoparietal cortices<br>• Continuous theta burst stimulation over the left temporoparietal junction |
| Brain stimulation—tDCS[11] | AH | Conventional tDCS with anodal stimulation of 2 mA at left dorsolateral prefrontal cortex and cathodal stimulation at left temporoparietal junction, for 20-minute session, two sessions per day with inter-session duration of 20–180 minutes, for 5–10 days |
| Psychological/Psychosocial management[2,3] | Improve coping strategies | Coping strategy enhancement, focus on reactions to AH, group therapy, distraction techniques like ear-plug, music, subvocalization |
| | Questioning the "reality" of the voices | Exploring the content, understanding relationship with mood and stress, CBT methods |
| | Subjective control over AH | CBT for content of AH (helpful in command AH) |
| | Disengagement from AH | Acceptance and mindfulness-based approaches, cognitive restructuring, and Socratic questioning |
| | Understanding the context of AH | CBT, psychodynamic approaches |
| | Improve self-esteem and self-compassion | Memory reinforcement, competitive memory training, supportive therapy, positive self-image, imagery, role-play, mindfulness, and compassionate mind training |
| | Specific traumatic memories/imagery related AH | Imagery rescripting, eye movement desensitization and reprogramming, and virtual reality-based approaches |
| | Interpersonal relationship with AH | Relative therapy, virtual reality-based approaches, and Avatar therapy |
| Others[2,3,16,17] | Symptoms of schizophrenia | • Yoga/Body-based therapies<br>• Music therapy<br>• Lifestyle changes<br>• Meditation is normally avoided |

(CBT: cognitive behavioral therapy; ECT: electroconvulsive therapy; mA: milliampere; rTMS: repetitive transcranial magnetic stimulation; tDCS: transcranial direct current stimulation; TMS: transcranial magnetic stimulation)

brainstem, and postsurgery recovery. Treatment is focused on the underlying cause.

- AH is associated with dysfunctions of the auditory pathway (such as hearing loss to auditory cortex dysfunction) and be elicited through sensory deprivation (also known as release hallucinations).
- AH may occur in 4–21% of the general population with no neuropsychiatric/medical illnesses. Although these experiences are mostly transients, difficult-to-treat AH may exist in such populations (about 4%).

## PHARMACOLOGICAL MANAGEMENT[2-4,7]

- Pharmacological management of difficult-to-treat AH in schizophrenia is similar to the management of positive symptoms. Details are given in the chapter "Management of Schizophrenia—Positive Symptoms".
- Some pharmacological add-on medications may include allopurinol, bexarotene, celecoxib, D-alanine, donepezil, D-serine, estradiol, famotidine, ginkgo biloba, glycine, lamotrigine, lithium, memantine, mianserin, minocycline, mirtazapine, N-acetylcysteine,

omega-3-fatty acids, ondansetron, propentofylline, raloxifene, riluzole, ritanserin, sarcosine, sodium benzoate, sodium valproate, tiapride, topiramate, and zotepine.[7,8]

- Few antipsychotics can also be used at higher dosages than recommended (supratherapeutic) with careful monitoring of adverse effects.
- The treatment dosage at which the AH reduces should be incorporated as continuous maintenance treatment. Relapse of AH may often be associated with poor adherence, and long-acting antipsychotics can be added to oral medications.

## BRAIN STIMULATION[2,7,9-12]

- Electroconvulsive therapy (ECT) has been used to reduce positive symptoms in schizophrenia and has also been utilized in refractory patients. ECT may be the first treatment choice when commanding AH increases suicidality or aggression (as in voices commanding towards suicide, self-harm, or harming others). Some evidence points toward reducing AH and other psychotic symptoms when used as an add-on therapy to antipsychotics, especially clozapine.
- Repetitive transcranial magnetic stimulation (rTMS) has been shown to reduce AH in selected cases. Different protocols (low-frequency, high-frequency, theta-burst) of rTMS at specific brain areas, such as the temporoparietal cortex, have been shown to affect AH differently.[2,9,12] Specifically, 1 Hz rTMS may reduce AH.[13] Newer protocols, such as continuous theta burst stimulation, may also be helpful for AH.[14]
- Recent evidence shows that add-on active transcranial direct current stimulation (tDCS) may be effective in up to 28% of patients with persistent AH.[15,16] Targeting the sensorimotor frontal-parietal network, cathodal stimulation at the left temporoparietal junction and left temporal area, and anodal stimulation at the left dorsolateral prefrontal cortex showed a significant reduction in AH. A minimum of 2 mA direct current administered twice daily for 5–10 days seems to be effective. An intersession interval of various durations (20 minutes to three hours) has been tried.

## PSYCHOLOGICAL/PSYCHOSOCIAL MANAGEMENT[1-3,17]

- Psychological treatment for difficult-to-treat AH can be mainly focusing, behavioral, cognitive, or a combination of these. In focusing treatments, the patient must focus on the form and content of the AH for a specified duration each day to "understand" the nature of the AH. Such an approach over a longer period (about 20 weeks) shows improvement in AH and the patient's coping mechanism and can temporarily reduce distress.
- Behavioral treatments aim at distraction/diversions techniques during active AH, such as interference/distraction with or without aversion techniques such as electrical shock (not ECT), thought-stopping technique/substitution, competing complex auditory input, performing motor tasks, time-out schedules (operant conditioning), listening to pleasant, and taped conversations/memories, with a variable focus at controlling or completely stopping the AH. These may be reinforced with relaxation techniques. More focused distraction techniques, such as earplugs, listening to music, subvocal counting, clenching fists, and raising eyebrows, have also yielded mixed and temporary results. Techniques such as keeping the mouth open, tongue biting, and singing/humming to reduce subvocalization during AH have been used. Distraction auditory techniques are often used only in one ear to counter deficit interhemispheric language transmission. Most have shown intermediate benefits and often reduce the frequency, duration, and distress associated with AH, but the effects seem to wear off after stopping such sessions. Overall, the use of earplugs has some long-term benefits.
- Cognitive approaches include similar distraction techniques with monitoring mood and AH, focusing on personal beliefs and, at times, challenging them in the context of the AH, realizing the meaning and significance of the content of AH. These approaches are reinforced with borrowed processes from individual therapy, supportive therapy, group therapy, relational aspects of the AH, psychodynamic approaches, development of social skills and newer coping strategies (coping strategy enhancement), Socratic questioning, integration of the experience of AH into everyday life, improving self-esteem and self-compassion, family involvement, trauma-focused therapy, rehabilitation, and crisis management. Again, these may lead to lesser distress and a decrease in AH, but the effects are often temporary.
- Increased self-control over AH is also advocated through direct methods such as visualization and

negotiation with the content of the AH, or indirectly regulating attention, locus of control, and affect regulation through an array of behaviors.

- Novel and theoretically complex approaches such as novel language therapy, didactic education and discussion sessions, a mix of personalizing previously described strategies such as stop techniques and distractions, such as hallucination-focused integrative therapy, mindfulness training, acceptance and commitment therapy, competitive memory training and compassionate mind training (both aimed at developing resilience), shared understanding of the AH by peers, imagery rescripting, eye movement desensitization and reprogramming, relative therapy (focusing on the relationship between patients and their AH), virtual-reality assisted therapy, and avatar therapy (computer-generated avatars aid to role-playing the voice of AH) have also been used with mixed results with some showing significant add-on benefits.[18,19] Specifically, in avatar therapy, a dialogue between the patient, therapist and "avatar" facilitates the patient to have a control over threatening AH, which can be toned down in intensity and derogatory content at a later stage.[18,20]
- Digital methods also have the potential for monitoring and treatment of difficult-to-treat AH.[20] Several components of AH may relate well to specific digital elements, such as ecological momentary intervention (providing reminders for coping mechanisms) in the self-management of intermittently occurring AH, digitalized autonomous interactive natural language processing mixed with virtual reality for the content and context of the AH, and language games to increase control over AH. The ability of technology to create hallucination-like stimuli which can be manipulated based on therapeutic needs is being explored through techniques like avatar therapy.

## Others[21,22]

- Yoga, specific and nonspecific exercises, and other body-based therapies such as tai-chi, qi-gong, and mindfulness can be utilized as add-on treatment options in those with refractory AH. Although direct evidence to reduce AH is lacking, overall improvement in symptoms of schizophrenia and social cognition may benefit the patients.
- However, these should be personalized and used only if deemed beneficial. There are few reports of exacerbation of psychosis following meditation.
- Music therapy and behavioral interventions may be helpful in difficult-to-treat AH and improve the quality of life.[23]
- General lifestyle changes may overall improve clinical symptoms and well-being and, in turn, help to reduce AH.

## REFERENCES


1. Shergill SS, Murray RM, McGuire PK. Auditory hallucinations: A review of psychological treatments. Schizophr Res. 1998;32:137-50.
2. Sommer IEC, Slotema CW, Daskalakis ZJ, Derks EM, Blom JD, van der Gaag M. The Treatment of Hallucinations in Schizophrenia Spectrum Disorders. Schizophr Bull. 2012;38:704-14.
3. Swyer A, Powers AR. Voluntary control of auditory hallucinations: phenomenology to therapeutic implications. Npj Schizophr. 2020;6:1-9.
4. Howes OD, McCutcheon R, Agid O, de Bartolomeis A, van Beveren NJ, Birnbaum ML, et al. Treatment-Resistant Schizophrenia: Treatment Response and Resistance in Psychosis (TRRIP) Working Group Consensus Guidelines on Diagnosis and Terminology. Am J Psychiatry. 2017; 174:216-29.
5. Sommer IEC, Koops S, Blom JD. Comparison of auditory hallucinations across different disorders and syndromes. Neuropsychiatry. 2012;2:57-68.
6. Waters F, Blom JD, Jardri R, Hugdahl K, Sommer IEC. Auditory hallucinations, not necessarily a hallmark of psychotic disorder. Psychol Med. 2018;48:529-36.
7. Taylor DM, Barnes TRE, Young AH. The Maudsley Prescribing Guidelines in Psychiatry. United States: John Wiley & Sons; 2021.
8. Karia S, Shah N, De Sousa A, Sonavane S. Tiapride for the Treatment of Auditory Hallucinations in Schizophrenia. Indian J Psychol Med. 2013;35:397-9.
9. Nathou C, Etard O, Dollfus S. Auditory verbal hallucinations in schizophrenia: current perspectives in brain stimulation treatments. Neuropsychiatr Dis Treat. 2019;15:2105-17.
10. Sreeraj VS, Arumugham SS, Venkatasubramanian G. Clinical Practice Guidelines for the Use of Transcranial Direct Current Stimulation in Psychiatry. Indian J Psychiatry. 2023;65:289-96.
11. Bose A, Shivakumar V, Agarwal SM, Kalmady SV, Shenoy S, Sreeraj VS, et al. Efficacy of fronto-temporal transcranial direct current stimulation for refractory auditory verbal hallucinations in schizophrenia: A randomized, double-blind, sham-controlled study. Schizophr Res. 2018;195:475-80.
12. Tikka SK, Siddiqui MA, Garg S, Gautam M. Clinical Practice Guidelines for the Therapeutic Use of Repetitive Transcranial Magnetic Stimulation in Neuropsychiatric Disorders. Indian J Psychiatry. 2023;65:270.

13. Li J, Cao X, Liu S, Li X, Xu Y. Efficacy of repetitive transcranial magnetic stimulation on auditory hallucinations in schizophrenia: A meta-analysis. Psychiatry Res. 2020;290:113141.
14. Chithra U, Samantaray S, Kumar V, K R, Maity K, E N, et al. Add-on accelerated continuous theta burst stimulation (a-cTBS) over the left temporoparietal junction for the management of persistent auditory hallucinations in schizophrenia: A case series. Brain Stimulat. 2022;15: 1511-2.
15. Rashidi S, Jones M, Murillo-Rodriguez E, Machado S, Hao Y, Yadollahpour A. Transcranial direct current stimulation for auditory verbal hallucinations: a systematic review of clinical trials. Neural Regen Res. 2020;16:666-71.
16. Fregni F, El-Hagrassy MM, Pacheco-Barrios K, Carvalho S, Leite J, Simis M, et al. Evidence-Based Guidelines and Secondary Meta-Analysis for the Use of Transcranial Direct Current Stimulation in Neurological and Psychiatric Disorders. Int J Neuropsychopharmacol. 2021;24:256-313.
17. Thomas N, Hayward M, Peters E, van der Gaag M, Bentall RP, Jenner J, et al. Psychological Therapies for Auditory Hallucinations (Voices): Current Status and Key Directions for Future Research. Schizophr Bull. 2014;40:S202-12.
18. Craig TK, Rus-Calafell M, Ward T, Leff JP, Huckvale M, Howarth E, et al. AVATAR therapy for auditory verbal hallucinations in people with psychosis: a single-blind, randomised controlled trial. Lancet Psychiatry. 2018;5:31-40.
19. Pontillo M, Crescenzo FD, Vicari S, Pucciarini ML, Averna R, Santonastaso O, et al. Cognitive behavioural therapy for auditory hallucinations in schizophrenia: A review. World J Psychiatry. 2016;6:372-80.
20. Thomas N, Bless JJ, Alderson-Day B, Bell IH, Cella M, Craig T, et al. Potential Applications of Digital Technology in Assessment, Treatment, and Self-help for Hallucinations. Schizophr Bull. 2019;45:S32-S42.
21. Sabe M, Sentissi O, Kaiser S. Meditation-based mind-body therapies for negative symptoms of schizophrenia: Systematic review of randomized controlled trials and meta-analysis. Schizophr Res. 2019;212:15-25.
22. Bangalore NG, Varambally S. Yoga therapy for Schizophrenia. Int J Yoga. 2012;5:85-91.
23. Ertekin Pinar S, Tel H. The Effect of Music on Auditory Hallucination and Quality of Life in Schizophrenic Patients: A Randomised Controlled Trial. Issues Ment Health Nurs. 2019;40:50-7.

CHAPTER 27

# Management of Negative Symptoms in Schizophrenia

*Rakshathi Basavaraju, Urvakhsh Meherwan Mehta, Jagadisha Thirthalli*

## INTRODUCTION

Negative symptoms in schizophrenia indicate a lack of or reduction in certain normal behaviors that are fundamental to intact functioning. They deserve special attention as they majorly contribute to long-term disability in schizophrenia, are frequently persistent and treatment resistant.

Negative symptoms are broadly divided into two psychopathological categories,[1,2] which are: (1) *Expressive deficits:* (i) Alogia characterized by poverty of speech and its content, lack of vocal inflections, and increased latency to respond verbally; (ii) affective flattening characterized by diminished range of emotional expressions and reactivity, poor eye contact, and paucity of nonverbal bodily gestures;[3] and (2) *Motivational deficits:* (i) Avolition/apathy characterized by diminished motivation to work, impoverished self-care and physical anergia; (ii) Anhedonia/asociality characterized by decreased interests in recreational activities, sexual activity, inability to form intimate relationships and reduced socialization.[3]

Negative symptoms are also classified into two clinically meaningful categories: (1) *Primary negative symptoms:* An inherent component of the schizophrenic illness which gives rise to enduring deficits; (2) *Secondary negative symptoms*: a result of another primary cause, namely, (i) positive psychotic symptoms, (ii) extrapyramidal symptoms (EPS) such as drug-induced parkinsonism, (iii) depression, (iv) social deprivation or lack of environmental stimulation, or (v) chronic substance/alcohol abuse.[4,5] Other than the conventional secondary negative symptoms described in literature, lately there have been mentions about unique instances where the negative symptoms can be secondary,[6-8] such causes are elaborated under the miscellaneous heading in **Flowchart 1**. This classification has treatment-related implications; hence, the clinician must arrive at this distinction during an assessment. Amongst established cases of schizophrenia, about 20% tend to have persistent primary negative symptoms.[9]

## ASSESSMENT OF NEGATIVE SYMPTOMS

A detailed clinical assessment is sufficient to assess the type and severity of negative symptoms. Expressive deficits can be reliably assessed with the patient interview alone. Equal or greater emphasis should be given to the account of the patient's primary caregivers in assessing the motivational deficits as it is often found that patients have poor insight into these deficits, and a patient interview alone may not give a reliable conclusion on the presence and severity of this domain. Simultaneously assessing the knowledge of caregivers about negative symptoms, the caregiving burden incurred by them, expressed emotions, role expectations of the patient by the family, the extent of accommodation and acceptance of the patient's negative symptoms by the family, and the financial condition of the family is also crucial in devising an individualized comprehensive management plan.

Select rating scales can supplement the clinical evaluation in assessing type and severity of negative symptoms and their components. The Scale for the Assessment of Negative Symptoms (SANS) can be used to assess the severity of the domains.[3] One can use the Schedule for the Deficit Syndrome (SDS)[10] to establish primary persistent negative symptoms. To rule out secondary negative symptoms due to depression, the Calgary Depression Scale in Schizophrenia (CDSS)[11] can be applied. This scale is specifically designed to diagnose depression in schizophrenia, the items comprising predominantly the cognitive and biological symptoms of depression to avoid overlap with negative symptoms of schizophrenia. Clinicians can also use Simpson Angus Rating Scale (SAS)[12] to quantify and differentiate drug-induced parkinsonism from primary negative symptoms.

**Flowchart 1:** Evaluation and management of negative symptoms of schizophrenia.

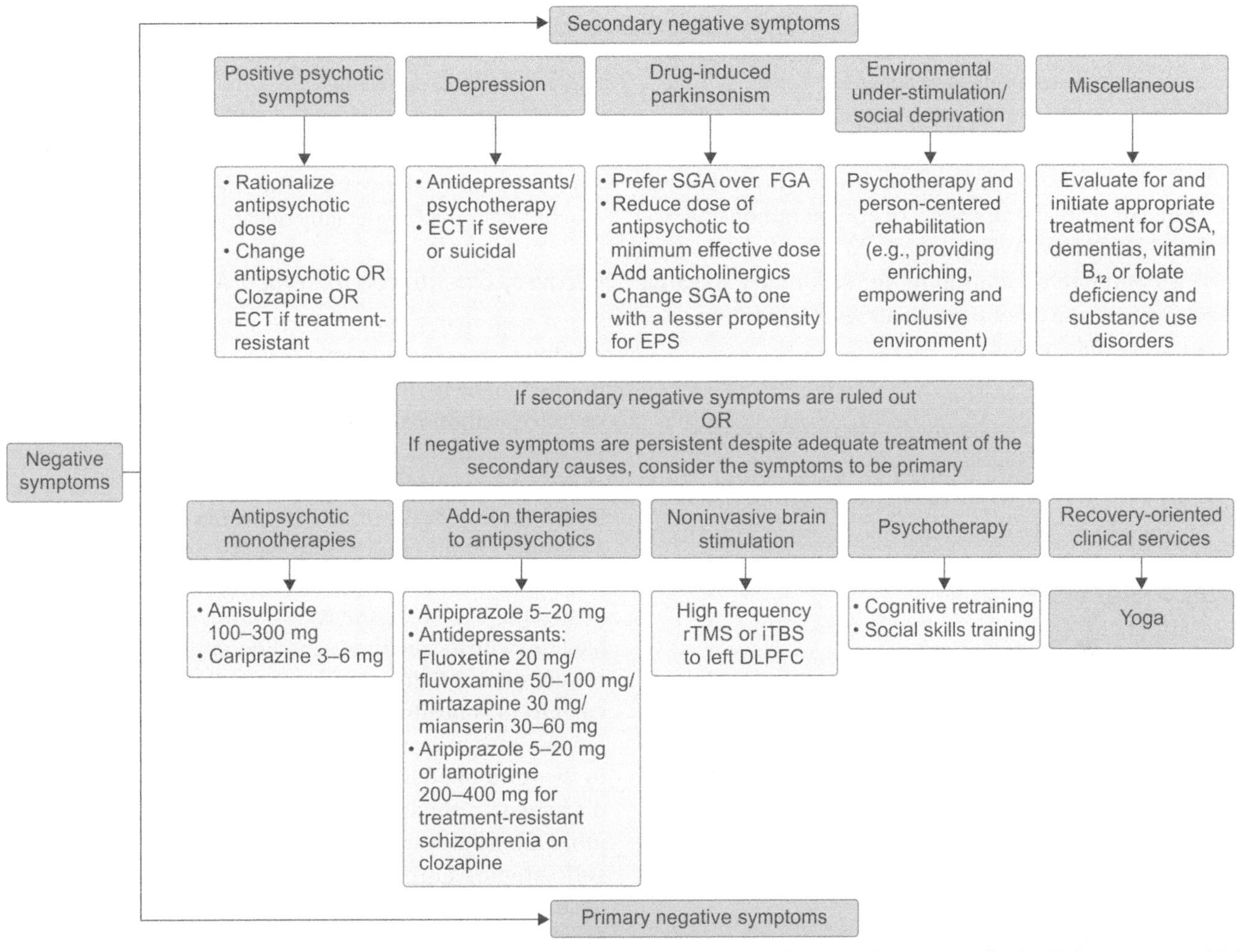


(ECT: electroconvulsive therapy; FGA: first generation antipsychotic; SGA: second generation antipsychotic; EPS: extrapyramidal symptoms; OSA: obstructive sleep apnea; rTMS: repetitive transcranial magnetic stimulation; iTBS: intermittent theta burst stimulation; DLPFC: dorsolateral prefrontal cortex)

After any intervention is offered to target negative symptoms, the impact of the intervention should be assessed at an interval of at least 3–6 months and generally not less than that to provide sufficient time for change in enduring deficits as well as to capture sustainability of changes.[13]

## MANAGEMENT

### Prevention of Negative Symptoms

Longer duration of untreated psychosis (DUP) is known to be associated with higher negative symptoms. It is debatable as to whether this is because patients with prominent negative symptoms seek help late, which suggests a reverse causal association between negative symptoms and longer DUP. However, experiments in which DUP was shortened through early detection programs have shown that shortening DUP prevents the development of negative symptoms over time.[14,15] Hence, it is crucial to treat first episode of schizophrenia as early as possible. Starting a second-generation antipsychotic instead of a first-generation antipsychotic is likely to prevent the occurrence of negative symptoms secondary to drug-induced EPS.

### Treatment of Negative Symptoms

#### *Pharmacology*

- *Secondary negative symptoms:* After thorough assessment, if the patient is diagnosed with secondary negative symptoms i.e., residual positive symptoms, EPS, depression, environmental under-stimulation, or other miscellaneous causes, the cause must be appropriately treated **(Flowchart 1)**.

- *Primary negative symptoms:* No treatment modalities for primary negative symptoms are backed by robust evidence. However, instead of offering no treatment, clinicians can attempt a few treatment options backed by some large, well-conducted trials, fairly (but not completely) controlling for secondary negative symptoms and a few meta-analyses. We mention a few such possible options:

*Monotherapies (antipsychotics):*

- *Amisulpiride 100–300 mg:*[16] There are only a few studies with a follow-up period of 6 months to 1 year. This period may be insufficient to comment on the sustainability of efficacy as well as safety in terms of the risk of psychotic relapse, especially in the lower dose range of 100–300 mg.
- Cariprazine 3–6 mg[17]

*Add-on therapies to antipsychotics:*

- Aripiprazole 5–20 mg[18]
- *Antidepressants:* Consider fluoxetine 20 mg/fluvoxamine 50–100 mg/mirtazapine 30 mg/mianserin 30–60 mg.[19,20]
- If the patient is treatment-resistant schizophrenia and is on clozapine, aripiprazole 5–20 mg[18] or lamotrigine 200–400 mg[21] can be added on.

There are many other pharmacological agents which are not discussed here. They are either studied in small, nonreplicated trials, have yielded inconsistent results in subsequent trials, or proved ineffective in large, well-conducted trials and meta-analyses.

### Noninvasive Brain Stimulation

Excitatory repetitive transcranial magnetic stimulation (rTMS) in the form of high frequency (10 Hz) conventional rTMS or intermittent theta burst stimulation (iTBS) over the left dorsolateral prefrontal cortex can be advised as an add-on therapy[22] for primary negative symptoms. Negative symptoms are not a standard indication for electroconvulsive therapy (ECT) in schizophrenia.

### Psychotherapy

Cognitive remediation[23] and social skills training[24] have some evidence for efficacy. Psychoeducation and family therapy aid the family in understanding and handling the negative symptoms of the patient better. Many cognitive behavioral therapies will aid in addressing disability and recovery in schizophrenia.[25]

### Alternative Forms of Therapy

Yoga has some evidence for being effective in the treatment of schizophrenia,[26] especially negative symptoms.[27]

### Recovery Orientation in Clinical Management

Since negative symptoms are a major contributor to disability in schizophrenia, rehabilitation is inevitable in the management of long-standing treatment-resistant negative symptoms.[28] As explained before, environmental under-stimulation and social deprivation are one of the causes of secondary negative symptoms, and many long-standing cases of schizophrenia will invariably be a complex combination of primary negative symptoms and a cascading chronic under-stimulation. Constant engagement of the patient in halfway homes or daycare facilities with a structured schedule, appropriate feedback/rewards for activities, and constant engagement of the caregivers is invaluable in providing a meaningful living for the patient and the family. Supported employment in the form of offering help in building curriculum vitae, placement in suitable jobs, constant training while on the job, and employer engagement can result in achieving self-esteem, ample integration into society, and a destigmatized identity leading to functional recovery.[29] Measures like disability assessment and certification not only bring financial respite to underprivileged families but also aid in assisted special employment of such patients. Psychotherapeutic and rehabilitative measures can go hand-in-hand in managing both primary as well as secondary negative symptoms. The above order implies no hierarchy of treatment efficacy. Clinicians can try any of the above sequentially or simultaneously as deemed feasible and suitable for a particular patient.

## REFERENCES

1. Strauss GP, Horan WP, Kirkpatrick B, Fischer BA, Keller WR, Miski P, et al. Deconstructing negative symptoms of schizophrenia: avolition-apathy and diminished expression clusters predict clinical presentation and functional outcome. J Psychiatr Res. 2013;47(6):783-90.
2. Galderisi S, Mucci A, Buchanan RW, Arango C. Negative symptoms of schizophrenia: new developments and unanswered research questions. Lancet Psychiatry. 2018;5(8):664-77.

3. Andreasen NC. The Scale for the Assessment of Negative Symptoms (SANS): conceptual and theoretical foundations. Br J Psychiatry Suppl. 1989;7:49-58.
4. Carpenter WT Jr, Heinrichs DW, Alphs LD. Treatment of negative symptoms. Schizophr Bull. 1985;11(3):440-52.
5. Kirkpatrick B. Developing concepts in negative symptoms: primary vs secondary and apathy vs expression. J Clin Psychiatry. 2014;75(Suppl 1):3-7.
6. Boufidis S, Kosmidis MH, Bozikas VP, Daskalopoulou-Vlahoyianni E, Pitsavas S, Karavatos A. Treatment outcome of obstructive sleep apnea syndrome in a patient with schizophrenia: case report. Int J Psychiatry Med. 2003;33(3):305-10.
7. Kulkarni G, Mehta UM, Das S, Arunachal G, Gunasekaran S, Chandra SR, et al. Novel CTSF Indel in a patient with Kufs disease and resistant schizophrenia: a case report. Schizophr Res. 2021;228:435-7.
8. Roffman JL, Lamberti JS, Achtyes E, Macklin EA, Galendez GC, Raeke LH, et al. Randomized multicenter investigation of folate plus vitamin B12 supplementation in schizophrenia. JAMA Psychiatry. 2013;70(5):481-9.
9. Bobes J, Arango C, Garcia-Garcia M, Rejas J, CLAMORS Study Collaborative Group. Prevalence of negative symptoms in outpatients with schizophrenia spectrum disorders treated with antipsychotics in routine clinical practice: findings from the CLAMORS study. J Clin Psychiatry. 2010;71(3):280-6.
10. Kirkpatrick B, Buchanan RW, McKenney PD, Alphs LD, Carpenter WT. The Schedule for the Deficit syndrome: an instrument for research in schizophrenia. Psychiatry Res. 1989;30(2):119-23.
11. Addington D, Addington J, Schissel B. A depression rating scale for schizophrenics. Schizophr Res. 1990;3(4):247-51.
12. Simpson GM, Angus JW. A rating scale for extrapyramidal side effects. Acta Psychiatr Scand Suppl. 1970;212:11-9.
13. Kirkpatrick B, Fenton WS, Carpenter WT, Marder SR. The NIMH-MATRICS Consensus Statement on Negative Symptoms. Schizophr Bull. 2006;32(2):214-9.
14. Waddington JL, Youssef HA, Kinsella A. Sequential cross-sectional and 10-year prospective study of severe negative symptoms in relation to duration of initially untreated psychosis in chronic schizophrenia. Psychol Med. 1995;25(4):849-57.
15. Melle I, Larsen TK, Haahr U, Friis S, Johannesen JO, Opjordsmoen S, et al. Prevention of negative symptom psychopathologies in first-episode schizophrenia: two-year effects of reducing the duration of untreated psychosis. Arch Gen Psychiatry. 2008;65(6):634-40.
16. Krause M, Zhu Y, Huhn M, Schneider-Thoma J, Bighelli I, Nikolakopoulou A, et al. Antipsychotic drugs for patients with schizophrenia and predominant or prominent negative symptoms: a systematic review and meta-analysis. Eur Arch Psychiatry Clin Neurosci. 2018;268(7):625-39.
17. Fleischhacker W, Galderisi S, Laszlovszky I, Szatmári B, Barabássy Á, Acsai K, et al. The efficacy of cariprazine in negative symptoms of schizophrenia: Post hoc analyses of PANSS individual items and PANSS-derived factors. Eur Psychiatry J Assoc Eur Psychiatr. 2019;58:1-9.
18. Galling B, Roldán A, Hagi K, Rietschel L, Walyzada F, Zheng W, et al. Antipsychotic augmentation vs. monotherapy in schizophrenia: systematic review, meta-analysis and meta-regression analysis. World Psychiatry. 2017;16(1):77-89.
19. Terevnikov V, Joffe G, Stenberg JH. Randomized controlled trials of add-on antidepressants in schizophrenia. Int J Neuropsychopharmacol. 2015;18:pyv049.
20. Möller HJ, Czobor P. Pharmacological treatment of negative symptoms in schizophrenia. Eur Arch Psychiatry Clin Neurosci. 2015;265(7):567-78.
21. Tiihonen J, Wahlbeck K, Kiviniemi V. The efficacy of lamotrigine in clozapine-resistant schizophrenia: a systematic review and meta-analysis. Schizophr Res. 2009;109(1-3):10-4.
22. Tseng PT, Zeng BS, Hung CM, Liang CS, Stubbs B, Carvalho AF, et al. Assessment of noninvasive brain stimulation interventions for negative symptoms of schizophrenia: a systematic review and network meta-analysis. JAMA Psychiatry. 2022;79(8):770-9.
23. Vita A, Barlati S, Ceraso A, Nibbio G, Ariu C, Deste G, et al. Effectiveness, core elements, and moderators of response of cognitive remediation for schizophrenia. JAMA Psychiatry. 2021;78(8):1-12.
24. Turner DT, McGlanaghy E, Cuijpers P, van der Gaag M, Karyotaki E, MacBeth A. A meta-analysis of social skills training and related interventions for psychosis. Schizophr Bull. 2018;44(3):475-91.
25. Nowak I, Sabariego C, Świtaj P, Anczewska M. Disability and recovery in schizophrenia: a systematic review of cognitive behavioral therapy interventions. BMC Psychiatry. 2016;16:228.
26. Bangalore NG, Varambally S. Yoga therapy for schizophrenia. Int J Yoga. 2012;5(2):85-91.
27. Rao NP, Ramachandran P, Jacob A, Joseph A, Thonse U, Nagendra B, et al. Add on yoga treatment for negative symptoms of schizophrenia: a multi-centric, randomized controlled trial. Schizophr Res. 2021;231:90-7.
28. Thirthalli J. Negative symptoms of schizophrenia: not all is negative! J Psychosoc Rehabil Ment Health. 2021;8:105-8.
29. Drake RE. Employment and schizophrenia: three innovative research approaches. Schizophr Bull. 2018;44(1):20-1.

CHAPTER 28

# Management of Aggression in Schizophrenia

*Dayal Narayan, Midhun Sidharthan*

## INTRODUCTION

Agitation is a state of physical and mental restlessness characterized by excessive motor activity, irritability, and inner tension. It is relatively common in patients with schizophrenia, with an estimated prevalence of 47.5%.[1] Agitation may progress to aggression and overtly violent behavior if not properly intervened at the right time. Hence, early identification and proper management of agitation and aggression are important for ensuring patient health and the safety of healthcare providers. **Flowchart 1** depicts the assessment and management of aggression in schizophrenia.

## ASSESSMENT

A prior diagnosis of schizophrenia does not exclude the possibility of other medical or surgical factors contributing to acute aggressive behavior **(Box 1)**. A focused medical assessment and essential relevant investigations to rule out such causes may be needed if the patient can be calmed with verbal de-escalation. This is particularly important in the subgroup of patients exhibiting certain clinical indicators.

There is no place for "routine" investigations in an emergency setting; tests should be chosen based on their potential immediate impact on management. Invasive investigations run the risk of further provoking a patient **(Box 2)**. Pregnancy should be anticipated and tested for in female patients of reproductive age. The geriatric population is particularly prone to serious

**Flowchart 1:** Assessment and management of aggression in schizophrenia.[6]

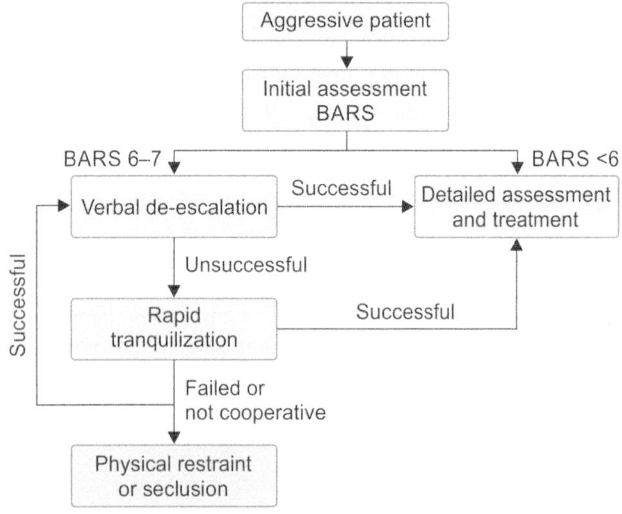


(BARS: Behavioral Activity Rating Scale)

**BOX 1:** ***Aggression in schizophrenia:*** Pointers to other causes.

- Substance intoxication/withdrawal
- Disorientation
- Memory problems
- Fever
- Excessive muscle rigidity
- Features of head injury
- Trauma
- Breathing difficulty
- Abnormal vital signs
- Seizures
- Incoordination
- Asymmetric pupil

**BOX 2:** Investigations in aggressive patients (as indicated clinically).

- Serum ammonia
- Serum CPK
- Serum electrolytes
- Complete blood count
- Blood glucose
- Liver function test
- Renal function test
- Neuroimaging (CT and MRI)
- Electroencephalography (EEG)

(CPK: creatine phosphokinase; CT: computed tomography; MRI: magnetic resonance imaging)

adverse reactions to antipsychotics and an increased risk of injuries during restraint. Akathisia can closely mimic and also coexist with psychotic aggression; therefore, it should be suspected, ruled out, or managed accordingly when identified. Adherence to the pertinent sections of the Mental Health Care Act is essential when managing an uncooperative patient displaying aggression.

The *Behavioral Activity Rating Scale* (BARS) is a 7-point scale used to measure agitation:

1. Difficult or unable to arouse
2. Asleep but responds normally to verbal or physical contact
3. Drowsy, appears sedated
4. Quiet and awake (normal level of activity)
5. Signs of overactivity (physical or verbal); calms down with instructions
6. Extremely or continuously active; does not require restraint
7. Violent behavior requiring restraint

This scale can be simplified to 4 levels:

1. *Not agitated*: Score 4
2. *Mildly agitated*: Score 5
3. *Moderately agitated*: Score 6
4. *Extremely agitated*: Score 7

This simplification makes it easier to identify and address different levels of agitation with appropriate treatments.[2]

## NONPHARMACOLOGICAL MANAGEMENT

Noncoercive approaches are preferred in clinical settings for managing aggression, thus avoiding premature use of restraints or involuntary medications. *Verbal de-escalation* is central to initial intervention in a patient who is aggressive or potentially aggressive. It is a communication-based approach to calming an agitated or aggressive patient, proceeding through three stages: (1) Engaging the patient verbally, (2) creating and maintaining a non-hostile relationship, and (3) helping the patient get out of the situation.[3]

The following factors are important determinants of successful verbal de-escalation:

- Ensure a safe environment by removing dangerous objects, providing adequate space, avoiding provocations/excess sensory stimulation, and ensuring an adequate number of trained staff.
- Ensure that the staff has appropriate skills and attitude.
- Be respectful and empathetic toward the patient.
- Take enough time; repeated engagement with the patient may be needed for desired results.
- *Keep a safe distance:* Stay two arm's length from the patient and avoid violating their personal space.
- *Be nonprovocative:* Use gentle body language and avoid sustained eye contact. Approach the patient from the sides or at an angle. Do not keep the fists clenched or hands concealed from the patient.
- *Be polite and introduce yourself:* Let the patient know you are there to help them. It is best if one person does the talking.
- *Use clear and simple language:* Speak in a calm and slow voice. Use small sentences and familiar vocabulary. Repeat things often and rephrase as needed.
- Be nonjudgemental; listen to the patient's wants and needs. Try to understand their perspective and respond in a respectful and supportive way.
- *Set limits:* Gently remind the patient about the consequences of their behavior in a non-threatening way.
- Give the patient choices about how to resolve the situation. If they are not willing to take medication, try to find other options that will work for them. Suggest to the patient that he may need medications to get adequate control, and ask him which route he prefers.
- *Explain your actions:* If you are forced to take coercive action, explain why you had to do so to the patient. This can help them to understand and accept your decision.
- *Provide space:* If the patient is delusional or fearful, give them adequate space to move.

## PHARMACOLOGICAL MANAGEMENT

Persistent aggressive behavior, despite de-escalation measures in the absence of clinical pointers toward medical causes for aggression, would necessitate appropriate pharmacological management **(Table 1)**.[4,5] Antipsychotics and benzodiazepines are commonly used for this purpose. The preferred route of administration would be parenteral, specifically intramuscular. This route offers advantages such as rapid onset of action, predictable bioavailability, and does not require patient cooperation (**Box 3** depicts for monitoring after rapid tranquilization). Oral treatment can be a feasible and equally effective option if patients cooperate following verbal de-escalation. Although the inhalational route is emerging with a few medications, it is not yet available in India. Intravenous haloperidol

**TABLE 1:** Pharmacological management of aggression.[4,5]

| *Medicines* | *Dose* | *Repeat after* | *Maximum dose per day* |
|---|---|---|---|
| *Parenteral* | | | |
| Haloperidol [intramuscular (IM)] | 5–10 mg | 15 minutes | 20 mg |
| Haloperidol + Promethazine (IM) | 5–10 mg + 25–50 mg | 30 minutes | 30 mg (haloperidol)<br>100 mg (promethazine) |
| Haloperidol + lorazepam (IM) | 5 mg + 2 mg | 1 hour | 30 mg (haloperidol)<br>4 mg (lorazepam) |
| Lorazepam (IM) | 2–4 mg | 2 hours | 12 mg |
| Olanzapine (IM) | 10 mg | 20 minutes | 30 mg |
| Zuclopenthixol (IM) | 50 mg | 24–48 hours | 150 mg |
| *Oral*[†] | | | |
| Haloperidol | 5–10 mg | 15 minutes | 20 mg |
| Lorazepam | 2 mg | 2 hours | 12 mg |
| Olanzapine | 5–10 mg | 2 hours | 20 mg |
| Risperidone | 2 mg | 2 hours | 6 mg |

[†]Tablet or liquid formulation

**BOX 3:** Monitoring after rapid tranquillization.

- Pulse rate, blood pressure, respiratory rate, and temperature should be monitored every 15 minutes for the first hour, then hourly until the patient wakes up and is ambulatory
- If uncooperative, watch for fever, reduced respiratory rate, and general physical well-being

**TABLE 2:** Seclusion and restraint.

| *If a threat to others* | *No immediate threat to others* | *Behavior poses an active threat to the patient's own safety* |
|---|---|---|
| Restraint or locked seclusion | Seclusion in a quiet, unlocked room | Restraint may be needed |

increases the risk of QT prolongation, particularly in the elderly. So it is advisable to avoid this route in patients with borderline prolonged QT intervals or those taking medications that may cause QT prolongation.

Newer pharmacological options approved for treating aggression in schizophrenia include sublingual dexmedetomidine and inhaled loxapine:

1. *Sublingual dexmedetomidine:* Initial dose is 120–180 μg; maximum daily dosage is 360 μg; two more additional doses 2 hours apart if agitation is not controlled by a single administration.
2. *Inhaled loxapine:* 10 mg/oral inhalation using an inhaler; only a single dose of a maximum of 10 mg/24 hours. Bronchospasm may develop in some patients.

## SECLUSION AND RESTRAINT

*Seclusion* and *restraint* should only be used as a last resort **(Table 2)**. When restraint is necessary, it should be used sparingly to minimize trauma, employing the least restrictive form of management while ensuring the patient's dignity and privacy. Trained staff should implement four-point restraint, employing appropriate personal protection methods against kicking, biting, spitting, etc. Vital signs, blood flow, and the restraint site (for indications of pain, heat, swelling, or wounds) should be monitored immediately upon application of restraints; subsequently, reassess every 15 minutes for 1 hour and every 30 minutes for the following 4 hours. Conduct brief and specific symptom evaluations when the patient is more cooperative. This approach will help optimize treatment and reduce the recurrence of aggressive behavior.

## REFERENCES

1. Mi W, Zhang S, Liu Q, Yang F, Wang Y, Li T, et al. Prevalence and risk factors of agitation in newly hospitalized schizophrenia patients in China: An observational survey. Psychiatry Res. 2017;253:401-6.

2. Swift RH, Harrigan EP, Cappelleri JC, Kramer D, Chandler LP. Validation of the behavioural activity rating scale (BARS): a novel measure of activity in agitated patients. J Psychiatr Res. 2002;36(2):87-95.
3. Richmond JS, Berlin JS, Fishkind AB, Holloman GH Jr, Zeller SL, Wilson MP, et al. Verbal De-escalation of the agitated patient: Consensus statement of the American Association for Emergency Psychiatry Project BETA De-escalation Workgroup. West J Emerg Med. 2012;13(1):17-25.
4. Wilson MP, Pepper D, Currier GW, Holloman GH Jr, Feifel D. The psychopharmacology of agitation: Consensus Statement of the American Association for Emergency Psychiatry Project BETA Psychopharmacology Workgroup. West J Emerg Med. 2012;13(1):26-34.
5. Baldaçara L, Diaz AP, Leite V, Pereira LA, Dos Santos RM, Gomes Júnior VP, et al. Brazilian guidelines for the management of psychomotor agitation. Part 2. Pharmacological approach. Braz J Psychiatry. 2019; 41(12):324-35.
6. Stowell KR, Florence P, Harman HJ, Glick RL. Psychiatric evaluation of the agitated patient: Consensus Statement of the American Association for Emergency Psychiatry Project BETA Psychiatric Evaluation Workgroup. West J Emerg Med. 2012;13(1):11-6.

CHAPTER

# 29 Management of Catatonia

NA Uvais, AM Ashfaq U Rahman

## FLOWCHART FOR MANAGEMENT OF CATATONIA (FLOWCHART 1)

A. *When to suspect catatonia:* Catatonia is a complex neuropsychiatric syndrome that can present with multiple signs and symptoms. It is seen in a variety of general medical conditions and severe psychiatric disorders. A diagnosis of catatonia should be considered whenever a patient presents with substantially altered levels of motor activity or abnormal behavior.[1]

B. *Diagnosis of catatonia:* A diagnosis of catatonia can be confidently made based on the clinical assessment of the patient, which includes history taking, clinical observation, elicitation of various signs, and physical

**Flowchart 1:** Management of catatonia.

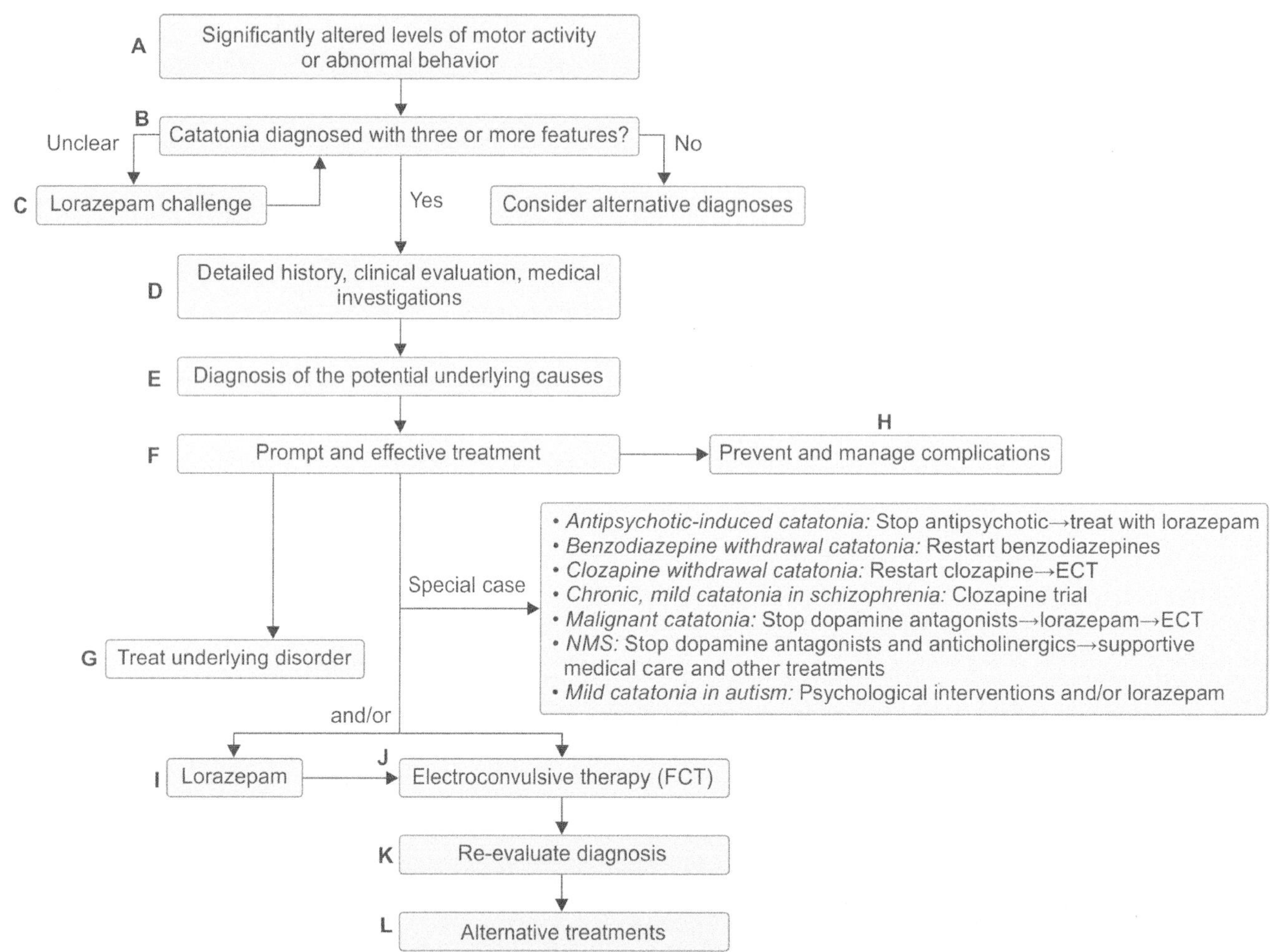

examination. A detailed history should be collected from the patient and/or caregivers to clarify the phenomenology, time course, and possible causes. Clinical observation of a patient suspected to have catatonia can reveal the following catatonic signs: stupor, agitation, posturing, mannerism, stereotypy, grimacing, impulsivity, combativeness, staring, and verbigeration. Catatonic signs such as mutism, negativism, echolalia, echopraxia, and ambitendency need to be elicited by environmental stimuli, whereas assessment of catalepsy, rigidity, and waxy flexibility requires physical examination. A diagnosis of catatonia can be made if three or more signs are present.[1] It is always better to use standardized rating instruments, such as the *Bush-Francis Catatonia Rating Scale* (BFCRS), while evaluating patients with catatonia to document various signs of catatonia, the longitudinal course, and treatment response.[2] An online link to BFCRS is provided here that includes useful brief descriptions and example videos of various catatonic signs (https://www.urmc.rochester.edu/MediaLibraries/URMCMedia/psychiatry/about/docs/BFCRS-with-Manual-links.pdf).

C. *Lorazepam challenge test:* In patients where there are ambiguities in diagnosing catatonic syndrome (i.e., if there are less than three signs of catatonia), a *lorazepam challenge test* can be performed to clarify the diagnosis. The recommended dose for a lorazepam challenge test is 1–2 mg intravenous/intramuscular or 2 mg oral lorazepam. After administering lorazepam, the patient should be reassessed after 5 minutes following intravenous lorazepam, 15 minutes following intramuscular lorazepam, or 30 minutes following oral lorazepam. A positive response is defined as a 50% reduction in the score in a standardized catatonia rating scale from the baseline score.[1]

D. *History, clinical evaluation, medical investigations:* In patients with suspected catatonia, a comprehensive approach involving detailed history taking, physical examination, and laboratory investigations is crucial to establish the diagnosis and identify potential underlying causes. Detailed information about the patient's medical, neurological, and psychiatric history should be taken to identify potential underlying causes of catatonia. Specifically, any history of exposure to or withdrawal from medications (e.g., benzodiazepines and clozapine), as well as recreational substances, should be explored.[1] Measuring plasma concentration of drugs and urine drug screening may be considered if available. Every patient presenting with a first episode of catatonia should receive a thorough clinical and laboratory evaluation for potential underlying medical disorders.[1]

- Clinical investigations such as laboratory investigations (including complete hemogram, liver and renal function tests, serum electrolytes, blood sugar, serum ammonia), brain imaging, electroencephalogram EEG, and cerebrospinal fluid (CSF) analysis should be judiciously ordered, based on the history and clinical examination findings, severity, and co-morbid medical and psychiatric illnesses. In patients with recurrent catatonia, clinicians should assess whether an adequate medical evaluation was done in the past and perform a detailed medical evaluation in the index episode to address potential complications of catatonia.[1]

E,F. *Diagnosis of the potential underlying causes and prompt treatment:* Following clinical evaluation and medical investigations, a potential underlying psychiatric or medical cause can often be identified in most patients with catatonia. Once a definitive diagnosis of catatonia is made, prompt and effective treatment should be initiated. Ideally, the treatment of catatonia should occur at a tertiary center where options for relevant investigations to rule out various medical causes of catatonia, as well as treatment options for catatonia and its potential complications, are available.[1] However, it is not always necessary to wait for medical investigation results to initiate treatment. In addition to treating catatonic features per se, the management of catatonic syndrome also involves the treatment of underlying causes and preventing and managing complications.

G. *Treatment of underlying causes:* Prompt and effective management of the underlying causes of catatonia is critical for a better prognosis. In emergency psychiatric settings, catatonia is most likely to occur in patients with bipolar disorder with psychotic features, psychotic depression, schizophrenia, and autism spectrum disorder. However, antipsychotics, especially D2 receptor antagonists, should be used with special caution in catatonia, considering the higher risk of neuroleptic malignant syndrome (NMS).[1] Catatonia can also be a presenting symptom of many general medical conditions, such as infectious, metabolic, autoimmune, and neurological disorders. In patients with catatonia secondary to general medical conditions, treatment of the general medical conditions should be prioritized over the treatment of catatonic features per se.

*Special clinical scenarios:*

- *Antipsychotic-induced catatonia:* Patients should be treated with lorazepam after discontinuing antipsychotic agents.
- *Benzodiazepine withdrawal catatonia:* Benzodiazepines should be restarted in these patients.
- *Clozapine withdrawal catatonia:* Clozapine should be restarted. If there is no response, electroconvulsive therapy (ECT) should be initiated.
- *Schizophrenia with chronic mild catatonia:* A trial of clozapine should be considered for treatment.
- *Malignant catatonia:* Treatment with lorazepam and/or ECT should be initiated after discontinuing dopamine antagonists.
- *Neuroleptic malignant syndrome:* Supportive medical care and other treatments should be provided after discontinuing dopamine antagonists and anticholinergics.
- *Autism with mild catatonia:* Treatment with psychological interventions and/or lorazepam may be considered.

H. *Prevention and management of complications:* In every patient with catatonia, clinicians should prioritize prevention and management of complications. Appropriate supportive measures and treatments are needed to maintain adequate hydration, nutrition, and oxygenation, as well as to prevent complications such as deep vein thrombosis, pulmonary embolism, aspiration pneumonia, pressure ulcers, and muscle contractures.[3]

I. *Lorazepam:* Lorazepam stands as the most evidence-based first-line treatment option for catatonia. It can be administered orally, nasogastrically, intramuscularly, or intravenously, typically in two to three divided doses per day. Most studies have used 1-4 mg of lorazepam per day, and some have recommended a maximum of 16–24 mg/day.[1] Initial parenteral administration of lorazepam may be more useful in patients with negativism, with a transition to oral administration as catatonia improves. Therapeutic response to lorazepam may appear within hours or take several days. An adequate trial may be considered once catatonic signs are adequately resolved, upward dose titration ceases due to adverse effects, or the maximum dose is reached (i.e., 6–24 mg/day).[1] For patients responding well to lorazepam, a slow taper of the dose over a few weeks should be considered.[1] However, some patients experiencing catatonia recurrence during tapering may require longer treatment with lorazepam. Positive responses to lorazepam in catatonia vary, ranging from 66 to 100% in studies.[1] Lorazepam is typically more effective in acute catatonia due to mood disorders. Patients having an inadequate response to an adequate trial of lorazepam should be considered for electroconvulsive therapy and other alternative treatment modalities.

J. *ECT:* ECT is considered one of the most effective treatments for catatonia, particularly when medications have failed. ECT should be considered when there is no significant improvement in catatonic signs even after 48–72 hours of a lorazepam trial with a dose of at least 6–8 mg/day, or as a first-line treatment when lorazepam is contraindicated.[1,3] Additionally, there is evidence supporting combination treatment with lorazepam and ECT in cases of suboptimal response to an initial lorazepam trial, as these treatments may synergistically enhance efficacy.[4] Bilateral ECT is typically preferred for the treatment of catatonia. In acute catatonia, ECT should be administered at least twice weekly. The total number of ECT sessions should be decided based on treatment response, associated risks, and side effects.

K. *Re-evaluate diagnosis:* In patients exhibiting poor response to benzodiazepines and/or ECT for catatonia, a re-evaluation of diagnosis is crucial. Various neurological conditions, such as movement disorders, speech disorders, seizure disorders, locked-in syndrome, and delirium, as well as psychiatric disorders, such as functional neurological disorders, malingering, and factitious disorders, may present with symptoms mimicking catatonia.[1] It is important to rule out such conditions before considering alternative treatment options.

L. *Alternative treatments:* For patients with catatonia who do not respond to benzodiazepines and/or ECT, alternative treatment options should be considered. These options are also relevant in patients who refuse ECT, lack access to ECT, or have contraindications for benzodiazepines or ECT. Numerous case reports have described various treatments that have shown beneficial results when added either as monotherapies or as augmentation agents to lorazepam treatment. Monotherapy treatments include amantadine, methylphenidate, carbamazepine, valproic acid, phenytoin, levetiracetam, zonisamide, bromocriptine, benztropine, and trihexyphenidyl.[1,3] Augmentation strategies to lorazepam treatment include memantine, minocycline, topiramate, and zolpidem.[1,3] Additionally, repetitive transcranial magnetic stimulation (rTMS) and transcranial direct-current stimulation (tDCS) over the bilateral dorsolateral prefrontal cortex have shown therapeutic benefits in patients with catatonia.[1]

## REFERENCES


1. Rogers JP, Oldham MA, Fricchione G, Northoff G, Ellen Wilson J, Mann SC, et al. Evidence-based consensus guidelines for the management of catatonia: Recommendations from the British Association for Psychopharmacology. J Psychopharmacol. 2023; 37(4):327-69.
2. Bush G, Fink M, Petrides G, Dowling F, Francis A. Catatonia. I. Rating scale and standardized examination. Acta Psychiatr Scand. 1996;93(2):129-36.
3. Coffey MJ, Catatonia: Treatment & Prognosis, Byrne PP, Marder S, Solomon D (Ed), UpToDate, Waltham, MA (Accessed on 1/6/2023)
4. Petrides G, Divadeenam KM, Bush G, Francis A. Synergism of lorazepam and electroconvulsive therapy in the treatment of catatonia. Biol Psychiatry. 1997;42(5):375-81.

CHAPTER 30

# Management of Delusional Disorder

*Shahul Ameen, Sreya Mariyam Salim*

## SECTION 1: EVALUATION

Check for modifiable risk factors of delusional disorder (DD), such as social isolation and sensory impairment. Exclude organicity, substance use, and prescribed medications as the cause of the delusions. Medications that can cause symptoms of delusional infestation (DI) include corticosteroids, stimulants, opiates, benzodiazepines, dopaminergic agents, ketoconazole, fluoroquinolones, and topiramate. Depression has been found in 21–56% of DD patients, and serious medical comorbidities in 66%, type 2 diabetes being the commonest. Baseline evaluations recommended in schizophrenia may be considered: pulse, blood pressure, weight, height, fasting blood glucose or glycated hemoglobin (HbA1C), lipid profile, complete blood count, electrolytes, renal and liver function tests, thyroid stimulating hormone (TSH), and pregnancy testing in women of childbearing potential.

## SECTION 2: MAINTAINING THERAPEUTIC ALLIANCE

Proper interviews can be therapeutic in themselves and can influence treatment adherence. The first step is to create a safe space for the patient's concerns through active listening and empathy. A delusion is a person's reality, and it is important to explore its personal meaning—its effects on work, mood, and social interactions; life factors that precipitated it; the patient's explanatory model, etc.[1] Be empathic while eliciting the details of the delusions' content. Avoid agreeing with or arguing about the delusion. Avoid confronting the falsehood of the claims, except during cognitive behavior therapy (CBT). Address the accompanying emotions and not the logic of the presented arguments. Reluctance to take antipsychotics may be countered with statements like "People with your condition often have elevated dopamine levels in the brain, and medications that correct them have been found to help". In DI, rather than discussing the underlying cause (infestation), affirm the distress and the severity of the experience, and inform that the symptoms can be ameliorated even if their source is not found.

## SECTION 3: ANTIPSYCHOTICS

According to a 2016 systematic review,[2] in 385 DD patients, antipsychotics achieved a good response in 33.6%; higher rates (39%) were noted with first-generation antipsychotics (FGAs) than second (28%); no specific antipsychotic had superiority over another. However, the authors found no randomized control trials to include in the review. A 2020 systematic review,[3] which included only studies that employed a clinician-rated scale, found FGAs to be only marginally superior; among the most used agents, risperidone (34.3%) and olanzapine (33.7%) had the highest response rates. In a cohort study of 9,076 DD patients,[4] 2,074 had at least one hospitalization for psychosis, the risk of which was 46% lower when any antipsychotic was used. Use of clozapine, any long-acting injectable, or oral olanzapine was associated with the lowest risk. A systematic review of 15 case series of 280 patients with DI found that aripiprazole had the highest complete remission rates (79%, $n = 14$).[5] A 2006 review found pimozide more effective than other antipsychotics in somatic DD;[6] however, pimozide is no longer regarded as a first-line antipsychotic as it increases the QT interval. Some studies have reported that, in general, the required doses in treating DD are lower than those needed for schizophrenia; others found that similar doses are necessary for both conditions. No specific guidelines exist on the duration of adequate trials or switching strategies for DD.

## SECTION 4: ANTIDEPRESSANTS

Antidepressants, especially selective serotonin reuptake inhibitors (SSRIs), might be helpful, especially in the somatic

**Flowchart 1:** Management of delusional disorder.

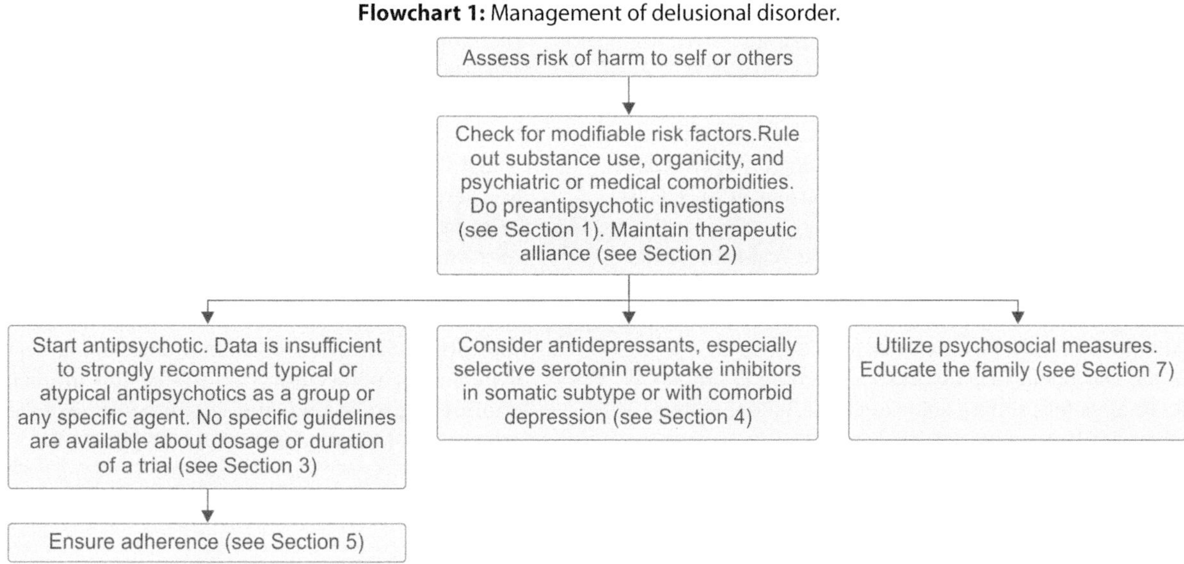


DD type, possibly by improving depressive symptoms or alleviating possible underlying serotonergic dysfunction. The systematic review of DI patients mentioned earlier found that in patients with comorbid depression, anxiety, or trichotillomania, SSRIs were the most effective among drug classes, with a complete remission rate of 79% and a partial remission rate of 43%.[5]

## SECTION 5: ENSURING ADHERENCE

Compared to schizophrenia, worse insight leading to worse adherence has been reported in DD. Measures to improve adherence include cost reduction, better social support, once-a-day dosing, and psychoeducation.

## SECTION 6: AGGRESSION AND SUICIDE

In managing aggression, deescalation strategies are generally preferred over pharmacotherapy.[7] The suicide risk rate is 8–21%, the highest being in those with somatic or persecutory delusions.

## SECTION 7: PSYCHOSOCIAL INTERVENTIONS

Cognitive behavior therapy helps identify and improve data gathering bias, interpersonal sensitivity, and reasoning style; teaches distress tolerance and coping skills; and encourages participation in enjoyable activities. It aims to facilitate an alternate model of thinking and acceptance, thus reducing the harmful consequences of delusions, such as distress, worry, and insomnia. Challenging the delusion is done only gently and after establishing a good therapeutic relationship.[8]

In a pilot study, emotional processing and metacognitive awareness intervention, a new brief treatment technique with three 1-hour sessions, significantly reduced delusional distress. It focused on increasing access to emotional experience, reducing verbal-linguistic processing (i.e., describing the current experience, as it is, nonjudgmentally, using experiential focus), and training in metacognitive awareness (i.e., labeling and noting down thoughts, feelings, sensations, images, and memories to recognize them as such and that they are not facts) to help the patients accept their experience without judgments.[9]

Teach the family to maintain a neutral stance towards the delusion and adopt empathic methods such as valuing the patient's opinion, being kind, respectful, and appreciative, and using distraction techniques. Family should also be taught to recognize and appropriately respond to impending signs of aggression.[1]

**Flowchart 1** summarizes the above recommendations.

## REFERENCES

1. González-Rodríguez A, Seeman MV. Addressing delusions in women and men with delusional disorder: Key points for clinical management. Int J Environ Res Public Health. 2020;17(12):4583.

2. Muñoz-Negro JE, Cervilla JA. A systematic review on the pharmacological treatment of delusional disorder. J Clin Psychopharmacol. 2016;36(6):684-90.
3. Muñoz-Negro JE, Gómez-Sierra FJ, Peralta V, González-Rodríguez A, Cervilla JA. A systematic review of studies with clinician-rated scales on the pharmacological treatment of delusional disorder. Int Clin Psychopharmacol. 2020;35(3): 129-36.
4. Lähteenvuo M, Taipale H, Tanskanen A, Mittendorfer-Rutz E, Tiihonen J. Effectiveness of pharmacotherapies for delusional disorder in a Swedish national cohort of 9076 patients. Schizophr Res. 2021;228:367-72.
5. Lu JD, Gotesman RD, Varghese S, Fleming P, Lynde CW. Treatments for primary delusional infestation: systematic review. JMIR Dermatol. 2022;5(1):e34323.
6. Manschreck TC, Khan NL. Recent advances in the treatment of delusional disorder. The Can J Psychiatry. 2006;51(2):114-9.
7. González-Rodríguez A, Seeman MV, Román E, Natividad M, Pagés C, Ghigliazza C, et al. Critical issues in the management of agitation, aggression, and end-of-life in delusional disorder: a mini-review. Healthcare. 2023;11(4):458.
8. O'Connell JE, Jackson HJ. Unusual conditions: delusional infestation: is it beyond psychological understanding and treatment? Time to rethink? Psychosis. 2017;10(1): 38-46.
9. Hepworth C, Startup H, Freeman D. Developing treatments of persistent persecutory delusions: the impact of an emotional processing and metacognitive awareness intervention. J Nerv Ment Dis. 2011;199(9):653-8.

# Rational Antipsychotic Polypharmacy: When, Where, and How to Use?

*Tess Maria Rajan, Muthukrishnan Venkatesan*

## INTRODUCTION

Antipsychotic polypharmacy (APP) is defined as the simultaneous prescription of more than one antipsychotic at a given time.[1] While most treatment guidelines do not recommend APP and suggest its use only in special circumstances, it is not uncommon. The median worldwide prevalence of APP use is around 19.2%, and in Asia, it is 32%; hence, understanding the rational use of APP is crucial.[1,2]

## COMMON INDICATIONS FOR APP[2-5]

- APP is commonly used in treatment-resistant schizophrenia when there is a poor or partial response to clozapine.
- In some cases, a second antipsychotic is added to mitigate certain side effects caused by the first antipsychotic. For instance, aripiprazole is often added to reduce antipsychotic-induced hyperprolactinemia.
- Patients may be briefly on APP while cross-titrating from one antipsychotic to another.
- APP is frequently used in the acute management of psychiatric conditions, where an injectable antipsychotic may be used for rapid tranquilization in addition to the regular oral antipsychotic.

## ANTIPSYCHOTIC POLYPHARMACY: GOOD CLINICAL PRACTICE[1,3,6]

- If a patient is being prescribed APP, the indication and further treatment plan should be clearly documented in the patient's clinical records.
- Before initiating APP, it is advisable to go through the following checklist.
    - Was the first antipsychotic tried at an adequate dose for an adequate duration?
    - Has compliance been ensured in cases where APP is used for partial response to the first antipsychotic? Have plasma levels of the first antipsychotic been checked for recommended levels, wherever possible?
    - Have other modalities of evidence-based pharmacological (e.g., long-acting injectables), neuromodulation (e.g., electroconvulsive therapy [ECT], psychological (e.g., cognitive behavior therapy [CBT] and psychosocial intervention for the given indication been tried?
    - Has a comorbid psychiatric or medical condition that could be contributing to the current picture been ruled out?
    - Is there a need to revisit the diagnosis?
- If a patient is on APP, it is ideal to regularly review the need for this combination by considering the benefits and risks for the patient.
- The choice of the second antipsychotic can be informed by their receptor profile (e.g., combining antipsychotics targeting different receptors for wider symptom coverage) and the side effect profile (e.g., avoiding antipsychotics with similar side effect profile to minimize the additive effect of risks).
- Patients on APP should regularly continue the recommended physical health monitoring for antipsychotics, including electrocardiogram (ECG), and they should be systematically monitored for antipsychotic-related side effects.

An algorithm to aid decision making with regards to the use of APP is discussed in **Flowchart 1**.

## EVIDENCE ON ANTIPSYCHOTIC POLYPHARMACY[3,7]

- There is some evidence of a reduction in the risk of hospitalization in APP. However, the evidence for this is limited and is derived mostly from combinations involving clozapine and long-acting injectables (LAIs).

**Flowchart 1:** Decision making algorithm for antipsychotic polypharmacy (APP).

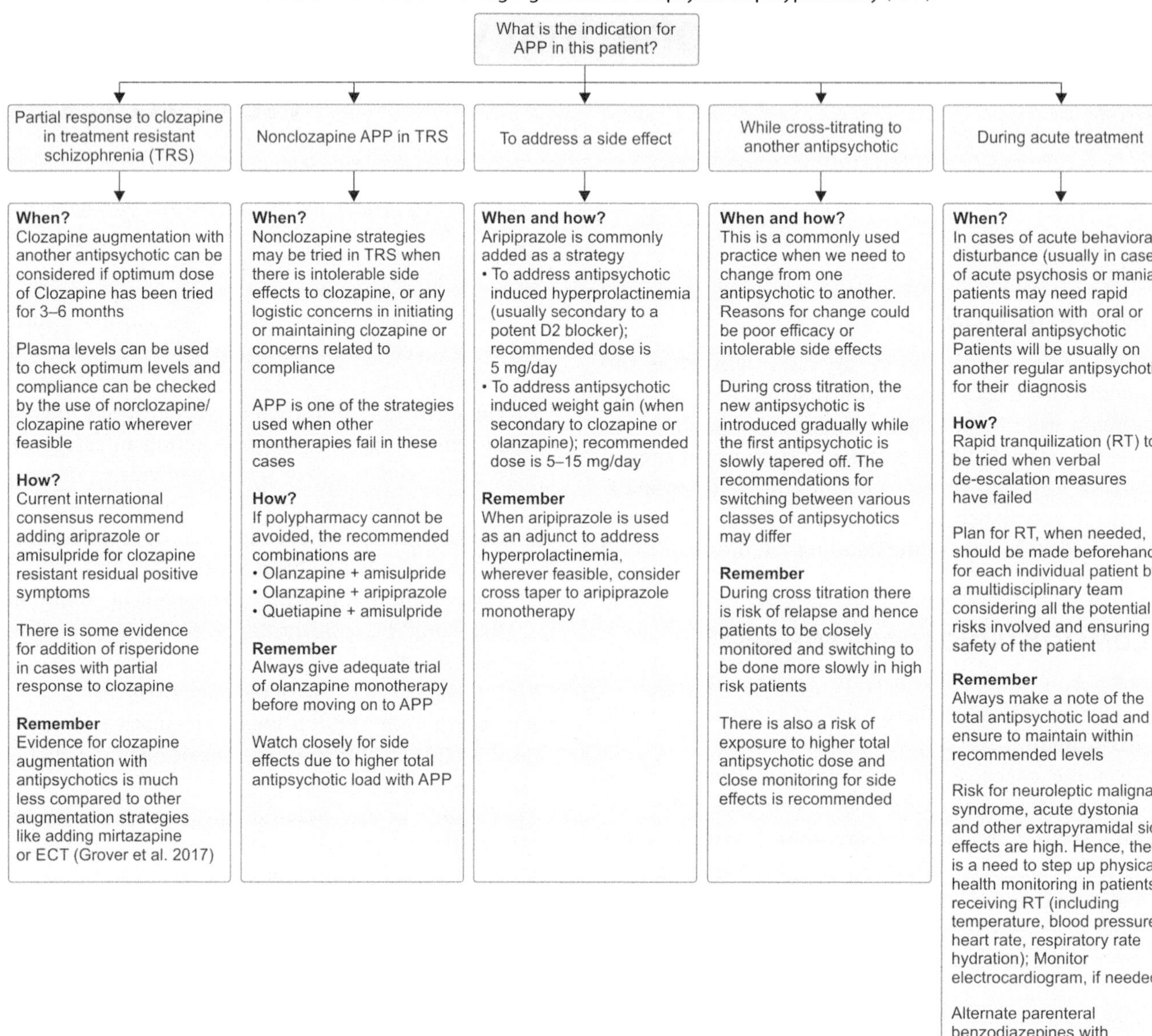


- There is more evidence of significant concerns related to the increased burden of side effects and high risk to patients from exposure to higher total antipsychotic doses.
- On the whole, APP is best avoided routinely and should be used after weighing the risks and benefits for each patient.

## REFERENCES

1. Lähteenvuo, M., Tiihonen, J. Antipsychotic Polypharmacy for the Management of Schizophrenia: Evidence and Recommendations. Drugs. 2021;81(11):1273-84.
2. Foster A, King J. Antipsychotic polypharmacy. Focus (Am Psychiatr Publ). 2020;18(4):375-85.

3. Taylor DM, Barnes TRE, Young AH. The Maudsley prescribing guidelines in psychiatry, 14th edition. New Jersey: John Wiley & Sons; 2021.
4. Grover S, Chakrabarti S, Kulhara P, Avasthi A. Clinical Practice Guidelines for Management of Schizophrenia. Indian J Psychiatry. 2017;59(Suppl 1): S19-S33.
5. Galletly C, Castle D, Dark F, Humberstone V, Jablensky A, Killackey E, et al. Royal Australian and New Zealand College of Psychiatrists clinical practice guidelines for the management of schizophrenia and related disorders. Aust N Z J Psychiatry. 2016;50(5): 410-72.
6. National Institute for Health and Care Excellence. (2014) Psychosis and schizophrenia in adults: prevention and management. www.nice.org.uk/guidance/cg178/chapter/1-Recommendations [Last accessed June, 2025].
7. Tiihonen J, Taipale H, Mehtälä J, Vattulainen P, Correll CU, Tanskanen A. Association of Antipsychotic Polypharmacy vs Monotherapy With Psychiatric Rehospitalization Among Adults With Schizophrenia. JAMA Psychiatry. 2019;76(5):499-507.

# How and When to Stop Treatment for Psychotic Disorders

*Gajanan Ganapati Sabhahit, Shivani Sivaramakrishnan, Suresh Bada Math*

## INTRODUCTION

Psychotic disorders include a range of diagnoses, from acute and transient psychotic disorders (ATPD) to schizophrenia and other chronic psychoses. Long-term treatment is generally recommended for these disorders. However, there is difficulty in accepting prolonged treatment among patients. Also, long-term use of psychotropic medications carries risks and side effects. While there are robust guidelines backed by research on starting these medications, there is a lack of clear protocols on when and how to stop them. This chapter aims to provide guidance on when not to stop treatment, when to consider stopping treatment, and how to stop treatment in psychotic disorders, based on existing research and consensus.

## WHEN NOT TO STOP TREATMENT?

It is challenging to determine when to stop treatment for psychotic disorders. However, it is easier for the clinician to identify when not to stop treatment. The following factors guide the reader on when not to stop treatment for psychotic disorders:

- Patient-related factors
- Illness-related factors
- Psychosocial factors

## PATIENT-RELATED FACTORS[1,2]

### Younger Age of Onset

Patients with an earlier onset, such as childhood schizophrenia, usually have a poorer prognosis. It is important not to stop treatment abruptly for these individuals. Continued treatment and support are essential to manage symptoms, prevent relapse, and promote overall well-being.

### Genetic Vulnerability and Family History

Patients with a genetic vulnerability or a family history of psychiatric illness are at a higher risk of developing psychotic disorders. Considering this increased susceptibility, maintenance treatment is advisable to manage symptoms effectively and minimize relapse risk.

### Poor Insight into Illness

A lack of insight is common in psychotic disorders. Patients with poor insight may not recognize the need for ongoing treatment or understand the consequences of discontinuing medication. Continuing treatment is essential to ensure symptom stabilization and prevent relapse in these cases.

### History of Noncompliance and Relapse

Patients with a prior history of noncompliance with medication or treatment are more likely to relapse. Stopping treatment prematurely for these individuals can increase the risk of symptom recurrence and functional impairment. Therefore, it is important to maintain treatment and closely monitor adherence to medication and therapy to ensure stability.

### Poor Social Support System

Patients lacking a strong social support system may struggle to manage their symptoms effectively. The absence of a supportive network can contribute to increased stress, isolation, and difficulty coping with the challenges of living with a psychotic disorder. In such cases, continued treatment provides ongoing support, therapy, and resources to improve overall well-being.

### History of Violence/Conflict with Law

Patients with a history of violence or those in conflict with the law may require ongoing treatment to manage aggression, impulsivity, or other behavioral symptoms associated with their psychotic disorder. Consistent treatment can help reduce harmful behaviors and improve the patient's ability to maintain healthy relationships and function within society.

### Occupational/Vocational Factors

Psychotic disorders can significantly impact occupational and vocational functioning. Discontinuing treatment for patients struggling with employment or vocational stability may exacerbate their difficulties in maintaining consistent work or achieving career goals. Continued treatment provides necessary support to manage symptoms and enhance their ability to function in a work setting.

## ILLNESS-RELATED FACTORS[1,3]

### Chronic Course of Illness

Psychotic disorders with a chronic course, characterized by persistent symptoms and frequent relapses, generally require ongoing treatment. Prematurely discontinuing treatment for individuals with a chronic illness can worsen symptoms and increase the risk of functional impairment. Maintaining treatment is essential to stabilize symptoms and promote long-term recovery.

### Severity of Illness

Individuals with severe psychotic disorders may require long-term or lifelong treatment to manage their symptoms adequately. Abruptly stopping treatment in severe cases can lead to rapid deterioration of functioning and a higher risk of relapse. Continuing treatment is crucial to maintain stability and enhance the patient's quality of life.

### Multiple Episodes

Patients who have experienced multiple episodes of psychosis are more likely to have recurrent relapses if treatment is stopped. Continuing treatment is crucial in these cases to prevent further episodes and maintain stability. Close monitoring, medication management, and psychosocial interventions are important for individuals with a history of multiple episodes.

### Persistent Psychopathology Despite Completion of Treatment Duration

In some cases, individuals may have persistent psychopathology despite completing the recommended duration of treatment. This indicates a need for ongoing treatment to address the residual symptoms, such as mild hallucinations, delusions, cognitive impairments, or persistent functional impairment. Extended treatment duration, medication adjustments, and additional therapeutic interventions may be necessary to improve overall outcomes.

### Predominant Negative Symptoms

Negative symptoms, such as social withdrawal, reduced motivation, or diminished emotional expression, can significantly impact daily functioning. When psychotic disorders predominantly present with these symptoms, continued treatment is vital to manage them and enhance functional recovery.

### Poor Interepisodic Functioning

Interepisodic functioning refers to the level of functioning between psychotic episodes. If patients experience significant impairment in functioning during these periods of symptomatic remission, treatment should not be stopped abruptly. Ongoing treatment can address residual impairments, improve social and occupational functioning, and reduce the risk of relapse.

### Comorbid Substance Use and Other Illnesses

When individuals with psychotic disorders also have substance use disorders or other mental health conditions, maintaining treatment is crucial. Treating these comorbid conditions alongside the psychotic disorder can enhance overall outcomes and reduce the risk of relapse and functional impairment.

### Comorbid Personality Disorder or Poor Premorbid Functioning

Patients with comorbid moderate-to-severe personality disorders or those with poor premorbid functioning may require ongoing treatment to manage their symptoms effectively. The complex nature of these conditions often necessitates integrated and comprehensive treatment approaches to address both the psychotic disorder and the comorbidities.

### Longer Duration of Untreated Illness

A longer duration of untreated illness is associated with a higher risk of chronicity and poorer outcomes. It is crucial to continue treatment for individuals with a longer duration of untreated illness to minimize the potential negative impact on their overall functioning and recovery.

### Treatment Resistance

In cases where the individual has shown resistance to multiple treatment interventions, stopping treatment abruptly is not advisable. Treatment-resistant psychotic disorders require ongoing management and exploration of alternative treatment options, such as augmentation strategies or psychosocial interventions, to optimize outcomes and quality of life.

## PSYCHOSOCIAL FACTORS

### High Expressed Emotions (Poor Family Support)

Highly expressed emotions in the family environment, such as hostility, criticism, and emotional overinvolvement, can increase stress and the risk of relapse in individuals with psychotic disorders. Poor family support can impede recovery and disrupt treatment progress. Continued treatment is crucial to provide support, psychoeducation, and therapeutic interventions to address family dynamics and enhance overall treatment outcomes.

### Severe Stress due to Personal, Vocational, Familial, and Other Factors

Severe stressors, such as traumatic events, significant life changes, job-related stress, discrimination, inadequate support, or ongoing stressful situations, can exacerbate symptoms and increase the risk of relapse in individuals with psychotic disorders. Treatment should not be stopped during periods of severe stress, as it is essential to provide support, coping strategies, and therapy to help individuals navigate and manage stress effectively.

### Psychosocial Disability

Psychotic disorders can result in psychosocial disability, which refers to limitations in functioning related to social interactions, relationships, and daily activities. Individuals with psychosocial disabilities require ongoing treatment to minimize the impact of their symptoms on their daily lives and to improve their overall functional abilities.

### Nonavailability of Psychosocial Treatment (Talk Therapy)

Access to psychotherapeutic interventions, such as talk therapy, is an important aspect of comprehensive treatment for psychotic disorders. If psychosocial treatment options are unavailable or inaccessible, discontinuing medications may be inappropriate. Efforts should focus on exploring alternative resources, adapting treatment approaches, or advocating for appropriate psychosocial interventions to support the individual's recovery.

## WHEN TO STOP TREATMENT?

The clinician may consider stopping treatment when the factors in **Boxes 1 to 3** are absent. In such

**BOX 1:** Patient-related factors that support continued treatment.

- Young age of onset
- Presence of family history/genetic vulnerability
- Poor insight into illness
- Prior history of noncompliance leading to relapse
- Poor social support system
- History of violence/conflict with law
- Occupational/vocational factors

**BOX 2:** Illness-related factors that support continued treatment.

- Age of onset
- Chronic course of the illness
- Severity of illness
- Multiple episodes
- Persistent psychopathology despite completion of treatment duration
- Predominant negative symptoms
- Poor interepisodic functioning
- Comorbid substance use and other illness
- Comorbid personality (moderate to severe) disorder or poor premorbid
- Longer duration of untreated illness
- Treatment resistance

cases, psychotropic medications can be tapered and discontinued. It is important for the clinician to assess the available healthcare services in the patient's community, their accessibility, and affordability for the family. These factors play an important role in minimizing morbidity in the event of a relapse. Good psychosocial support from the patient's community and family further supports the clinician's decision to consider stopping treatment when **(Boxes 1 to 3)** factors are absent.

## HOW TO STOP TREATMENT?[4-6]

Clearly, guidelines are currently lacking on "how" to stop treatment for psychotic disorders. However, it is established that chronic use of psychotropic medications leads to neuroadaptation, and abrupt discontinuation can lead to withdrawal syndrome, rebound psychosis, or relapse of preexisting symptoms. **Box 4** outlines important steps to follow when ceasing treatment for psychotic disorders. These steps provide guidance on what to consider before stopping and how to stop treatment for psychotic disorders.

**BOX 3:** Psychosocial factors that support continued treatment.

- High negative expressed emotions (poor family support)
- Severe stress due to personal, vocational, familial and other factors
- Psychosocial disability
- Nonavailability of psychosocial treatment (talk)

**BOX 4:** Steps to follow in stopping the treatment for psychotic disorders.

- Reconfirm the diagnosis and treatment
- Assess for the absence of factors as stated above
- Identify the barriers and mitigation strategies
- Note the primary support system in family/society
- Identify the accessible primary, secondary and tertiary healthcare facilities
- Educate the patient and his support system on early warning signs (EWS)
- *Collaborative decision making:* Have a dialogue with the patient and his/her support system regarding the discontinuation of treatment
- Inform the local health care system for wellness visits to ensure patient's optimum functioning [community health officers (CHO)/accredited social health activists (ASHA) workers]
- Have a planned routine
- Document the communication and communicate the documentation
- Gradually taper the medication dose over 4–10 weeks
- Observe for early warning signs during dose taper—if no signs present, taper and stop the medication
- Schedule a follow-up visit after 2–4 weeks of stopping medication
- Ensure a healthy lifestyle
- Encourage sleep hygiene approaches
- Avoid substance use

## CONCLUSION

The decision to discontinue treatment of psychotic disorders is a complex and individualized process that requires careful consideration and collaboration among the patient, their healthcare providers, and support network. While discontinuation may be a desired goal for some, prioritizing the patient's well-being and safety is important throughout the process. Close monitoring and gradual tapering of medication, along with the implementation of alternative therapies and support systems, can help mitigate the potential risks associated with treatment cessation. It is crucial to acknowledge that stopping treatment should only be done under the guidance of qualified professionals to ensure the best possible outcomes for the individual's long-term mental health.

## REFERENCES


1. Galletly C, Castle D, Dark F, Humberstone V, Jablensky A, Killackey E, et al. Royal Australian and New Zealand College of Psychiatrists clinical practice guidelines for the management of schizophrenia and related disorders. Aust N Z J Psychiatry. 2016;50(5):410-72.
2. Townsend M, Pareja K, Buchanan-Hughes A, Worthington E, Pritchett D, Brubaker M, et al. Antipsychotic-related stigma and the impact on treatment choices: A systematic review and framework synthesis. Patient Prefer Adherence. 2022;16:373-401.
3. Goff DC, Falkai P, Fleischhacker WW, Girgis RR, Kahn RM, Uchida H, et al. The long-term effects of antipsychotic medication on clinical course in schizophrenia. Am J Psychiatry. 2017;174(9):840-9.
4. Keks N, Schwartz D, Hope J. Stopping and switching antipsychotic drugs. Aust Prescr. 2019;42(5):152-7.
5. Hauser K, Koerfer A, Kuhr K, Albus C, Herzig S, Matthes J. Outcome-relevant effects of shared decision making: A systematic review. Dtsch Arztebl Int. 2015;112(40):665-71.
6. Tranter R, Healy D. Neuroleptic discontinuation syndromes. J Psychopharmacol. 1998;12(4):401-6.

CHAPTER 33

# Management of Nicotine Dependence Comorbid with Mood and Anxiety Disorders

*Arpit Parmar, Amit Singh, Arghya Pal*

## INTRODUCTION

Tobacco use is the most common form of psychoactive substance use in India. As per the National Mental Health Survey 2016, around 20.9% of the general adult population of India suffers from tobacco use disorder.[1] Around 28.6% of the Indian population uses tobacco in any form. Smokeless tobacco use is more common (21.4%) than smoking form (10.7%). Additionally, the lifetime and current prevalence of mood disorders are 5.6 and 2.8%, respectively. Anxiety disorders are also prevalent: Phobia: 1.9%, other anxiety disorders: 1.3%, OCD: 0.8%, and PTSD: 0.2%.

- Long-term quit rates for tobacco use are generally low, especially among those with comorbid mental illnesses. For example, a large nationwide study reported the past month quit rates for individuals with a past month mental illness diagnosis are as follows: 0% for schizophrenia, 29.2% for social phobia, 32.9% for panic disorder, 26% for major depression, 22% for dysthymia, and 33.3% for simple phobia. In comparison, the quit rate among those with no mental illness is as high as 42.5%.[2]
- Comorbid anxiety or mood disorder may be a vulnerability factor associated with the initiation and maintenance of tobacco use or the development of tobacco dependence; hence, these individuals may find it challenging to quit.[3] In addition, some evidence suggests that individuals with these comorbid conditions experience more severe nicotine withdrawal symptoms.

## ASSESSMENT

- The first step for managing tobacco use is a comprehensive assessment of tobacco use, comorbid conditions, and other psychosocial aspects.
    - The following aspects of tobacco use need to be enquired into:
        - Past tobacco use history (age of initiation of tobacco use, age at daily use started, different types of tobacco products used, the pattern of use)
        - Current smoking/smokeless tobacco use
        - Comorbid use of areca/betel nut
        - Primary tobacco form (smoking or smokeless)
        - Perceived benefits of tobacco use (such as social benefits)
        - *Past abstinent attempts:* History of past quit attempts, reasons for such attempts, any significant abstinent attempt (those lasting more than a month), withdrawal symptoms experienced during the attempts, use of pharmacotherapy, use of nonpharmacological techniques, and reasons for relapse.
    - Structured assessment tools are used widely to assess the level of nicotine dependence and provide an objective measurement of progress made during treatment. The *Fagerstrom Test for Nicotine Dependence* (FTND) is widely used to assess tobacco use in patients with comorbid mood/anxiety disorders.[4] The FTND involves asking six questions:
        1. If the smoking occurs within five, 5–30, or 31–60 minutes after waking up.
        2. Difficulty in abstaining from places where smoking is forbidden.
        3. Number of cigarettes smoked per day.
        4. If the first cigarette in the morning is the most difficult to give up.
        5. Frequent tobacco use in the morning.
        6. Smoking even when bedridden.

The FTND has also been adapted to be used for smokeless tobacco users. Other scales include: the *Tiffany Questionnaire for Smoking Urges* and the *Minnesota Nicotine Withdrawal Scale*.[5,6]

- *Relationship of tobacco use with mood and anxiety disorders:*
  - Some patients with mood/anxiety disorders may report that the initiation or maintenance of their tobacco use is associated with alleviating or reducing their underlying psychiatric symptoms (i.e., *self-medication hypothesis*).[7]
  - Some of these symptoms may be incorrectly attributed to the underlying psychiatric conditions and may be part of the tobacco withdrawal syndrome. Such symptoms may improve in some days to weeks following abstinence from tobacco.[7]
  - Some examples of tobacco withdrawals mimicking mood/anxiety disorders are as follows:
    - Symptoms of dysphoria, insomnia, irritability, anxiety, difficulty concentrating, restlessness, weight gain, and increased appetite may mimic major depressive disorder or dysthymia.
    - Symptoms of irritability, restlessness, impaired concentration, and insomnia may resemble hypomania or mania.

## MANAGEMENT

- Various approaches have been developed to treat cooccurring disorders or dual-diagnosis patients.[8] However, the *integrated treatment approach* has the best evidence compared to the sequential or parallel treatment. In an integrated treatment approach, both tobacco use and comorbid anxiety/mood disorders are considered primary but interrelated and are treated in an integrated manner. **Flowchart 1** shows the overall algorithm.
- Pharmacological and non-pharmacological interventions are provided simultaneously.[8] Current guidelines recommend the use of a combination of medicines and psychotherapy.
- Nonpharmacological approaches include psychoeducation, motivational interviewing (MI), relapse prevention, and cognitive behavior therapy (CBT).
  - Psychoeducation helps provide better insights into the relationship between tobacco use and anxiety and mood symptoms. Additionally, it can help provide resources for tobacco cessation.
  - Providing MI to people in the precontemplation or contemplation stage may help engage those who are unmotivated to quit in treatment. Motivation levels are generally high in dual-diagnosis patients.[9] Hospitalization for psychiatric issues is also considered an important time to address comorbid tobacco use. The provision of MI along with nicotine replacement therapy (NRT) during psychiatric inpatient discharge helps reduce rehospitalization rates and improves cessation rates.

**Flowchart 1:** Algorithm for management of tobacco use comorbid with anxiety disorders (AD) or mood disorders (MD).

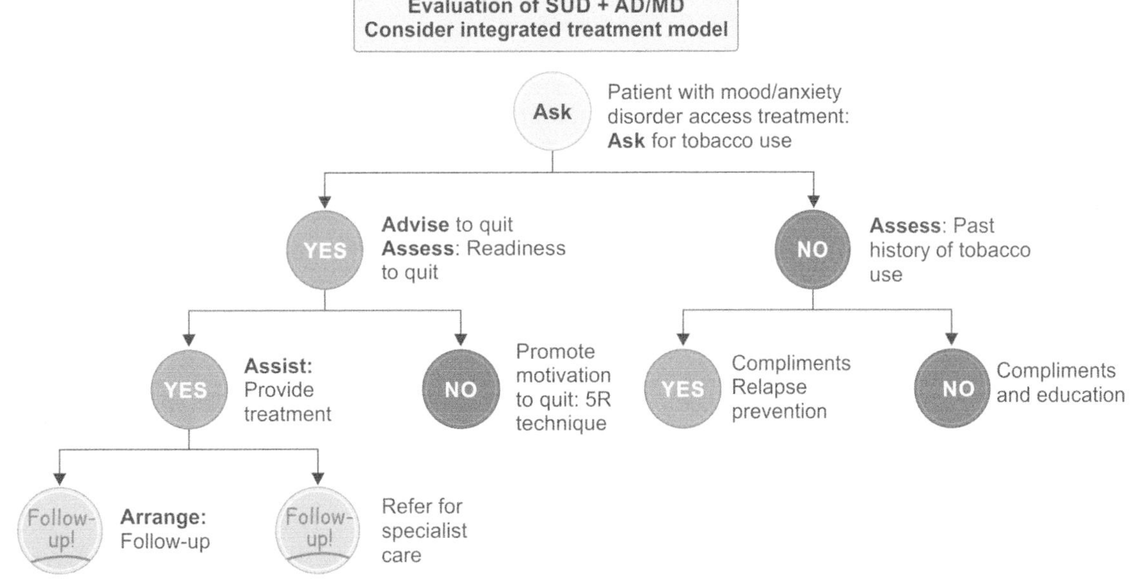


(SUD: substance use disorder)

- Behavioral interventions such as relapse prevention therapy, aimed at high-risk situation identification and coping, and CBT are more effective during the preparation, action, and maintenance stages of change.[10]
- The WHO recommends using that 5As model for brief intervention and the 5Rs model to increase motivation to quit **(Table 1)**.[11]

- Current guidelines recommend the use of pharmacotherapy for all patients unless contraindicated. Three medications are found to be consistently effective for smoking cessation: All forms of NRT, bupropion sustained release, and varenicline **(Table 2)**. Usually, combination therapy using two agents is more effective than a single agent.
- The treatment of tobacco dependence in patients with mood and anxiety disorders is relatively less studied. The majority of these studies include patients with a history of depression, with very few on patients currently experiencing depression. Additionally, most

**TABLE 1:** 5A's and 5R's model of tobacco cessation intervention.

| ***The 5A's model to help patients ready to quit*** | | ***The 5R's model to increase motivation to quit*** | |
|---|---|---|---|
| *Ask* | Systematically identify all tobacco users at every visit | *Relevance* | Indicate how quitting tobacco is personally relevant/important for the patient |
| *Advise* | Advise all users that they need to quit tobacco | *Risks* | Encourage the patient to identify the personally relevant negative consequences associated with tobacco use |
| *Assess* | Determine the readiness to quit tobacco | *Rewards* | Establish the potentially beneficial effects of quitting tobacco use by asking the patient |
| *Assist* | Assist the patient in making a quit plan | *Roadblocks* | Ask the patient to identify potential roadblocks to quitting tobacco use |
| *Arrange* | Arrange a follow-up contact or refer to a specialist support | *Repetition* | Repeat assessment of motivation. If still poor, repeat the intervention at a later date |

**TABLE 2:** Pharmacotherapy for tobacco dependence.

| ***Medication*** | ***Dose*** | ***Side effects*** | ***Contraindications*** | ***Comments*** |
|---|---|---|---|---|
| Nicotine gum | 2–4 mg per dose up to 14 pieces per day | Nausea, indigestion, gingival soreness, and mouth ulceration | Hypersensitivity, poorly controlled cardiac illness, recent MI, or stroke | *Other available formulations:* Nicotine lozenge, patch, inhaler, nasal spray |
| Bupropion | 150 mg for three days, followed by 150 mg BD for up to 12 weeks | Insomnia, dry mouth, hypertension, restlessness, agitation, lowering of seizure threshold | Hypersensitivity, use of concomitant MAOIs, uncontrolled seizures, severe liver disease, pregnancy and lactation | • Can be used with SSRI/TCAs if required<br>• Use cautiously in anxiety disorders, as it may cause agitation or anxiety |
| Varenicline | Start with 0.5 mg/day for 3 days, then 0.5 mg BD for the next 4 days, then 1 mg BD for the next 12 weeks | Nausea, vivid dreams, and seizure risk | Hypersensitivity, use with caution in patients with pre-existing mental illnesses | No increased risk of cardiovascular events. No increased risk of neuropsychiatric side effects |
| Nortriptyline | Start with 25 mg/day, increasing gradually to 75–100 mg/day for 12–24 weeks | Drowsiness, dry mouth, constipation, blurred vision, palpitations, tachycardia, and urinary retention | Hypersensitivity, patients recovering from MI, use of concomitant MAOIs, or linezolid | Not FDA approved, it may have beneficial effects on tobacco-induced dysphoria |

(FDA: Food and Drug Administration; MI: myocardial infarction; MAOIs: monoamine oxidase inhibitors)

smoking cessation trials exclude patients with current major depression/anxiety disorders. Studies that do include patients with current depression show mixed results. Some of the important findings are as follows:

- Some evidence suggests that antidepressant medications may have beneficial effects on tobacco-induced mood symptoms. Studies indicate that a history of major depression in the past is not associated with greater effectiveness of nortriptyline. Nortriptyline reduces the initial dysphoria experienced by patients during the acute withdrawal stage.[12]
- SSRI antidepressants (such as fluoxetine) are ineffective for tobacco cessation and might be even counterproductive, as a study reported higher smoking rates in fluoxetine-treated participants compared to the placebo group.[13-15]
- An RCT compared varenicline 1 mg twice daily with a placebo given for 12 weeks in 525 smokers with stably treated current/past major depression and found that more patients with varenicline stopped smoking. In addition, varenicline did not worsen anxiety or depression symptoms.[16] A recent RCT suggested that varenicline is associated with fewer withdrawal-related depressive symptoms and is effective in smoking cessation in depressed individuals.[17]
- A meta-analysis of 17 RCTs concluded that varenicline is not associated with increased rates of agitation, aggression, suicidality, or depression. However, patients with a current or past history of depression or anxiety disorders have an increased chance of developing neuropsychiatric side effects.[18]
- Very little is known about the effectiveness of varenicline for smoking cessation in anxiety disorder patients. In one comparative study, NRT, varenicline, and combination NRT reported increased abstinence during the initial phase of treatment. There were no differences in psychiatric side effects (notably, 21% of the patients had a comorbid anxiety disorder).
- Bupropion should be used cautiously in patients with existing anxiety disorders as it is associated with agitation and anxiety. One recent RCT suggested significantly reduced quit rates among those with depressive symptoms compared to those without depressive symptoms (7% vs. 17.3%).[19]
- Buspirone, in the dose of up to 60 mg, is associated with higher abstinence rates in smokers with anxiety disorders.[20]

## CONCLUSION

Tobacco use and addiction rates are higher among patients with mental illnesses compared to the general population, particularly among those with mood and anxiety disorders. The literature suggests that tobacco users with these comorbidities have lower quit rates than the general population. Studies also indicate that such cooccurring conditions should be treated using an integrated rather than parallel or sequential approach. Medications such as NRT, bupropion, and varenicline can be useful in cooccurring disorders. Most tobacco cessation guidelines recommend a combination approach using pharmacotherapy and psychosocial interventions. There is a need to study these approaches in more detail in the context of dual diagnosis using naturalistic designs.

## REFERENCES


1. Gururaj G, Varghese M, Benegal V, Rao G, Pathak K, Singh L, et al. National Mental Health Survey of India, 2015-16: Prevalence, Pattern and Outcomes. [online]. Available from http://indianmhs.nimhans.ac.in/Docs/Report2.pdf [Last accessed June, 2025].
2. Lasser K, Boyd JW, Woolhandler S, Himmelstein DU, McCormick D, Bor DH. Smoking and mental illness: A population-based prevalence study. JAMA. 2000;284(20):2606-10.
3. MacKowick KM, Lynch MJ, Weinberger AH, George TP. Treatment of Tobacco Dependence in People with Mental Health and Addictive Disorders. Curr Psychiatry Rep. 2012;14(5):478.
4. Heatherton TF, Kozlowski LT, Frecker RC, Fagerstrom K-O. The Fagerström Test for Nicotine Dependence: a revision of the Fagerström Tolerance Questionnaire. Br J Addict. 1991;86(9):1119-27.
5. Cappelleri JC, Bushmakin AG, Baker CL, Merikle E, Olufade AO, Gilbert DG. Revealing the multidimensional framework of the Minnesota nicotine withdrawal scale. 1991;21(5):749-60.
6. Tiffany ST, Drobes DJ. The development and initial validation of a questionnaire on smoking urges. Br J Addict. 1991;86(11):1467-76.
7. Wai JM, Shulman M, Nunes EV, Hasin DS, Weiss RD. Co-occurring Mood and Substance Use Disorders. Textb Addict Treat. 2021;1297-313.
8. Ziedonis DM, Hitsman B, Beckham JC, Zvolensky M, Adler LE, Audrain-McGovern J, et al. Tobacco use and cessation

in psychiatric disorders: National Institute of Mental Health report. Nicotine Tob Res. 2008;10(12):1691-715.
9. Du Plooy JL, Macharia M, Verster C. Cigarette smoking, nicotine dependence, and motivation to quit smoking in South African male psychiatric inpatients. BMC Psychiatry [Internet]. 2016;16(1):1-7.
10. Ouellet-Plamondon C, Mohamed NS, Sharif-Razi M, Simpkin E, George TP. Treatment of Comorbid Tobacco Addiction in Substance Use and Psychiatric Disorders. Curr Addict Reports. 2014;1(1):61-8.
11. Fiore MC, Baker TB. Treating Smokers in the Health Care Setting. N Engl J Med. 2011;365(13):1222-31.
12. Hall SM, Reus VI, Muñoz RF, Sees KL, Humfleet G, Hartz DT, et al. Nortriptyline and cognitive-behavioral therapy in the treatment of cigarette smoking. Arch Gen Psychiatry. 1998;55(8):683-907.
13. Saules KK, Schuh LM, Arfken CL, Reed K, Kilbey MM, Schuster CR. Double-blind placebo-controlled trial of fluoxetine in smoking cessation treatment including nicotine patch and cognitive-behavioral group therapy. Am J Addict. 2004;13(5):438-46.
14. Howes S, Hartmann-Boyce J, Livingstone-Banks J, Hong B, Lindson N. Antidepressants for smoking cessation. Cochrane database Syst Rev. 2020;4(4).
15. Spring B, Doran N, Pagoto S, McChargue D, Cook JW, Bailey K, et al. Fluoxetine, smoking, and history of major depression: A randomized controlled trial. J Consult Clin Psychol. 2007;75(1):85-94.
16. Tulloch HE, Pipe AL, Els C, Clyde MJ, Reid RD. Flexible, dual-form nicotine replacement therapy or varenicline in comparison with nicotine patch for smoking cessation: a randomized controlled trial. BMC Med. 2016;14(1).
17. Doran N, Dubrava S, Anthenelli RM. Effects of Varenicline, Depressive Symptoms, and Region of Enrollment on Smoking Cessation in Depressed Smokers. Nicotine Tob Res [Internet]. 2019;21(2):156-62.
18. Gibbons RD, Mann JJ. Varenicline, smoking cessation, and neuropsychiatric adverse events. Am J Psychiatry. 2013;170(12):1460-7.
19. Zhang H, Gilbert E, Hussain S, Veldhuizen S, Le Foll B, Selby P, et al. Effectiveness of Bupropion and Varenicline for Smokers With Baseline Depressive Symptoms. Nicotine Tob Res. 2023;25(5):937-44.
20. Cinciripini PM, Lapitsky L, Seay S, Wallfisch A, Meyer WJ, Van Vunakis H. A placebo-controlled evaluation of the effects of buspirone on smoking cessation: differences between high- and low-anxiety smokers. J Clin Psychopharmacol. 1995;15(3):182-91.

# Management of Nicotine Dependence Comorbid with Psychotic Disorders

*Yatan Pal Singh Balhara, Dinesh M*

## INTRODUCTION

The prevalence of nicotine-containing products use among individuals with psychotic disorders has been consistently found greater than the general population. Many studies have reported rates two to three times higher than the general population (60–90% vs. 23–30%).[1]

Compared to general population, persons with psychotic disorders have a higher incidence of metabolic syndrome, coronary artery disease, stroke, chronic obstructive pulmonary disease, and lung cancer—conditions in which nicotine-containing product use plays a causal role. These health conditions contribute to an increased risk of premature mortality among persons with psychotic disorders.[2-6]

While persons with psychotic disorder and nicotine use disorders have a higher propensity to use nicotine products more heavily, they are two to five times less likely to quit nicotine-containing products as compared to the general population. Moreover, they have more severe levels of nicotine dependence and experience greater withdrawal symptoms when attempting to quit.[6-9]

While there has been progress in developing nicotine-containing product cessation interventions for persons with psychotic disorders, long-term quit rates remain low compared to those without mental disorders. Additionally, quit rates among persons with psychotic disorders are even lower than among those with most other mental disorders.[6,7]

## MANAGEMENT OF NICOTINE DEPENDENCE IN PERSONS WITH PSYCHOTIC DISORDERS

Management of nicotine dependence in persons with psychotic disorders requires a systematic approach that includes screening, assessment, and treatment.

- *Screening:* Given the high prevalence of use of nicotine products among persons with psychotic disorders, it is imperative to screen all such patients for use of nicotine products. Alcohol, Smoking, and Substance Involvement Screening Test (ASSIST), developed by WHO, can be used for screening purposes and to ascertain the risk levels associated with use of nicotine products **(Table 1)**.
- *Assessment:* The assessment includes history taking, clinical examination, and laboratory investigations. A detailed history covering the following should be obtained:
  - Age of initiation of use of nicotine containing products
  - Type of nicotine containing products used—smoking and smokeless
  - Amount consumed—usual dose, maximum dose
  - Last use
  - Withdrawal features following cessation or reduction in use
  - Craving for nicotine
  - Tolerance to the effects of nicotine
  - Increasing precedence of nicotine use over other aspects of life
  - Evidence of loss of control
  - Complications due to use of nicotine containing products
  - Continued use despite of harm due to use of nicotine containing products

The clinical examination should corroborate the findings form patient's history. It should also include assessment for signs indicative of regular use of nicotine-containing products, such as staining of teeth and fingertips. In addition, signs of involvement of any bodily system due to an underlying medical condition attributable to use of nicotine-containing products should be looked for. The assessment should also include assessment of motivation to quit.

**TABLE 1:** Medications used for management of nicotine dependence comorbid with psychotic disorders.

| | | ***Dosing*** | | |
|---|---|---|---|---|
| ***Medicine*** | ***General principle/ mechanism of action*** | ***Smoking <20 cigarettes/day***[15] | ***Smoking >20 cigarettes/day or smoking within 30 minutes of waking up***[15] | ***Side effects*** |
| *Nicotine replacement therapy*[15]—licensed for age >12 years, pregnant, and breastfeeding women | | | | |
| • Transdermal patch<br>• 24-hour formulation (21 mg, 14 mg, and 7 mg)<br>• 16-hour formulation (25 mg, 15 mg, and 10 mg) | The general principle of replacement therapies is to present the patient with a safer and more therapeutically manageable form of the drug that directly alleviates the signs and symptoms of withdrawal and craving | Start with 14 mg/15 mg or 7 mg/10 mg | Start with 21 mg or 25 mg | Skin irritation, insomnia, and vivid dreams |
| Gum (2 mg, 4 mg, and 6 mg) | | One piece of 2 mg hourly to prevent craving | One piece of 4 mg or 6 mg hourly to prevent craving. No more than 15 pieces 4 mg/day | Mouth irritation, jaw soreness, heartburn, hiccups, or nausea |
| Lozenge (1 mg, 2 mg, and 4 mg) | | One 1 mg hourly to prevent craving | One 2 mg or 4 mg hourly to prevent craving. Usually not >15 lozenges/day | Mouth irritation, hiccups, nausea, or heartburn |
| Nasal spray (0.5 mg/T) | | One spray in each nostril when craving; not more than twice per hour, maximum 64 sprays/day | | Nasal and throat irritation, rhinitis, sneezing, cough, or teary eyes |
| Inhalator (15 mg) | | No >6 cartridges of 15 mg/day | | Mouth and throat irritation |
| Oral spray (1 mg/T) | | 1–2 sprays when craving; not more than twice per hour; maximum 64 sprays/day | | |
| Mouth strips (2.5 mg) | | One strip of 2.5 mg hourly to prevent craving; not more than 15 strips/day | | |
| Sublingual tablet (2 mg) | | 1–2 tablets hourly to prevent craving | 2 tablets hourly to prevent craving; not >40 tablets/day | |
| *Non-nicotine replacement therapy (non-NRT)*[12,15]—Age >18 years | | | | |
| Varenicline | $\alpha_4\beta_2$ nicotinic acetylcholine receptor partial agonist | Initially 0.5 mg OD for first 3 days, then 0.5 mg BD for next 4 days and increased to 1 mg BD daily for 12 weeks | | Nausea, insomnia, vivid dreams, headache, skin rash (<3%) |
| Bupropion sustained release | Norepinephrine and dopamine reuptake inhibitor | 150 mg OD for first 6 days, then 150 mg BD from day 7–12 weeks | | Insomnia, agitation, dry mouth, headache, dizziness, taste changes |
| Nortriptyline | Tricyclic antidepressant | 75–100 mg/day and length of treatment is 8–12 weeks | | Dry mouth, constipation, dizziness |
| Clonidine | Alpha 2 adrenergic receptor agonist | 0.15–0.75 mg/day | | Dizziness, hypotension |

The information form history and clinical examination shall guide the diagnosis, which can be made using either the ICD-11 or DSM-5 criteria. The severity assessment of nicotine dependence can be carried out using the Fagerstrom Test for Nicotine Dependence-smoking and smokeless forms (FTND and FTND-ST). Laboratory investigations are carried out based on the findings from history and clinical examination. While point-of-care test kits are available to detect nicotine in body fluids, these may not be routinely required during the management of nicotine dependence.

- *Treatment:* Absolute tobacco quit rates are somewhat lower in individuals who use nicotine-containing products and also have a psychiatric illness. However, evidence indicates that the same medications are effective for tobacco users with and without psychiatric comorbidity.[10]

## Pharmacological Approaches

Food and Drug Administration (FDA) has approved medications for smoking-cessation, including nicotine replacement therapy (NRT) in the form of transdermal patches, gum, nasal spray, inhaler, and lozenges, as well as sustained release (SR) bupropion and varenicline.[11,12] Nortriptyline and clonidine, although not approved by the FDA, are clinically used for smoking-cessation.[12-14]

For patients with comorbid psychiatric disease, varenicline or combination NRT was found to be more efficacious than placebo or single NRT or bupropion SR alone.[10,15-18]

Studies evaluating the effects of NRT or bupropion SR with or without behavioral intervention in persons with psychotic disorders was found to be associated with decrease in amount and frequency of nicotine products use with better abstinence and quit rate compared to placebo.[19-31]

Despite concerns regarding treatment of those with concomitant mental illness with varenicline and bupropion SR, evidence suggests that these medications are safe in this population. As an example, in a trial including over 8,000 patients with psychiatric disorders, treatment with varenicline and bupropion SR did not increase the risk of neuropsychiatric adverse effects compared with NRT.[32]

Whatever medication is chosen, patients with severe mental illness may benefit from a longer duration of pharmacotherapy to achieve prolonged abstinence **(Table 2)**.[33]

# DRUG INTERACTIONS BETWEEN MEDICINES USED FOR CESSATION OF USE OF TOBACCO PRODUCTS AND MEDICINES USED FOR TREATMENT OF PSYCHOTIC DISORDERS

Since integrated treatment approach is followed mainly for management of nicotine dependence in persons with psychotic disorders, it is important to be aware about the effect on antipsychotic drug levels due to cessation of nicotine products as well as interaction with the medicines used for cessation **(Table 3)**.

**TABLE 2:** Interaction of first line medicines used for cessation of use of nicotine products with commonly prescribed antipsychotic medicines.

| *Pharmacotherapy* | *Interactions* | *Action* |
|---|---|---|
| NRT[15] | No known clinically relevant interaction with psychotropic medications | No dose adjustments needed |
| Bupropion SR[38] | Inhibits CYP2D6 and increases the serum levels of haloperidol, risperidone, thioridazine | May need lower dose |
| Varenicline[15,39] | No known clinically relevant interaction with psychotropic medications | No dose adjustments needed |

(NRT: nicotine replacement therapy; SR: sustained release)

**TABLE 3:** Impact of cessation of use of nicotine products on commonly used antipsychotic medicines.

| *Medicine* | *Effect of cessation of use of tobacco product* | *Impact on dosage required on cessation of nicotine product* |
|---|---|---|
| Chlorpromazine[34] | Serum levels rise | May need lower dose |
| Clozapine[35] | Serum levels rise significantly | An average 25% dose reduction may be required |
| Fluphenazine[36] | Serum levels rise significantly | 25% dose reduction may be required |
| Haloperidol[37] | Serum levels may rise | May need lower dose |
| Olanzapine[35] | Serum levels rise significantly | An average 25% dose reduction may be required |

## Nonpharmacological Approaches

A systematic review revealed that nonpharmacological approaches when combined with pharmacological treatment increased the chance of abstinence and quit rate than when used alone. Interventions such as 5A, brief intervention, motivational interviewing, motivational enhancement therapy (MET), relapse prevention therapy (RPT), and cognitive behavioral therapy were effective. Also, individual supportive psychotherapy, group therapy and family therapy were also found to play a role.[40]

Telephone support and quitlines, text messaging, web-based services, and social media support have also been found to be helpful.

## Neuromodulation

The repetitive transcranial magnetic stimulation (rTMS) has received FDA clearance as a smoking cessation aid for cigarette smokers. A meta-analysis showed that, comparing with sham rTMS, active rTMS significantly decreased the average daily number of cigarettes smoked and the FTND score.[41]

# CONCLUSION

To conclude, persons with psychotic disorders using nicotine products should be encouraged to quit. They should receive a combination of pharmacotherapy and behavioral interventions for at least 12 weeks which can be extended for a period of another 12 weeks to increase the chance of 1 year abstinence.[15,17]

# REFERENCES


1. Dervaux A, Laqueille X. Smoking and schizophrenia: epidemiological and clinical features. Encephale. 2008;34:299-305.
2. Brown S, Inskip H, Barraclough B. Causes of excess mortality in schizophrenia. Br J Psychiatry. 2000;177:212-7.
3. Hennekens CH, Hennekens AR, Hollar D, Casey DE. Schizophrenia and increased risks of cardiovascular disease. Am Heart J. 2005;150:1115-21.
4. Hser YI, McCarthy WJ, Anglin MD. Tobacco use as a distal predictor of mortality among longterm narcotic addicts. Prev Med. 1994;23:61-9.
5. Hurt RD, Offord KP, Croghan IT, Gomez-Dahl L, Kottke TE, Morse RM, et al. Mortality following inpatient addictions treatment. Role of tobacco use in a community-based cohort. JAMA. 1996;275:1097-103.
6. Mackowick KM, Lynch MJ, Weinberger AH, George TP. Treatment of tobacco dependence in people with mental health and addictive disorders. Curr Psychiatry Rep. 2012;14:478-85.
7. Lasser K, Boyd JW, Woolhandler S, Himmelstein DU, McCormick D, Bor DH. Smoking and mental illness: A population-based prevalence study. JAMA. 2000; 284:2606-10.
8. Grant BF, Hasin DS, Chou SP, Stinson FS, Dawson DA. Nicotine dependence and psychiatric disorders in the United States: Results from the National Epidemiologic Survey on Alcohol and Related Conditions. Arch Gen Psychiatry. 2004;61:1107-15.
9. Hitsman B, Moss TG, Montoya ID, George TP. Treatment of tobacco dependence in mental health and addictive disorders. Can J Psychiatry. 2009;54:368-78.
10. Evins AE, Cather C, Laffer A. Treatment of tobacco use disorders in smokers with serious mental illness: toward clinical best practices. Harv Rev Psychiatry. 2015;23:90-8.
11. Fiore MC, Jaen CR, Baker TB. Treating tobacco use and dependence: 2008 update. US: US Department of Health and Human Services; 2008.
12. US Department of Health and Human Services. Quick Reference Guide for Clinicians: Treating Tobacco Use and Dependence. Washington (DC): US Department of Health and Human Services; 2000.
13. Jiloha RC. Pharmacotherapy of smoking cessation. Indian J Psychiatry. 2014;56:87-95.
14. Tønnesen P, Tonstad S, Hjalmarson A, Lebargy F, Van Spiegel PI, Hider A, et al. A multicentre, randomized, double-blind, placebo-controlled, 1-year study of bupropion SR for smoking cessation. J Intern Med. 2003;254:184-92.
15. Taylor DM, Barnes TRE, Young AH. The Maudsley Prescribing Guidelines in Psychiatry, 14th edition. United States: John Wiley & Sons; 2021.
16. Leone FT, Zhang Y, Evers-Casey S, Evins AE, Eakin MN, Fathi J, et al. Initiating pharmacologic treatment in tobacco-dependent adults. An official American Thoracic Society Clinical Practice Guideline. Am J Respir Crit Care Med. 2020;202:e5-e31.
17. Cather C, Pachas GN, Cieslak KM, Evins AE. Achieving smoking cessation in individuals with schizophrenia: Special considerations. CNS Drugs. 2017;31:471-81.
18. Wu Q, Gilbody S, Peckham E, Brabyn S, Parrott S. Varenicline for smoking cessation and reduction in people with severe mental illnesses: systematic review and meta-analysis. Addiction. 2016;111:1554-67.
19. Hartman N, Leong GB, Glynn SM, Wilkins JN, Jarvik ME. Transdermal nicotine and smoking behavior in psychiatric patients. Am J Psychiatry. 1991;148:374-5.
20. Ziedonis DM, George TP. Schizophrenia and nicotine use: Report of a pilot smoking cessation program and review of neurobiological and clinical issues. Schizophr Bull. 1997;23:247-54.
21. Addington J, El Guebaly N, Campbell W, Hodgins DC, Addington D. Smoking cessation treatment for patients with schizophrenia. Am J Psychiatry. 1998;155:974-6.

22. Dalack GW, Becks L, Hill E, Pomerleau OF, Meador-Woodruff JH. Nicotine withdrawal and psychiatric symptoms in cigarette smokers with schizophrenia. Neuropsychopharmacology. 1999;21:195-202.
23. Dalack GW, Meador-Woodruff JH. Acute feasibility and safety of a smoking reduction strategy for smokers with schizophrenia. Nicotine Tob Res. 1999;1:53-7.
24. Dalack GW, Ritter LM, Meador-Woodruff JH. Nicotine replacement and smoking suppression in schizophrenia. Biol Psychiatry. 2000;47:S48.
25. Chou KR, Chen R, Lee JF, Ku CH, Lu RB. The effectiveness of nicotine-patch therapy for smoking cessation in patients with schizophrenia. Int J Nurs Stud. 2004;41:321-30.
26. Evins AE, Cather C, Deckersbach T, Freudenreich O, Culhane MA, Olm-Shipman CM, et al. A doubleblind placebo-controlled trial of bupropion sustained-release for smoking cessation in schizophrenia. J Clin Psychopharmacol. 2005;25:218-25.
27. Evins AE, Cather C, Rigotti NA, Freudenreich O, Henderson DC, Olm-Shipman CM, et al. Two-year follow-up of a smoking cessation trial in patients with schizophrenia: Increased rates of smoking cessation and reduction. J Clin Psychiatry. 2004;65:307-11.
28. Evins AE, Deckersbach T, Cather C, Freudenreich O, Culhane MA, Henderson DC, et al. Independent effects of tobacco abstinence and Bupropion- SR on cognitive function in schizophrenia. J Clin Psychiatry. 2005;66:1184-90.
29. Evins AE, Mays VK, Rigotti NA, Tisdale T, Cather C, Goff DC. A pilot trial of bupropion added to cognitive behavioral therapy for smoking cessation in schizophrenia. Nicotine Tob Res. 2001;3:397-403.
30. George TP, Vessicchio JC, Termine A, Bregartner TA, Feingold A, Rounsaville BJ, et al. A placebo controlled trial of Bupropion- SR for smoking cessation in schizophrenia. Biol Psychiatry. 2002;52:53-61.
31. Ahluwalia JS, Harris KJ, Catley D, Okuyemi KS, Mayo MS. Sustained-release bupropion for smoking cessation in African Americans: A randomized controlled trial. JAMA. 2002;288:468-74.
32. Anthenelli RM, Benowitz NL, West R, St Aubin L, McRae T, Lawrence D, et al. Neuropsychiatric safety and efficacy of varenicline, Bupropion, and nicotine patch in smokers with and without psychiatric disorders (EAGLES): a double-blind, randomised, placebo-controlled clinical trial. Lancet. 2016;387:2507-20.
33. Evins AE, Cather C, Pratt SA, Pachas GN, Hoeppner SS, Goff DC, et al. Maintenance treatment with varenicline for smoking cessation in patients with schizophrenia and bipolar disorder: a randomized clinical trial. JAMA. 2014;311:145-54.
34. Desai HD, Seabolt J, Jann MW. Smoking in patients receiving psychotropic medications: a pharmacokinetic perspective. CNS Drugs. 2001;15:469-94.
35. Tsuda Y, Saruwatari J, Yasui-Furukori N. Meta-analysis: the effects of smoking on the disposition of two commonly used antipsychotic agents, olanzapine and clozapine. BMJ Open. 2014;4:e004216.
36. Ereshefsky L, Jann MW, Saklad SR, Davis CM, Richards AL, Burch NR. Effects of smoking on fluphenazine clearance in psychiatric inpatients. Biol Psychiatry. 1985;20:329-32.
37. Jann MW, Saklad SR, Ereshefsky L, Richards AL, Harrington CA, Davis CM. Effects of smoking on haloperidol and reduced haloperidol plasma concentrations and haloperidol clearance. Psychopharmacology (Berl). 1986;90:468-70.
38. Englisch S, Morgen K, Meyer-Lindenberg A, Zink M. Risks and benefits of Bupropion treatment in schizophrenia: a systematic review of the current literature. Clin Neuropharmacol. 2013;36:203-15.
39. Yousefi MK, Folsom TD, Fatemi SH. A review of varenicline's efficacy and tolerability in smoking cessation studies in subjects with schizophrenia. J Addict Res Ther. 2011;S4:3045.
40. Rajalu BM, Jayarajan D, Muliyala KP, Sharma P, Gandhi S, Chand PK, et al. Non-pharmacological interventions for smoking in persons with schizophrenia spectrum disorders —A systematic review. Asian J Psychiatr. 2021;56:102530.
41. Zangen A, Moshe H, Martinez D, Barnea-Ygael N, Vapnik T, Bystritsky A, et al. Repetitive transcranial magnetic stimulation for smoking cessation: a pivotal multicenter double-blind randomized controlled trial. World Psychiatry. 2021;20:397-404.

# Management of Comorbid Cannabis Use Disorder in Psychotic and Bipolar Disorder Patients

*Amit Singh, Arpit Parmar, Arghya Pal*

## INTRODUCTION

- Cooccurring cannabis use disorder (CUD) often accompanies patients diagnosed with psychosis or bipolar disorder (BD). For example, among individuals experiencing first episode psychosis (FEP), the prevalence of cannabis use is about 64%, while that of CUD is 30%.[1] Moreover, approximately 26% of all patients with schizophrenia may have additional comorbid CUD.[2] Compared with the general population, individuals with severe psychotic disorders are 3.5 times more likely to engage in heavy cannabis use and are 4.6 times more likely to use cannabis for recreational purposes.[3]
- In BD, the lifetime prevalence of cannabis use is high, ranging from 52% to 71%, while the lifetime prevalence of CUD falls within the range of 3.3% to 7.2%.[4] Another study reported that approximately 24% of patients with BD use cannabis.[5] A systematic review and meta-analysis found strong associations between cooccurring CUD and bipolar illness in individuals in clinical settings, with a prevalence of cannabis use at 20%.[6]
- The association between cannabis use and psychosis/BD is intricate and bidirectional. Each condition can intensify the other's impact. Cannabis use is linked to earlier psychosis onset and increased risk of transition to psychosis in clinically high-risk individuals. The early age of onset of cannabis use and the severity and frequency of use increases the risk of developing psychosis. Cannabis use also has a detrimental impact on the severity of psychotic symptoms, adherence to treatment, relapse risk and hospitalizations, as well as clinical and functional outcomes of individuals experiencing FEP.[7]
- The presence of comorbid cannabis use can result in symptoms that resemble, overlap, obscure, or worsen the presentation of psychosis/BD, thereby adding complexity to the diagnosis and clinical management.

**Flowchart 1:** Management of comorbid cannabis use disorder in psychosis and bipolar disorder.

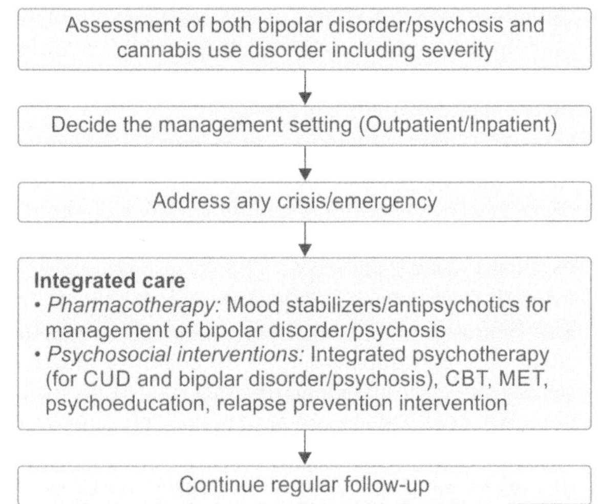


(CUD: cannabis use disorder; CBT: cognitive-behavioral therapy; MET: motivational enhancement therapy)

- Cannabis use cessation has been linked to better clinical and functional outcomes as well as a lower relapse risk in FEP.[8] Similarly, in BD patients experiencing manic/mixed episodes, cannabis use cessation improves clinical and functional outcomes, making it similar to never users.[7]
- Managing CUD in individuals with psychosis/BD requires a comprehensive approach that addresses both conditions simultaneously. The approach should be individualized one, tailored to the specific needs and circumstances of the affected person. Here are some key considerations regarding managing CUD in BD/psychosis **(Flowchart 1)**.

## ASSESSMENT

- A crucial first step in effective management involves conducting a thorough assessment, which encompasses a detailed exploration of the individual's psychiatric condition, CUD, and any other cooccurring health conditions.

- Physical examination and mental status examination offer insights into several aspects, including the patient's current psychopathological state, their substance use condition (whether they are currently intoxicated or experiencing withdrawal), and their level of motivation.
- Urine toxicology can be used to verify cannabis use, and use of other substances.
- The severity of both CUD and psychosis/BD should be ascertained, as it will help guide in deciding the locus of care and treatment priority.
- It is vital to determine the temporal association between psychosis/BD and CUD—whether they cooccur independently or if cannabis use has triggered symptoms of BD/psychosis. Distinguishing cannabis-induced psychosis from primary psychotic disorders is crucial for treatment planning.[9]
- Continuously assess psychiatric symptoms and their connection to cannabis use or abstinence over time. Most cannabis-induced BD/psychosis symptoms usually begin to improve within hours or days after cannabis use has stopped.
- Structured instruments should be used wherever possible as they aid in tracking the change in clinical presentation and symptom severity with treatment. The Young Mania Rating Scale or the Bech–Rafaelsen Mania Scale is commonly used for mania, and Bipolar Depression Rating Scale can be used for bipolar depression. Similarly, the Brief Psychiatric Rating Scale (BPRS) can be used to rate psychotic symptoms in dual diagnosis.[10]

## TREATMENT

- Integrated substance use and psychosis treatment provided at a mental healthcare setting may be preferable as it is associated with better treatment outcomes than care provided in a parallel or sequential manner.[11] An integrated treatment approach involves addressing both BD/psychosis and CUD simultaneously, rather than as separate issues and in the same setting and by the same care-provider team.
- A combination of medication, addiction counseling, and psychotherapy is advised for favorable long-term outcomes.

### Pharmacological

- Pharmacological treatment for comorbid BD/psychosis and CUD involves treatment for both. Medications commonly used to manage BD/psychosis, such as mood stabilizers (e.g., lithium and valproate) and antipsychotics, can still be prescribed to reduce symptoms of comorbid conditions.
- As untreated psychosis or mood states are risk factors for continuing cannabis use, treating these disorders may reduce cannabis use in the affected individuals and make them suitable for psychological interventions.
- There is currently poor evidence to support one antipsychotic over another or first versus second-generation antipsychotics when treating schizophrenia with comorbid CUD, either in relation to superiority in reducing cannabis use or improving psychiatric symptoms.[12]
- A single small trial suggests that clozapine may be superior to other antipsychotics in reducing cannabis use in comorbid CUD and schizophrenia, while risperidone may be better compared to olanzapine in reducing craving for cannabis. Olanzapine, clozapine, and risperidone showed superiority for the reduction of psychotic symptoms compared to some other drugs. Side effects followed known patterns.[12]
- No trials have examined the effectiveness of pharmacological treatment options for comorbid BD and CUD.[4,13]
- For cannabis withdrawal symptoms, medications can also be prescribed for symptomatic management. Benzodiazepines and zolpidem can be given for insomnia.
- There are no specific medications approved for treating CUD. Besides, there is no evidence to support any available pharmacological treatment as potentially beneficial for CUD.

### Nonpharmacological

- Psychosocial treatment approaches, including cognitive-behavioral therapy (CBT), motivational enhancement therapy (MET), and their combination, have the best evidence of effectiveness in reducing cannabis use frequency and severity of cannabis dependence.[14]
- Limited research has explored nonpharmacological strategies for addressing the cooccurring BD and CUD. However, interventions such as group CBT, integrated

therapy, and relapse prevention therapy have shown promise in potentially decreasing hospitalizations, increasing abstinence, promoting medication adherence, reducing addiction severity, and improving mood-related symptoms.[15]

- In FEP plus CUD, CBT was shown to be effective in reducing cannabis use severity, positive psychotic symptoms, response duration, and improved clinical and functional outcomes. The key components of the therapy involved motivation enhancement strategies, CBT for cannabis abstinence, symptom management, improvement in psychosocial functioning, and relapse prevention.[8]
- Brief interventions such as motivational interviewing (MI) added to standard care in cannabis users suffering from psychosis has been shown to reduce cannabis use and enhance the confidence to change cannabis use, at least in short term. MI was well accepted by patients and should be integrated into routine clinical practice to reduce cannabis use.[16,17]
- Patients with psychosis and CUD who develop stronger therapeutic alliances with their therapists during MI and CBT interventions tend to have significantly more improvements in global functioning.[17]
- Group psychological interventions based on CBT and MI in patients with FEP with comorbid cannabis dependence can enhance subjective quality of life.[18]
- Regular follow-up and monitoring are necessary to evaluate treatment progress, adjust interventions as needed, and provide ongoing support. This may involve routine psychiatric assessments, urine drug screenings, and monitoring for any potential side effects of medications.[19]

## REFERENCES


1. Foglia E, Schoeler T, Klamerus E, Morgan K, Bhattacharyya S. Cannabis use and adherence to antipsychotic medication: a systematic review and meta-analysis. Psychol Med. 2017;47:1691-705.
2. Hunt GE, Large MM, Cleary M, Lai HMX, Saunders JB. Prevalence of comorbid substance use in schizophrenia spectrum disorders in community and clinical settings, 1990-2017: Systematic review and meta-analysis. Drug Alcohol Depend. 2018;191:234-58.
3. Hartz SM, Pato CN, Medeiros H, Cavazos-Rehg P, Sobell JL, Knowles JA, et al. Comorbidity of severe psychotic disorders with measures of substance use. JAMA Psychiatry. 2014;71:248-54.
4. Tourjman SV, Buck G, Jutras-Aswad D, Khullar A, McInerney S, Saraf G, et al. Canadian Network for Mood and Anxiety Treatments (CANMAT) Task Force Report: A systematic review and recommendations of cannabis use in bipolar disorder and major depressive disorder. Can J Psychiatry. 2023;68:299-311.
5. Pinto JV, Medeiros LS, Santana da Rosa G, Santana de Oliveira CE, Crippa JA de S, Passos IC, et al. The prevalence and clinical correlates of cannabis use and cannabis use disorder among patients with bipolar disorder: A systematic review with meta-analysis and meta-regression. Neurosci Biobehav Rev. 2019;101:78-84.
6. Hunt GE, Malhi GS, Cleary M, Lai HMX, Sitharthan T. Prevalence of comorbid bipolar and substance use disorders in clinical settings, 1990-2015: Systematic review and meta-analysis. J Affect Disord. 2016;206: 331-49.
7. Zorrilla I, Aguado J, Haro JM, Barbeito S, López Zurbano S, Ortiz A, et al. Cannabis and bipolar disorder: does quitting cannabis use during manic/mixed episode improve clinical/functional outcomes? Acta Psychiatr Scand. 2015;131:100-10.
8. González-Ortega I, Echeburúa E, Alberich S, Bernardo M, Vieta E, de Pablo GS, et al. Cognitive behavioral therapy program for cannabis use cessation in first-episode psychosis patients: A 1-year randomized controlled trial. Int J Environ Res Public Health. 2022;19:7325.
9. Basu D, Basu A, Ghosh A. Assessment of clinical co-morbidities. Indian J Psychiatry. 2018;60:S457-65.
10. Lykke J, Hesse M, Austin SF, Oestrich I. Validity of the BPRS, the BDI and the BAI in dual diagnosis patients. Addict Behav. 2008;33:292-300.
11. SAMHSA. Substance Use Disorder Treatment for People with Co-occurring Disorders. Rockville: Substance Abuse and Mental Health Services Administration; 2020.
12. Krause M, Huhn M, Schneider-Thoma J, Bighelli I, Gutsmiedl K, Leucht S. Efficacy, acceptability and tolerability of antipsychotics in patients with schizophrenia and comorbid substance use. A systematic review and meta-analysis. Eur Neuropsychopharmacol. 2019;29: 32-45.
13. González-Pinto A, Goikolea JM, Zorrilla I, Bernardo M, Arrojo M, Cunill R, et al. Clinical practice guideline on pharmacological and psychological management of adult patients with bipolar disorder and comorbid substance use. Adicciones. 2022;34:142-56.

14. Gates PJ, Sabioni P, Copeland J, Le Foll B, Gowing L. Psychosocial interventions for cannabis use disorder. Cochrane Database Syst Rev. 2016;2016:CD005336.
15. Gold AK, Otto MW, Deckersbach T, Sylvia LG, Nierenberg AA, Kinrys G. Substance use comorbidity in bipolar disorder: A qualitative review of treatment strategies and outcomes. Am J Addict. 2018;27:188-201.
16. Bonsack C, Gibellini Manetti S, Favrod J, Montagrin Y, Besson J, Bovet P, et al. Motivational intervention to reduce cannabis use in young people with psychosis: a randomized controlled trial. Psychother Psychosom. 2011;80:287-97.
17. Parmar A, Sarkar S. Brief interventions for cannabis use disorders: A review. Addict Disord Treat. 2017; 16:80-93.
18. Berry K, Gregg L, Lobban F, Barrowclough C. Therapeutic alliance in psychological therapy for people with recent onset psychosis who use cannabis. Compr Psychiatry. 2016;67:73-80.
19. Madigan K, Brennan D, Lawlor E, Turner N, Kinsella A, O'Connor JJ, et al. A multi-center, randomized controlled trial of a group psychological intervention for psychosis with comorbid cannabis dependence over the early course of illness. Schizophr Res. 2013;143:138-42.

CHAPTER 36

# Approach to Delirium: Diagnosis and Management

*Sandeep Grover, Chandrima Naskar*

## INTRODUCTION

- Delirium is a complex neuropsychiatric syndrome that results due to one or more structural or physiological abnormalities affecting the brain directly or indirectly.
- It can be called a state of potentially reversible "acute brain failure" precipitated by various causes **(Table 1)**, in vulnerable individuals (Predisposing factors, **Table 1**).
- It has a high prevalence, especially among inpatient admissions, patients in intensive care units (ICUs), those receiving palliative care and among the elderly, with a prevalence reported as high as 80%.[1]
- It is often associated with multiple adverse outcomes in the form of increases in the duration of hospital stay, higher mortality, and persistent cognitive impairment, increases in the healthcare cost, significant distress among the caregivers when the patient is symptomatic and distress among the patients after recovery.[2] Thus, it is important to confidently identify and manage delirium in a timely manner.

## DIAGNOSIS

- Delirium is generally characterized primarily as a disorder of attention and awareness that has an acute onset, and fluctuating course with evening worsening of symptoms. There is in general agreement between the International Classification of Diseases, Eleventh Edition (ICD-11) and Diagnostic and Statistical Manual, Fifth Revision (DSM-5), with certain differences in description **(Table 2)**.
- It is usually short lasting, with an average duration of delirium lasting 1–4 days in different treatment settings.

### Scales to Assess Delirium

- Even though delirium has a high prevalence, clinicians often face difficulty in identifying delirium. For the ease of screening and diagnosing delirium, various scales have been developed. The most common among these are Confusion Assessment Method (CAM) and its variants, and Delirium Rating Scale-Revised-98 (DRS-R-98).
- Other than screening and diagnosing delirium, there are many other scales to assess the level of consciousness, subtyping delirium, and assessing cognitive functioning, etc. **(Table 3)**.
- CAM and CAM-ICU have now been updated and these are not only useful for screening but can also be used for grading the severity of delirium.

**TABLE 1:** Predisposing, precipitating, and perpetuating factors of delirium.[3]

| *Predisposing* | *Precipitating* | *Perpetuating* |
|---|---|---|
| • Advanced age | • Surgical stress | • Uncontrolled pain |
| • High comorbidity | • Acute infections/sepsis | • Persisting infection |
| • Frailty | • Dehydration | • Invasive devices |
| • Dementia | • Electrolyte imbalance | • Physical restraints |
| • Depression | • Acute kidney injury | • Immobility |
| • History of delirium | • Liver dysfunction | • Blood transfusion |
| • Visual/hearing impairment | • Alcohol/drug withdrawal | • Polypharmacy/high-anticholinergic burden |
| • Alcohol abuse | • Seizures | • Environmental factors |
| • Illicit drug/opioid/BZD use | • Heart failure | • Deep sedation |
| • Poor nutrition | • Prolonged mechanical ventilation | • Infusion of BZD/opioid |
| • Low educational level | • Severe illness | • Lack of communication with family |

(BZD: benzodiazepine)

**TABLE 2:** Nosological differences.

| *Point* | *DSM-5* | *ICD-11* |
|---|---|---|
| Diagnostic criteria | • A disturbance in attention and awareness<br>• Represents a change from baseline attention and awareness<br>• An additional disturbance in cognition | • Disturbance of attention, orientation, and awareness<br>• Significant confusion or global neurocognitive impairment<br>• Represents a change from baseline functioning<br>• Transient symptoms that may fluctuate<br>• Often includes disturbance of behavior and emotion<br>• May include impairment in multiple cognitive domains; disturbance of the sleep-wake cycle |
| Exclusion | • Symptoms must not be better accounted for a pre-existing of developing neurocognitive d/o<br>• Excludes "a severely reduced level of arousal", such as coma | • Symptoms must not be better accounted for a pre-existing developing neurocognitive disorder<br>• Does not specifically exclude coma |
| Subtypes | *Etiology based:*<br>• Substance withdrawal delirium<br>• Medication-induced delirium<br>• Delirium due to another medical condition<br>• Delirium due to multiple etiologies<br>*Psychomotor activity based:*<br>• Hyperactive<br>• Hypoactive<br>• Mixed<br>*Duration based:*<br>• *Acute:* Lasting a few hours or days<br>• *Persistent:* Lasting weeks or months | *Etiology based:*<br>• Disease classified elsewhere<br>• Psychoactive substances including medications<br>• Multiple etiological factors<br>• Other specified cause<br>• Unspecified or unknown cause |

(DSM-5: Diagnostic and Statistical Manual, Fifth Revision; ICD-11: International Classification of Diseases, Eleventh Edition)

**TABLE 3:** Scales to assess delirium.[4]

| *Domain to be assessed* | *Tools available* |
|---|---|
| Assessment of level of consciousness | Richmond Agitation Sedation Scale |
| Screening instruments | • *4AT:* Arousal, Attention, Abbreviated Mental Test-4, Acute change<br>• Confusion Assessment Method (CAM)<br>• Confusion Assessment Method for ICU (CAM-ICU)<br>• Memorial Delirium Assessment Scale (MDAS)<br>• Saskatoon Delirium Checklist (SDC)<br>• *DSS:* Delirium Severity Scale-Revised 98 (DRS-R-98)<br>• Resident's Assessment Instrument-Acute Care (RAI-AC)<br>• Delirium-o-meter |
| Severity of delirium | • CAM-ICU-7<br>• DRS-R-98<br>• MDAS<br>• DRS-R-98<br>• Delirium Severity Interview (DSI) |
| Differentiating delirium from dementia | Cognitive Performance Scale-2, RAI-AC |
| Premorbid cognitive disturbances | Short Informant Questionnaire for Cognitive Decline in Elderly (Short-IQCODE) |
| To assess cognitive symptoms in delirium | • Mini Mental Status Examination (MMSE)<br>• Clock drawing<br>• Cognitive test for delirium (CTD)<br>• Digit span test |

*Contd...*

*Contd...*

| *Domain to be assessed* | *Tools available* |
|---|---|
| Motoric subtyping | • Delirium motor checklist<br>• Delirium Motor Severity Scale (DMSS)<br>• 4 item abbreviated Delirium Motor Severity Scale (DMSS-4) |
| Etiology | Delirium etiology checklist |
| Pediatric delirium | • CAM-Pediatric<br>• CAM-ICU-p<br>• CAM-preschool<br>• Pediatric Anesthesia Emergence Delirium Scale (PAEDS)<br>• Cornell Assessment of Pediatric Delirium (CAPD) |
| Distress with delirium experience | Delirium Experience Questionnaire |

**TABLE 4:** Multicomponent intervention.[5]

| | |
|---|---|
| Reorientation | Orient patient to time, place, and situation, discuss their fear, apprehensions, and queries. Involve family to develop a sense of connection and security |
| Cognition | Engage in conversations, books, and puzzles |
| Mobility | Sitting up, early ambulation, and physical therapy |
| Sensorium | Glasses, hearing aids, and interpreter assistance |
| Sleep | Eye masks, earplugs, minimize unnecessary disruptions during the targeted sleep period, and optimize light and dark exposure to regulate sleep-wake pattern |
| Agency and independence | Minimize duration of physical restraint, review the necessity of urinary catheter, nasogastric tube, multiple intravenous access and minimize the number of invasive devices |
| Nutrition and hydration | Assist with eating and drinking |

## Assessing the Factors Contributing to the Delirium

- *From history and examination:*
  - A thorough review of the signs, symptoms, level of distress experienced by the patient, the derangements in the investigations, and the medications that he/she is receiving including their anticholinergic effect.
  - Even minor derangements like a 1–2 point reduction in the serum sodium level can precipitate and prolong delirium in an individual who is the vulnerable due presence of multiple predisposing factors such as old age and preexisting dementia.
- *From laboratory evaluation:* A detailed evaluation of the metabolic parameters is essential.
- *Investigations:*
  - Complete blood count, liver function test, renal function test, thyroid function test, etc.
  - Urine screening (both routine and toxicology screen)
  - Electrocardiogram is necessary before starting antipsychotics.
  - Additional investigations—vitamin $B_{12}$/folate, other nutritional deficiencies
  - *Neuroimaging:* If there is neurodeficit, history of fall, and presence of seizure

## MANAGEMENT

- Management of delirium includes both its prevention and treatment. Nonpharmacological management is considered to be the first-line strategies for treatment and prevention of delirium.
- Current research suggests that nonpharmacological multicomponent interventions such as environmental, behavioral, and communication-related changes have the maximum effectiveness in both preventing and reducing the duration of delirium **(Table 4)**.
- Management of delirium in the ICU will involve additional steps **(Table 5)**.

**TABLE 5:** ABCDEF model.[6]

| | |
|---|---|
| A | *Assess, prevent, and manage pain:* Non-opioid pain management preferred, regional anesthesia if needed<br>Analgesia based sedation like Fentanyl infusion |
| B | *Spontaneous breathing trial and spontaneous awakening trials (SBT and SAT)*<br>• Faster removal from mechanical ventilation (MV)<br>• Daily attempts at SAT and SBT |
| C | *Choice of sedation*<br>• Avoid benzodiazepines<br>• Targeted light sedation, when necessary<br>• Dexmedetomidine in postcardiac-surgery patients, during MV weaning |
| D | *Delirium monitoring and management:*<br>• Routine CAM/CAM-ICU/DRS-R-98 monitoring<br>• Assess and ensure maintenance of the sleep-wake cycle<br>• *Nutritional support, adequate hydration, least restrictive treatment:* Minimum invasive devices, restraint for the least possible duration |
| E | *Early mobilization:*<br>• Physical and occupational therapy assessment<br>• Progress through the movement of limbs, sitting, standing, walking, and then activities of daily living |
| F | *Family engagement and empowerment:*<br>• Cognitive stimulation, participation in mobilization<br>• Reorientation to the time, place, person, sequence of events, and progression of illness<br>• Providing emotional support<br>• Family can be allowed to take part in multidisciplinary rounds |

(CAM: confusion assessment method; ICU: intensive care unit; DRS-R-98: Delirium Rating Scale-Revised-98)

**TABLE 6:** Evidence of usefulness of pharmacotherapy in delirium.

| *Medication* | *Prevention* | *Treatment* |
|---|---|---|
| Haloperidol | – | +/– |
| Dexmedetomidine | + | – |
| Melatonin/Ramelteon | + | – |
| Quetiapine | – | +/– |
| Other antipsychotics | – | +/– |

## Nonpharmacological

The nonpharmacological approaches for treatment of delirium are summarized in **Table 4**.

## Pharmacological

- Pharmacological measures have shown limited efficacy in treating delirium **(Table 6)**,[7] and their use should be limited to patients who are severely disturbed, agitated and uncooperative with treatment.
- For pharmacological management of delirium, start with a low dose of one of the drugs and increase the dose with close monitoring of improvement of symptoms of delirium as well as their side effects like QT prolongation (>450 ms).
- Once the delirium starts improving, maintain the effective dose for about 2–3 days before tapering.
- The recommended doses for various antipsychotics are:
  - Haloperidol, oral/IV (0.25–0.5 mg, may repeat every 20–30 minutes, not to exceed 3–5 mg in 24 hours)
  - Risperidone (0.5–1 mg twice daily)
  - Olanzapine (2.5–5 mg twice daily)
  - Quetiapine (12.5–25 mg twice daily)
- Due to the risk of torsades de pointes, intravenous haloperidol should be administered in monitored settings only.
- If a patient is not severely agitated but is having difficulty in sleep onset, melatonin 3–6 mg at night can be prescribed.
- Benzodiazepines should be considered for the management of delirium occurring due to alcohol or benzodiazepine withdrawal **(Flowchart 1)**.

**Flowchart 1:** Approach to a patient presenting with symptoms suggestive of delirium.

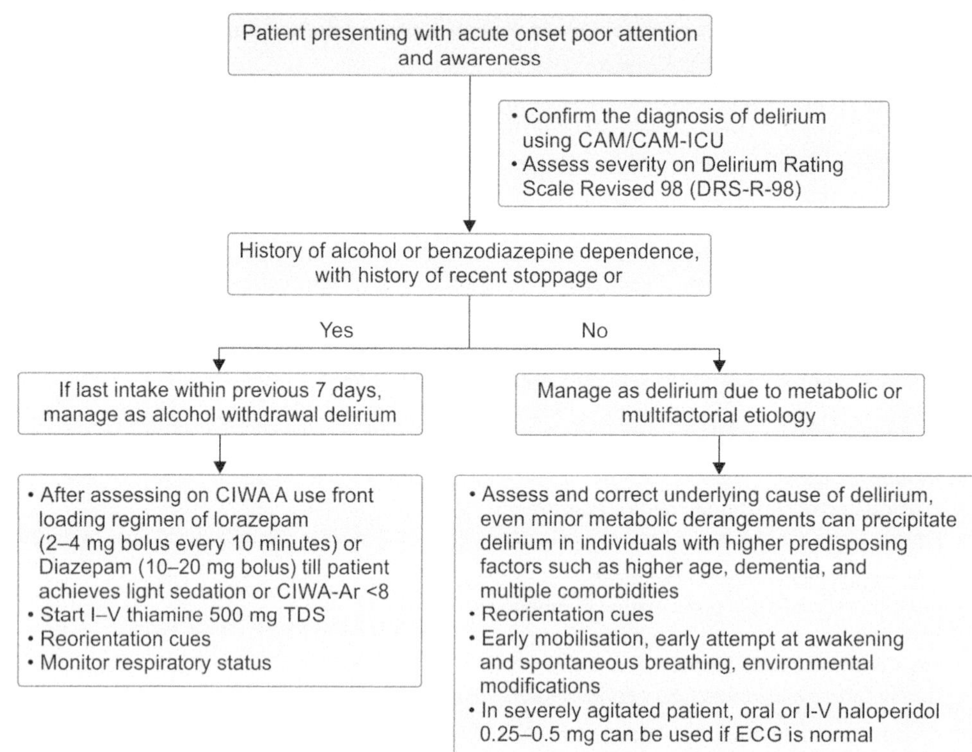


(CAM: confusion assessment method; ICU: intensive care unit; IV: intravenous; ECG: electrocardiogram; CIWA-Ar: Clinical Institute Withdrawal Assessment-Alcohol, revised)

## REFERENCES


1. Grover S, Kathiravan S, Dua D. Delirium Research in India: A Systematic Review. J Neurosci Rural Pract. 2021;12(2):236-66.
2. Bellelli G, Brathwaite JS, Mazzola P. Delirium: A Marker of Vulnerability in Older People. Front Aging Neurosci. 2021;13:626127.
3. Wilson JE, Mart MF, Cunningham C, Shehabi Y, Girard TD, MacLullich AMJ, et al. Delirium. Nat Rev Dis Primers. 2020;6(1):90.
4. Grover S, Kate N. Assessment scales for delirium: A review. World J Psychiatry. 2012;2(4):58-70.
5. Chou ST, Pogach M, Rock LK. Less pharmacotherapy is more in delirium. Intensive Care Med. 2022;48:743-5.
6. Trogrlić Z, van der Jagt M, Bakker J, Balas MC, Ely EW, van der Voort PH, et al. A systematic review of implementation strategies for assessment, prevention, and management of ICU delirium and their effect on clinical outcomes. Crit. Care. 2015;19:157.
7. Kim MS, Rhim HC, Park A, Kim H, Han KM, Patkar AA, et al. Comparative efficacy and acceptability of pharmacological interventions for the treatment and prevention of delirium: A systematic review and network meta-analysis. J Psychiatr Res. 2020;125:164.

CHAPTER 37

# Differential Diagnosis of Dementia

*Siddharth Sarkar, Vaibhav Patil, Preethy Kathiresan*

## INTRODUCTION AND DIFFERENTIALS OF DEMENTIA

Dementia is categorized as a neurocognitive disorder (NCD) in the Diagnostic and Statistical Manual of Mental Disorders (DSM-5).[1] According to the DSM-5, a major NCD is one in which there has been a clear and significant decline in cognitive function in one or more cognitive domains (complex attention, executive function, learning and memory, language, perceptual-motor, or social cognition), as demonstrated by (1) concern expressed by the patient, a knowledgeable informant, or the clinician; and (2) a significant impairment in cognitive performance. These cognitive deficits make it difficult for the person to be independent in daily activities (requiring at least some support with complex instrumental daily living activities like managing medications or paying bills). The cognitive deficits do not occur exclusively in the context of delirium and are not better explained by another psychiatric condition like schizophrenia and major depressive disorder.

The cognitive functions affected in dementia are also affected in chronic psychiatric disorders such as depression, schizophrenia, etc. Dementia also leads to affective and behavioral changes that may present as a primary psychiatric disorder. Thus, it is important to rule out psychiatric conditions that can mimic dementia-like symptoms, such as depression, delirium, schizophrenia, malingering, factitious disorder, and side effects of psychotropic medications such as benzodiazepines **(Flowchart 1)**.[2] Apart from these, the other differentials

**Flowchart 1:** Common differential diagnosis of dementia.

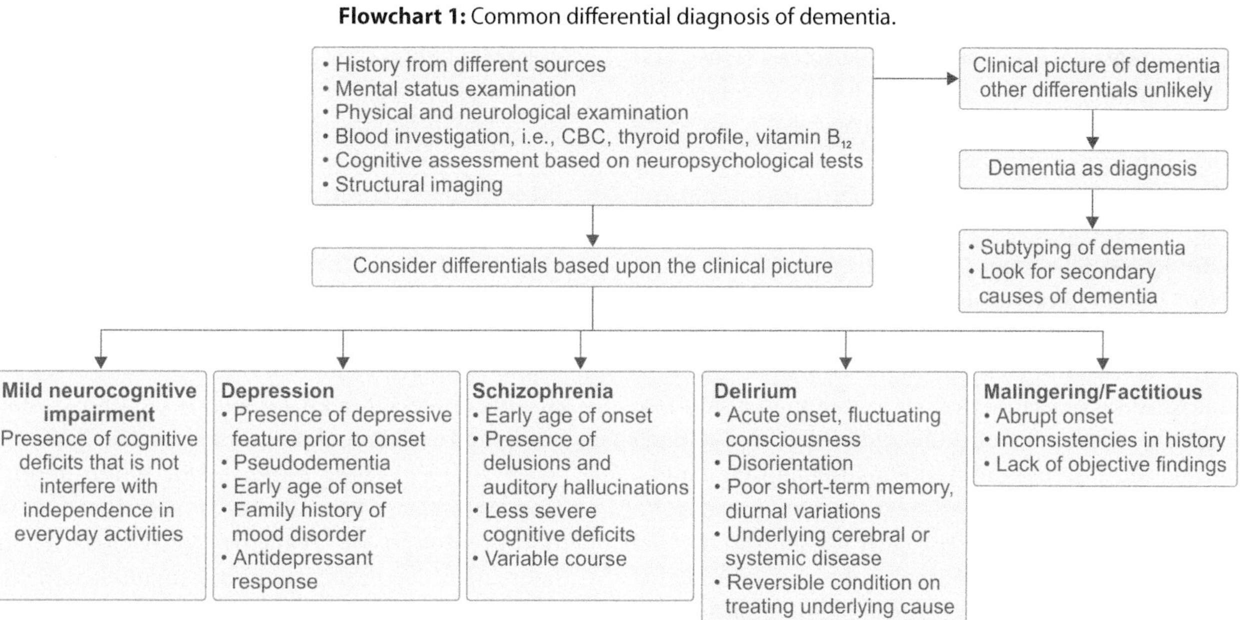


*Note:* The above schematic is not exhaustive, and represent common differentials in clinical setting.
(CBC: complete blood count)

of dementia include mild neurocognitive impairment and cognitive decline is secondary to medical conditions. The following list is not exhaustive, and there may be other conditions presenting with gradual and stable cognitive decline.

- *Depression:* It is one of the common differentials for dementia. Some patients may present with cognitive impairment in the background of depressive disorder, often referred to as "pseudodementia". Patients with pseudodementia typically have depressive features before the onset of cognitive symptoms, have an earlier age of onset compared to those with dementia, an acute onset of cognitive decline with rapid progression, maintain insight into their symptoms, and have a family history of mood disorder or a personal history of multiple prior depressive episodes, and variations in cognitive symptoms in line with changes in depressive symptoms. A detailed neuropsychiatric assessment, including neuropsychological and psychiatric evaluation, is necessary for diagnosis. Focal neurological deficits are absent, and mental status assessment and task performance show variable results. Aphasia, apraxia, and agnosia are common in dementia but uncommon in pseudodementia. These patients typically respond well to antidepressants.
- *Delirium:* Delirium is a common, complex neuropsychiatric disorder with a high prevalence among elderly hospitalized patients, manifesting as global cognitive impairment and other behavioral phenomena. Delirium and dementia can coexist, and delirium may act as a risk factor for the development of dementia. It is typically characterized by an acute onset (hours or days) of clouded consciousness and disturbed cognition, which fluctuates in nature. Other associated clinical features include variable activity levels, changes in the sleep-wake cycle, and perceptual alterations (illusions and hallucinations). The underlying etiological causes include cerebral or systemic diseases, exposure to drugs or toxins, intoxication or withdrawal, or a combination of these factors. Delirium can be differentiated from dementia based on its acute onset, fluctuating consciousness, disorientation, poor short-term memory, presence of visual hallucinations in the early stages, and diurnal fluctuations with preceding underlying etiological conditions. Delirium is a reversible condition, and treatment depends on identifying and treating the underlying cause.
- *Schizophrenia:* Schizophrenia is one of the most common severe mental disorders, characterized by delusions, hallucinations, disorganized speech, disorganized behavior, and negative symptoms. Since personality and behavioral changes are common in both disorders, it can be difficult to differentiate them, particularly the behavioral variant of frontotemporal dementia from schizophrenia. Schizophrenia typically begins early in life, usually before 25 years of age. The most common hallucinations in schizophrenia are auditory, whereas in dementia, psychotic symptoms appear in the advance stages and hallucinations are usually visual. Cognitive deficits are present in schizophrenia but are generally less severe than those in dementia. Schizophrenia has a variable course, whereas dementias are progressive.
- *Malingering and factitious disorder:* It is important to differentiate these disorders from dementia as patients may intentionally produce or feign memory loss for external gain or to assume a sick role. Detailed history taking can reveal erratic patterns and inconsistencies in symptoms, along with a lack of objective evidence such as neurocognitive deficits on neuropsychological tests or neuroimaging findings consistent with dementia.
- *Substance-induced cognitive decline:* Certain substances, such as benzodiazepines, inhalants, and cannabis, can lead to cognitive decline. Benzodiazepines are the most commonly prescribed sedative-hypnotics and are highly prevalent among elderly patients. They impair aspects of cognition such as attention and memory, and chronic use may lead to cognitive decline. In short-term users, the effects include decreased alertness, impaired psychomotor performance, confusional state, and anterograde amnesia, whereas dementia is characterized by global cognitive decline. These effects are usually reversible with short- to medium-term use of benzodiazepine. While cognitive deficits can occur at any age, elderly individuals are at higher risk, and the progression of substance-induced cognitive decline is slower compared to the rapid progression seen in dementia.
- *Mild neurocognitive impairment:* While dementia is diagnosed when there is interference with independence in everyday activities, in mild neurocognitive impairment, the cognitive deficits do not interfere with independence in everyday activities.
- *Cognitive decline secondary to medical causes:* Certain medical conditions can lead to temporary cognitive

decline, which may improve once the underlying medical cause is addressed. For example, postoperative cognitive dysfunction (POCD) is a condition that can occur after surgery and usually improves over a few months. However, patients who develop POCD are at a higher risk of developing dementia in the future. The patient's history and clinical condition can provide valuable clues to differentiate dementia from these conditions.

## SUBTYPES OF DEMENTIA

Among patients diagnosed with dementia, identifying the type of dementia can help target treatment, especially in cases of secondary dementia where the cause is treatable. There are several types of dementia based on etiology **(Flowchart 2)**. Primary dementia refers to conditions where dementia is the main illness, whereas secondary dementia occurs due to another disease or condition. Examples of primary dementia include Alzheimer disease, Lewy body dementia, vascular dementia, and frontotemporal dementia. Secondary dementias include conditions such as dementia due to Parkinson's disease, NCD due to HIV infection, NCD due to Prion disease, and alcohol-related dementia.[3]

### Primary Dementias

In the case of primary dementia, clinical features can help distinguish different types of dementia in the early stages, However, as cognitive impairment broadens in the later stages, it may become difficult to distinguish between the types. Some diagnostic pointers for the type of dementia based on the clinical picture are as follows:

1. *Alzheimer's dementia:* The clinical picture usually shows insidious onset and gradual progression of symptoms. Memory impairment and difficulty in learning new things are the most common early features, while visuospatial and language deficits occur as the disease progresses. In severe stages, parkinsonian-like extrapyramidal signs and symptoms may appear. Behavioral and psychological symptoms can also occur.
2. *Vascular dementia:* The clinical picture is usually stepwise deterioration. The cognitive decline depends on the location and the extent of the cerebrovascular event. There is unequal distribution of deficits in higher cognitive functions, with some functions affected more than others. There will be a temporal relation between the cerebrovascular event and onset of cognitive impairment. Evidence of cerebrovascular disease will be present.
3. *Frontotemporal dementia:* This heterogenous group of dementias is characterized by circumscribed atrophy of the frontal and temporal regions, with an insidious onset and gradual progression. There are two main types—the behavioral variant and the language variant. In the behavioral variant, prominent changes in social behavior or personality occur, including disinhibition, apathy, loss of sympathy, perseveration in speech, and compulsive or ritualistic behavior. In the language variant, there can be difficulty finding

**Flowchart 2:** Types of dementias.

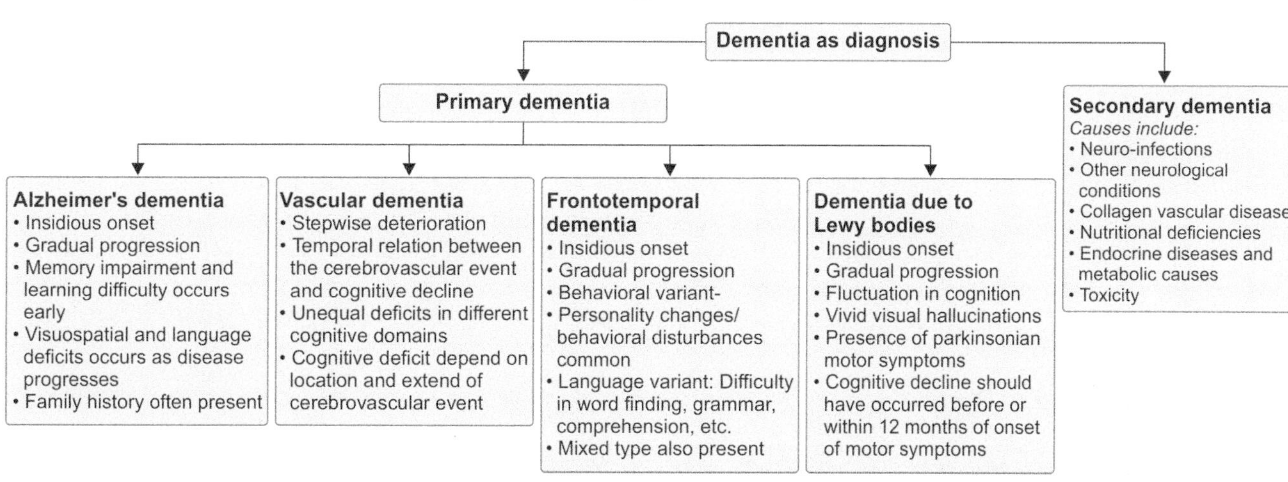

words, frequent pauses, impaired naming, difficulty in comprehension, agrammatism, and/or impaired speech production. Learning and memory are relatively spared.

4. *Dementia due to Lewy bodies (DLB):* This type also has an insidious onset and gradual progression. It is characterized by fluctuations in cognition with pronounced variation in attention and alertness, recurring or long-lasting vivid visual hallucinations, and motor features of parkinsonism such as tremors, rigidity, and slowness of movement. DLB should be diagnosed if dementia precedes or occurs within 12 months of the onset of motor symptoms. If it occurs after 12 months of the onset of motor symptoms, it is diagnosed as dementia due to Parkinson's disease. The other challenge that occurs in diagnosis of DLB is that because of the clinical picture of fluctuating cognition, it is often difficult to differentiate it from delirium. Also, patients with DLB are at higher risk of developing superimposed delirium. While delirium is an acute condition and DLB develops gradually, clinically, it is often difficult to differentiate.

## Secondary Dementias

There are various etiological possibilities for secondary dementia. A detailed history, careful clinical examination, and appropriate investigations can help to identify the cause for secondary dementia.

Some of the causes for secondary dementias are as follows:

- *Neuroinfections:* HIV-associated dementia, tuberculosis, syphilis, Creutzfeldt-Jacob disease, and Whipple's disease
- *Other neurological conditions:* Normal pressure hydrocephalus, multiple sclerosis, brain tumors, and Huntington disease
- *Collagen vascular disease:* Systemic lupus erythematosus and sarcoidosis
- *Nutritional deficiencies:* Vitamin $B_{12}$ deficiency, thiamine deficiency, and folate deficiency
- *Endocrine diseases and metabolic causes:* Hypothyroidism, Cushing's syndrome, hepatic insufficiency, renal insufficiency, and Wilson's disease
- *Toxicity:* Alcohol, heavy metal toxicity, and secondary to radiotherapy

## REFERENCES

1. Diagnostic and Statistical Manual of Mental Disorders: DSM-5, 5th edition. United States: American Psychiatric Association; 2013.
2. Bottino C, Pádua AC, Smid J, Areza-Fegyveres R, Novaretti T, Bahia VS. Differential diagnosis between dementia and psychiatric disorders: Diagnostic criteria and supplementary exams Recommendations of the Scientific Department of Cognitive Neurology and Aging of the Brazilian Academy of Neurology. Dement Neuropsychologia. 2011;5:288-96.
3. Weiner MF, Lipton AM. The American Psychiatric Publishing textbook of Alzheimer disease and other dementias. United States: American Psychiatric Publishing; 2009.

CHAPTER 38

# Pharmacological Management of Dementia: Cognitive Symptoms

*Rohit Verma, Panna Sharma*

## INTRODUCTION

- The term dementia originates from the Latin word "*dementatus*", which means "out of one's mind". The International Classification of Diseases version 10 defines dementia as a syndrome due to brain disease, typically chronic or progressive nature. It involves the disturbance of multiple higher cortical functions, including memory, thinking, orientation, orientation, comprehension, calculation, learning capacity, language, and judgment.
- *Etiology:* Neurodegenerative disorders, vascular diseases, multiple sclerosis, brain tumor, hypothyroidism, hypercalcemia, infections, traumatic factors, chronic alcohol abuse, vitamin deficiencies, etc.
- The most prevalent neurodegenerative disorder is Alzheimer's disease (AD), accounting for 70–80% of dementia cases, while vascular diseases contribute to 5–20% of cases.
- Cognitive impairment is a hallmark feature of dementia, affecting nearly all cognitive domains, including complex attention, executive function, learning and memory, language, perceptual motor skills, and social cognition.
- *Pathogenesis:*
  - Abnormal processing, misfolding, and the accumulation of specific proteins such as amyloid beta, tau, alpha-synuclein, and TDP-43 contribute to the pathology of various neurodegenerative disorders.
  - Cholinergic neural circuits play a crucial role in cognitive functions such as attention, memory, and emotions. In AD, there is a notable loss of cholinergic neurons, particularly in the nucleus basalis of Meynert. This reduction in cholinergic function correlates with the cognitive decline in AD.
  - The number of glutamatergic neurons is also significantly reduced in AD, particularly in the cerebral cortex and the hippocampus, leading to cognitive decline.

## ASSESSMENT TOOLS

*Some of the instruments for assessment of cognitive impairment are:*

- Mini Mental State Examination (MMSE)
- Hindi Mental Status Examination (HMSE)
- Addenbrooke's Cognitive Examination (ACE-III)
- Montreal Cognitive Assessment (MoCA)
- Alzheimer's Disease Assessment Scale-cognitive (ADAS-cog)
- California Verbal Learning Test (CVLT)
- Rey Auditory Verbal Learning Test (RAVLT)
- Wechsler Memory Scale (WMS)
- Rey-Osterrieth Complex Figure (ROCF)
- Wisconsin Card Sorting Task (WCST)
- Verbal Fluency Test (VFT)
- Boston Naming Test (BNT)
- Judgment of Line Orientation (JLO)

## MEDICATIONS TO MANAGE COGNITIVE IMPAIRMENT IN DEMENTIA

Several medications developed over the years have played an important role in ameliorating cognitive deficits, which are discussed here:[1]

- The progressive memory decline in AD has been linked to the selective impairment of cholinergic neurotransmission. Cholinergic neurotransmission occurs when acetylcholine (ACh), released from the presynaptic neuron, binds to nicotinic or muscarinic postsynaptic ACh receptors. The human brain has two major forms of cholinesterase (ChE) enzymes: acetylcholinesterase (AChE) and butyrylcholinesterase (BuChE). AChE is found in the synaptic cleft (in a soluble form) and synaptic membranes (in a membrane-bound form), while BuChE is mainly associated with glial cells.

- Medications acting as cholinesterase inhibitors (ChEIs) primarily inhibit the enzyme AChE, thereby reducing the breakdown of ACh.
- ChEIs are classified as reversible, irreversible, or pseudoreversible. Reversible ChEIs are commonly used for therapeutic purposes, while irreversible and pseudoreversible ChEIs are often used in pesticides and biowarfare (nerve agents). These are very effective in improving cognitive symptoms in Dementia.[2]
    - *Donepezil:* Reversible noncompetitive AChE inhibitor
    - *Galantamine:* Reversible competitive AChE inhibitor
    - *Rivastigmine:* Pseudoirreversible dual AChE and BuChE inhibitor
- ChEIs have the potential to induce centrally mediated cholinergic adverse events such as nausea and vomiting if the dose is increased too rapidly or in excessively large increments. To avoid these, the usual practice is to adopt a "start low and go slow" approach.
- Glutamate is a major excitatory neurotransmitter in the brain. One of the receptors activated by glutamate is the N-methyl-D-aspartate (NMDA) receptor, essential for functions such as neural transmission, learning, memory processes, and neuronal plasticity.
- N-methyl-D-aspartate receptor (NMDAR) is a voltage-gated cation channel that, in its physiological

**Flowchart 1:** Treatment algorithm for cognitive symptoms of AD.

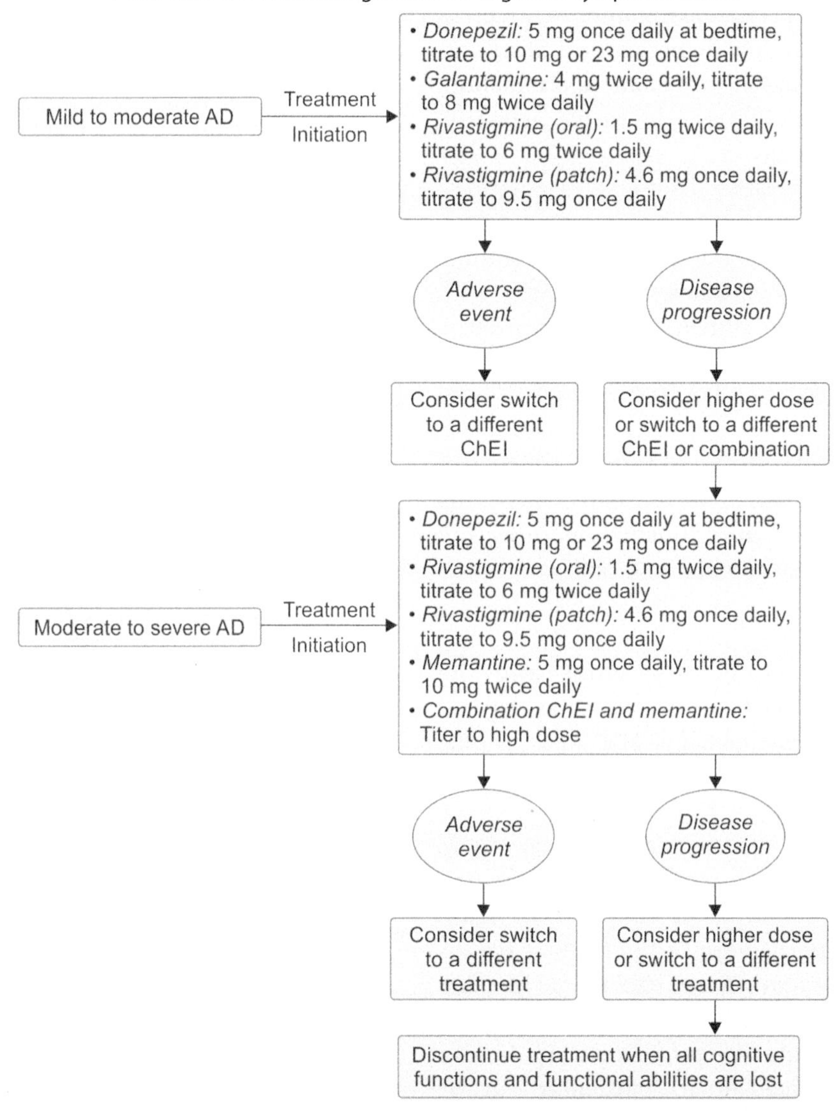

non-stimulated state, is blocked by magnesium ions. Upon stimulation, magnesium is displaced, allowing calcium influx through the channel and activation of the neuron. In AD, it is estimated that there is pathological overstimulation of the receptor, leading to a chronically active state. While physiological NMDAR activity is essential for normal neuronal function, an excessive activation of NMDAR is associated with neuronal loss/damage, contributing to dementia. Thus, it is imperative to maintain an optimal balance that reduces NMDAR activity without affecting healthy physiological function.

- *Memantine:* Noncompetitive antagonist of extrasynaptic NMDAR.

- *Combination treatment:* Both glutamatergic and cholinergic mechanisms play crucial roles in the induction and maintenance of long-term potentiation, highlighting their significance in cognitive function. Studies suggest that the addition of memantine to ChEIs helps prevent further cognitive deterioration.
- *Other pharmacological treatment*: Various pharmacological treatment strategies have been employed to address cognitive deficits, but none have demonstrated robust evidence to warrant recommendation in treatment guidelines. Examples include cholinergic enhancers, European herbs and natural essential oils (such as *Salvia officinalis* and *Melissa officinalis*), *Ginkgo biloba*, nonsteroidal anti-inflammatory drugs (NSAIDs), estrogens, selegiline, vitamin E, nootropics (e.g., olacetam, piracetam, and aniracetam), ergot alkaloids (e.g., dihydroergotoxine mesylate), and α1-adrenergic receptor antagonist (e.g., nicergoline).

## CONCLUSION

There are few large-scale studies for the treatment of cognitive impairment in dementias apart from AD. The majority of beneficial evidence is for ChEIs and NMDAR antagonists in AD, and to some extent in Lewy body dementia. While ChEIs are recommended for mild to severe forms of impairment, memantine has modest evidence, mostly as an adjunct in severe impairment only **(Flowchart 1)**. Medications should be initiated as early as possible, and dose titration should be done slowly. The pharmacological management approach should always be complemented with psychosocial therapy, which remains the mainstay of management. Emerging neuromodulation techniques show promise and may provide newer insights into treatment approaches for improving cognitive functioning in dementia.

## REFERENCES

1. Perng CH, Chang YC, Tzang RF. The treatment of cognitive dysfunction in dementia: a multiple treatments meta-analysis. Psychopharmacology (Berl). 2018;235(5):1571-80.
2. Tisher A, Salardini A. A comprehensive update on treatment of dementia. Semin Neurol. 2019;39(2):167-78.

CHAPTER 39

# Pharmacological Management of Noncognitive Symptoms of Dementia

*Lokesh Kumar Singh, P Lakshmi Nirisha*

## INTRODUCTION

Dementia is a neurodegenerative disorder characterized by cognitive symptoms and noncognitive symptoms. >70% of individuals with dementia have noncognitive symptoms, which are also known as *behavioral and psychological symptoms of dementia* (BPSD).Click or tap here to enter text.[1,2] Noncognitive symptoms are characterized by behavioral and psychiatric symptoms associated with dementia; these may also present as primary symptoms, such as psychotic symptoms in Lewy body dementia (LBD). They often correlate with the progression of the illness and hence are equally important as cognitive symptoms.

## NONCOGNITIVE SYMPTOMS OF DEMENTIA

- Depression and anxiety
- Psychosis
- Agitation and aggression
- Wandering, pacing, hoarding
- Repetitive shouting
- Inappropriate sexual behavior
- Sleep disturbances
- Apathy

## BRIEF DESCRIPTION OF NONCOGNITIVE SYMPTOMS OF DEMENTIA

- *Psychosis or psychotic symptoms:* The prevalence of psychosis or psychotic symptoms varies widely, ranging from 10 to 80%.[3-5] Paranoid delusions are common in Alzheimer's dementia (AD), particularly in severe stages, while visual hallucinations are commonly seen in LBD.
- *Agitation and aggression:* Agitation and aggression are commonly seen in patients with dementia, more so as the illness progresses. The prevalence of agitation and aggression varies across different types of dementia: 30–50% in AD, 30% in LBD, and 40% in frontotemporal dementia (FTD) and vascular dementia (VaD). Factors associated with aggression and agitation could be illness-related, i.e., disease progression, acute and chronic pain, and sleep disturbances. Additionally, sensory impairment, delirium, infections, and other psychiatric manifestations such as depression, anxiety, and psychosis can play a role. Substance use and medications are other important causes that can contribute to agitation.
- *Sleep disorders:* Dementia is frequently associated with sleep disorders. In AD, 40% of patients experience sleep and circadian rhythm disturbances. In LBD, 90% of patients have sleep disturbances. FTD often leads to poorer sleep quality, shorter sleep duration, daytime hypersomnia, delayed circadian phase, and sundowning. In VaD, obstructive sleep apnea is commonly seen. Sleep disturbances can also result from the adverse effects of medications, such as acetylcholinesterase inhibitors. Comorbidity of primary sleep disorders is also high in patients with dementia.[6,7]
- *Depression:* Among patients with dementia, 40% experience depression. It is noteworthy that in dementia patients, mood disturbances manifest differently than typical low mood; instead, they may present with anxiety, irritability, agitation, accompanied by disturbances in biological functions.[8]
- *Anxiety:* The incidence of anxiety symptoms varies widely, ranging from 8 to 71%, while anxiety disorders occur in 5 to 21% of dementia cases. Anxiety is more common in AD, VaD, FTD, and Parkinson's disease dementia, and are more common in the early stages of dementia.[9]
- *Inappropriate sexual behavior (ISB):* Inappropriate sexual behavior in dementia can manifest as inappropriate touching of genitals, inappropriate speech, sexual disinhibition, and hypersexuality. Its prevalence ranges between 7 and 25%.[10,11]

- *Wandering and pacing:* Wandering and pacing are common behaviors seen in persons with dementia and can cause significant distress to caregivers. If their movement is restricted, they may exhibit aggression. When a patient is on medications such as antipsychotics, it is important to consider the possibility of akathisia and discontinue the offending drug. Nonpharmacological interventions are often preferred over psychotropics as the primary line of treatment.[12]
- *Hoarding:* Hoarding behavior, i.e., collecting unnecessary objects or items that have lost their utility, is common in patients with dementia. While its exact prevalence is unknown, it is frequently seen in the behavioral variant of FTD. *Diogenes syndrome*, which includes excessive hoarding and severe self-neglect, has been observed in patients with dementia, particularly FTD. Attempting to discard or remove hoarded objects can lead to aggression and anxiety in elderly individuals with dementia[13]. Treatment for hoarding primarily involves behavioral strategies, with psychotropic medications reserved for cases of severe anxiety and aggression. Clear recommendations for psychotropics in hoarding behavior are lacking **(Table 1)**.

## MANAGEMENT OF NONCOGNITIVE SYMPTOMS OF DEMENTIA (FLOWCHART 1 AND TABLE 2)

### Assessment

- *Detailed clinical history:* Review the clinical course of the illness, medical comorbidities, substance use, psychiatric illness, and medications.
- Patient's subjective experiences need evaluation whenever possible.
- *Objective behavior:* Caregiver report or observation.
- Assess the comfort of the patient.

### Scales for Assessment of Noncognitive Symptoms of Dementia

Tools help set a baseline and measure the response to treatment.

- *Neuropsychiatric inventory (NPI):* Most commonly used scale, has 12 items.
  - Based on the caregiver report.
  - Includes all domains of BPSD.
  - It is type-specific.
- *Behavioral Pathology in Alzheimer's Disease Rating Scale (BEHAVE-AD)*
  - Informant-based assessment
  - Mainly designed for AD
  - It has two parts: Part 1—focuses on symptomatology and part 2—the rating of the symptoms.
  - The domains covered are paranoid and delusional ideation; hallucinations; activity disturbances; aggression; diurnal variation; mood; and anxieties and phobia

## GENERAL PRINCIPLES OF PRESCRIBING PSYCHOTROPICS FOR NONCOGNITIVE SYMPTOMS OF DEMENTIA

- *Assessment:* Identify and evaluate the symptoms, including stage of dementia, behavioral analysis of other symptoms, general medical and preexisting

**TABLE 1:** Factors contributing to and influencing the presentation of noncognitive symptoms of dementia (NCSD).

| *Biological factors* | *Psychological factors* | *Environmental factors* |
|---|---|---|
| Type of dementia | *Unmet needs:* The loss of ability to express needs or goals | Overstimulation or understimulation |
| *Stage of dementia:* Severity corresponds to the neurodegeneration | *Premorbid neuroticism:* The tendency to respond to challenges with exaggerated negative emotions such as anxiety, depression, and anger | Lack of activity |
| Comorbidities | History of post-traumatic stress disorder | Lack of a set routine |
| Acute medical conditions such as infection | Loss of purpose, loss of control | Unfamiliarity with the surroundings |
| Pain | Problematic caregiver communication styles | |
| History of psychiatric illnesses: Mood disorders or psychotic illness | | |
| Substance use and withdrawal | | |

**Flowchart 1:** Steps to follow for evaluation of NCSD.

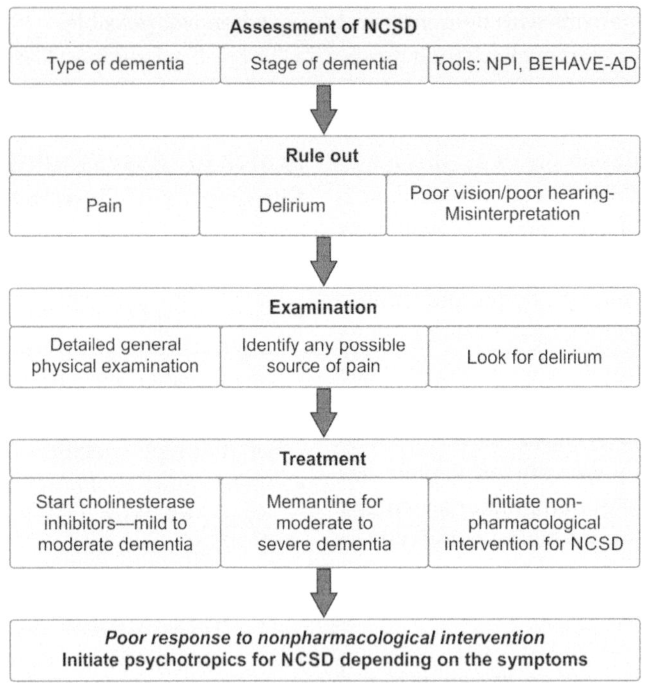


(NCSD: noncognitive symptoms of dementia; NPI: neuropsychiatric inventory; BEHAVE-AD: Behavioral Pathology in Alzheimer's Disease Rating Scale)

**TABLE 2:** Summary of management of various NCSDs.

| | ***Pharmacological management*** | ***Duration of treatment*** | ***Precautions*** |
|---|---|---|---|
| Psychosis | • Low-dose antipsychotics<br>• Risperidone/aripiprazole/olanzapine/quetiapine<br>• Clozapine/quetiapine in LBD | Trial of 4 weeks<br>• Response present: 4 months duration, attempt tapering<br>• Poor or no response: Reassess and change antipsychotic | • FGAs are only in the case of acute aggression<br>• And low-dose haloperidol in delirium<br>• Avoid FGAs otherwise – the risk of EPS and other adverse effects<br>• In case of psychosis and Psychotic symptoms in LBD, Clozapine/quetiapine is to be administered in view decreased risk of EPS |
| Depression and anxiety | • *Mild to moderate depression:* Nonpharmacological intervention<br>• *Previous history of depression/severe depression:* SSRIs are the first choice of drugs<br>*However, nonpharmacological interventions take precedence*<br>• ECT to be considered in case of severe depression with risk of harm to self/others, and in case of poor response to Antidepressants | • No clear duration of treatment, review the risks versus benefits of continuing the antidepressants<br>• Taper and stop drug watch for worsening of symptoms and discontinuation syndrome | • Monitor adverse effects—sedation, hyponatremia, anticholinergic side effects<br>• Avoid high doses of medications |

*Contd...*

*Contd...*

| | ***Pharmacological management*** | ***Duration of treatment*** | ***Precautions*** |
|---|---|---|---|
| Agitation | • Nonpharmacological management should be attempted first. Assess for antecedents such as pain, discomfort due to environmental factors, medications, and drug withdrawal<br>• If not manageable with behavioral strategies, and agitation is persistent<br>Then consider *SSRIs as first-line psychotropic agents* | • No clear duration of treatment, review the risk vs benefits of continuing the antidepressants<br>• Taper and stop drug watch for worsening of symptoms and discontinuation syndrome | • Antipsychotics should not be routinely used—no utility in agitation in dementia<br>• Watch for paradoxical worsening of agitation if using benzodiazepines |
| Aggression | Verbal deescalation is to be attempted before administering medication<br>• Low-dose first-generation antipsychotics for acute management of aggression<br>• Low-dose SGAs as described for psychosis management for a longer duration of treatment | • Assess the requirement periodically<br>• Attempt tapering after a few weeks of a decrease in symptoms | FGAs should not be used continuously only for acute aggression management |
| *Sleep disorders:* Insomnia/night terrors | The first line focuses on sleep hygiene<br>*Medications:*<br>• *Melatonin:* 3–6 mg, beneficial in improving the quality of sleep<br>• *Trazodone:* 25–50 mg (benefits sleep and can consider if there is comorbid depression too)<br>• *Mirtazapine:* Up to 15 mg<br>• Nonbenzodiazepines (Z-drugs)<br>– Zolpidem 5 mg at night<br>– Zaleplon 5 mg | Use medications for a short-term period | • Watch for excess sedation<br>• Risk of falls<br>• Dependence on sedative hypnotics and risk of withdrawal to be watched for |
| Inappropriate sexual behavior (ISB) | *First line:* Nonpharmacological—behavioral strategies to be adopted<br>*Medications:*<br>• *Antidepressants:* SSRIs are beneficial in addressing disinhibition, hypersexuality<br>• *Hormonal treatments:*<br>– *Antiandrogens:*<br>- Medroxyprogesterone acetate in women<br>- Finasteride is a 5α-reductase inhibitor in men<br>- Estrogens<br>• *Antipsychotics:* Atypical antipsychotics in low dose | No clear duration of treatment, assess risk vs benefit periodically, and then consider withdrawing the drug in a 6–8 week duration | • Weigh risks vs benefits before initiating medication for ISB<br>• Hormonal treatments are not used routinely |
| Hoarding/pacing | • Behavioral management is primary<br>• Psychotropics have little role and often have shown to have no benefit in the symptoms of pacing and hoarding in dementia<br>• SSRIs may be given in hoarding only if there is comorbid obsessive-compulsive disorder (OCD) | | |

**Flowchart 2:** Psychotropics, indications in NCSD.

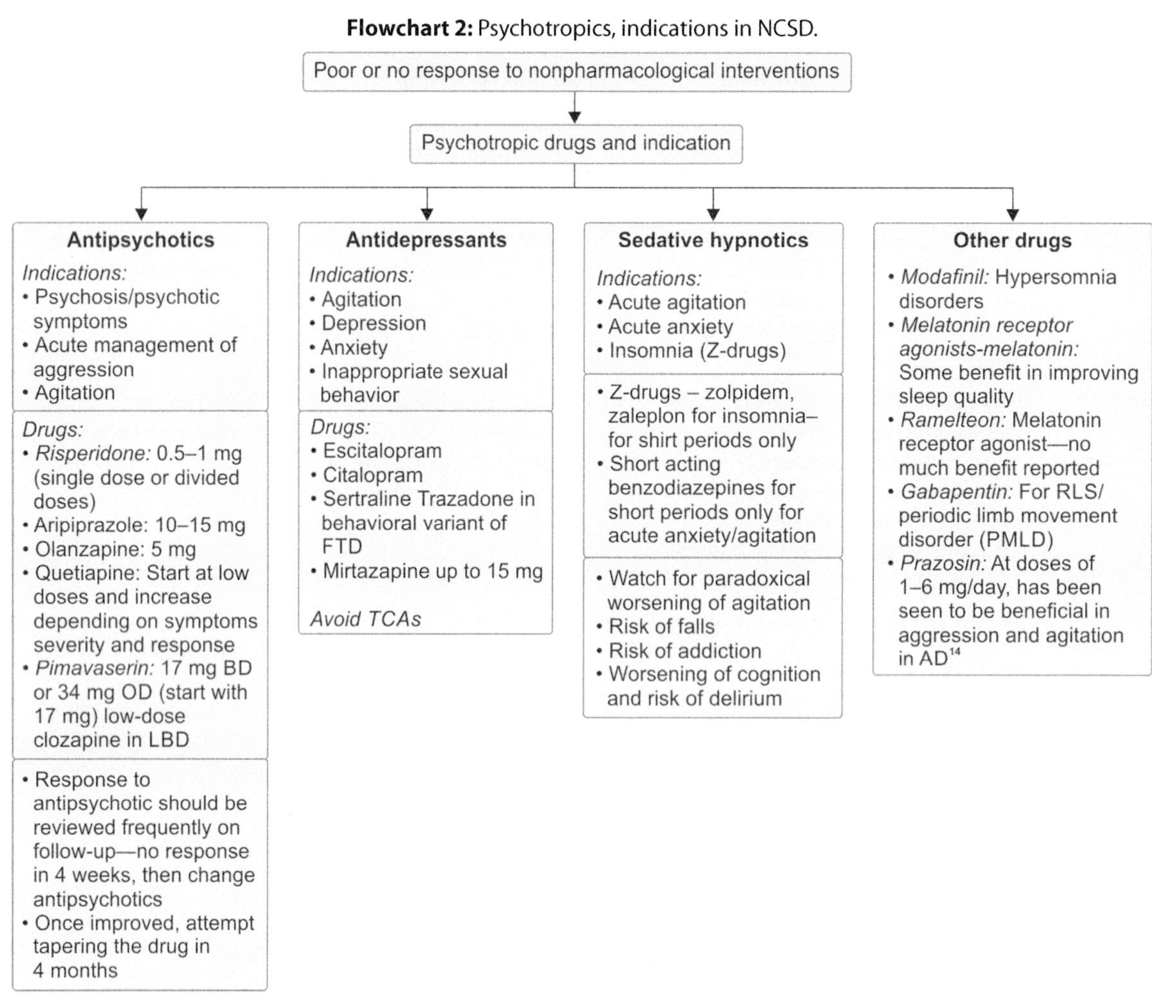


(FTD: frontotemporal dementia; LBD: Lewy body dementia; NCSD: noncognitive symptoms of dementia; PMLD: periodic limb movement disorder; RLS: restless leg syndrome; TCA: tricyclic antidepressant)

psychiatric comorbidities, and treatment history, including current and past medications, and their effects.

- Review other medications that may contribute to these symptoms.
- Prioritize nonpharmacological interventions as the first-line management for noncognitive symptoms.
- Involve caregivers in treatment planning.
- Consider pharmacological interventions only when nonpharmacological interventions fail or when non-cognitive symptoms are severe and pose a risk of harm to the patient or caregivers.
- Start at low doses and titrate gradually.
- Monitor closely for adverse effects and adjust treatment accordingly **(Flowchart 2)**.

## CONCLUSION

Noncognitive symptoms of dementia are seen commonly observed across all types of dementia. Treatment strategies should prioritize initiating acetylcholinesterase inhibitors as first-line management for NCSD. Psychotropic medications should be considered only if symptoms cause distress to the patient and caregiver after ruling out other factors such as pain, infection, and discomfort. If psychotropics are initiated, start at low doses and review periodically for adverse effects. Once symptoms improve, assess the risks vs benefits and consider tapering off the medications.

## REFERENCES


1. Selbæk G, Engedal K, Bergh S. The prevalence and course of neuropsychiatric symptoms in nursing home patients with dementia: A Systematic Review. J Am Med Dir Assoc. 2013;14(3):161-9.
2. Management of non-cognitive symptoms associated with dementia. Drug Ther Bull. 2014;52(10):114-8.
3. Leroi I, Voulgari A, Breitner JCS, Lyketsos CG. The epidemiology of psychosis in dementia. Am J Geriatr Psychiatr. 2003;11(1):83-91.
4. Chen J, Bell S, Brain C. The incidence of dementia-related psychosis in people with dementia: Results from a survey of 302 U.S. healthcare providers. Alzheimer's Dementia. 2020;16(S6).
5. Ismail Z, Creese B, Aarsland D, Kales HC, Lyketsos CG, Sweet RA, et al. Psychosis in Alzheimer disease — mechanisms, genetics and therapeutic opportunities. Nat Rev Neurol. 2022;18(3):131-44.
6. Ooms S, Ju YE. Treatment of sleep disorders in dementia. Curr Treat Options Neurol. 2016;18(9):40.
7. Rose KM, Lorenz R. Sleep disturbances in dementia: what they are and what to do. J Gerontol Nurs. 2010 May;36(5):9-14.
8. Kitching D. Depression in dementia. Aust Prescr. 2015;38(6):209-11.
9. Kwak YT, Yang Y, Koo MS. Anxiety in dementia. Dement Neurocogn Disord. 2017;16(2):33.
10. Sarangi A, Jones H, Bangash F, Gude J. Treatment and management of sexual disinhibition in elderly patients with neurocognitive disorders. Cureus. 2021;13(10): e18463.
11. De Giorgi R, Series H. Treatment of inappropriate sexual behavior in dementia. Curr Treat Options Neurol. 2016;18(9):41.
12. Desai AK, Grossberg GT. Recognition and management of behavioral disturbances in dementia. Prim Care Companion CNS Disord. 2001;3(3).
13. Finney CM, Mendez MF. Diogenes syndrome in frontotemporal dementia. Am J Alzheimers Dis Other Demen. 2017;32(7):438-43.
14. Davies SJ, Burhan AM, Kim D, Gerretsen P, Graff-Guerrero A, Woo VL, et al. Sequential drug treatment algorithm for agitation and aggression in Alzheimer's and mixed dementia. J Psychopharmacol. 2018;32(5):509-23.

CHAPTER 40

# How to Assess Suicidal Behavior?

Rahul Patley, Suchandra Harihara, Manjunatha Narayana

## INTRODUCTION

Addressing suicide risk is a paramount concern in the field of mental health, necessitating meticulous assessment and intervention. It is imperative to acknowledge that suicide risk can manifest across a range of mental illnesses, including depression, bipolar disorder, psychosis, post-traumatic stress disorder (PTSD), substance use disorders, and others.[1] The identification and assessment of suicide risk demand constant vigilance to ensure the safety and well-being of individuals grappling with these conditions.

It is essential for mental health practitioners to recognize that suicidal thoughts and behaviors can emerge amidst various clinical presentations. While specific mental disorders such as bipolar disorder and major depressive disorder may exhibit a higher correlation with suicide risk, it is crucial to understand that the potential for suicide exists across the entire spectrum of psychiatric conditions.[1] This realization underscores the need for a comprehensive and systematic approach to suicide risk assessment that transcends specific diagnostic categories.

By comprehending the intricate interplay between mental health conditions and suicide risk, healthcare professionals can cultivate heightened awareness and adopt a proactive stance in identifying individuals who may be at an elevated risk of self-harm or suicide. Through vigilant assessment and appropriate intervention, it becomes possible to save lives and extend crucial support to those in distress.

In the forthcoming chapter, we will delve into the fundamental components of psychiatry history taking, emphasizing its pivotal role in the identification of suicide risk. By exploring pivotal aspects such as the patient's background, psychiatric history, and present clinical presentation, we can gain a holistic understanding of their unique circumstances and potential risk factors. This knowledge, combined with a systematic approach to conducting a mental status examination, empowers healthcare professionals to effectively evaluate and address suicide risk.

## ASSESSMENT

### Establishing Rapport

Building a trusting and empathetic relationship with the patient is essential. Begin the assessment by creating a safe and nonjudgmental environment, ensuring privacy, and expressing genuine concern for the patient's well-being. Provide adequate time for the individuals to open up.

### Gathering General Information

Start the history taking process by collecting basic demographic details, such as age, gender, marital status, and occupation **(Box 1)**. This information provides a foundation for understanding the patient's background and potential risk factors.

### Presenting Complaint

Allow the patient to share their primary concerns, symptoms, or distressing experiences. Encourage them to openly express their emotions, thoughts, and any recent life events that may have contributed to their current state.

### Exploring Contributing Factors

Inquire about factors that may increase suicide risk, including:

- *Psychiatric history:* Evaluate the presence of any previous suicide attempts, psychiatric diagnoses (especially bipolar disorders, mood disorders, substance abuse, or personality disorders), and family history of suicide. Remember that the presence of past or family history of suicide, and the presence of psychiatric disorders are risk factors for suicide. Medical illnesses such as terminal illness and physical disability are also associated with increased suicide risk.

**BOX 1:** Demographics and suicide.[2,3]

- *Age:*
  - Highest risk among the 15–29 years age group
  - Common in the elderly as well and is associated with lack of family support, boredom and loneliness, depression, chronic physical illness, and substance abuse
- *Gender:*
  - Suicide attempts are seen in women more than in men
  - Numbers and rates of suicide fatalities are consistently higher among men
  - Higher risk is due to marital problems, interpersonal problems with husband and in-laws, domestic violence, and divorce
- *Educational status:*
  - Maximum are educated up to secondary level. <5% of suicides are seen in graduates or those with higher education
- *Occupation:*
  - Unemployed, daily-wage laborers, housewives, and self-employed persons
- *Marital status:*
  - Considerably high suicide rates have been reported for those who are separated, divorced, or widowed when compared to those who were married or never married at all
- *Socioeconomic status:*
  - Lower economic status, especially those with an annual income of less than one lakh

- *Recent stressors:* Identify recent life events (e.g., loss of a loved one, job loss, or relationship problems) that may have triggered or exacerbated the patient's distress.[4]
- *Social support:* Assess the quality and availability of the patient's support system, including friends, family, or significant others. Literature has shown that good social support is a strong protective factor for those individuals with suicide risk and vice versa.
- *Access to lethal means:* Easy access to lethal means increases the risk of suicide. Determine if the patient has access to firearms, medications, or other potentially lethal methods.

### Evaluating Protective Factors

Identify protective factors that may mitigate suicide risk, including:

- *Social support:* Assess the presence of a strong network of supportive individuals who can provide emotional support and practical assistance.
- *Coping skills:* Evaluate the patient's ability to effectively manage stress, problem-solving skills, and engage in healthy coping mechanisms.
- *Treatment engagement:* Determine if the patient is currently receiving psychiatric care or has a history of positive response to treatment interventions.

## MENTAL STATUS EXAMINATION

Conduct a thorough mental status examination (MSE) to assess the patient's overall mental state. Pay particular attention to mood, affect, thought content, and cognition. Note any signs of hopelessness, helplessness, or persistent suicidal thoughts during the examination.

### Appearance and Behavior

Observe the patient's appearance, noting any changes in grooming, hygiene, or self-care. Look for signs of psychomotor agitation or retardation, restlessness, or behaviors indicative of impulsivity or hopelessness.

### Speech

Assess the patient's speech for abnormalities such as slowed speech, paucity of speech, or changes in volume. Note any indications of sadness, despair, or feelings of worthlessness expressed in their speech content.

### Mood and Affect

Evaluate the patient's mood, paying attention to indications of sadness, hopelessness, or despair. Assess the congruence between their reported mood and the expressed affect. Note any signs of heightened distress, irritability, or anhedonia (loss of interest or pleasure).

### Thought Process and Content

Explore the patient's thought process for signs of cognitive distortions, negative thinking patterns, or hopelessness. Assess for the presence of suicidal thoughts, plans, or intent. Inquire about the frequency, intensity, and duration of these thoughts. Note any evidence of cognitive constriction or hopelessness in their thought content.

### Perception

Ask about the presence of any perceptual disturbances related to suicide, such as auditory hallucinations commanding self-harm and visual images of self-harm. Assess the patient's interpretation and beliefs regarding these experiences.

## Insight and Judgment

Evaluate the patient's insight into their current mental state, including their understanding of the potential consequences of suicidal thoughts and actions. Assess their ability to recognize the need for help and engage in safety planning. Inquire about their judgment and decision-making when faced with distressing situations.

## Assessing Suicide Ideation

The following are the questions that can be asked to assess suicidality **(Box 2)**.

**BOX 2:** Questions to assess suicidality.

**Q1. What are your thoughts regarding the future?**
Many patients maintain optimism for improvement despite experiencing severe symptoms, but it is concerning when they feel hopeless and believe that things will never improve

**Q2. Have you ever had the feeling that life was not worth living?**
When someone feels hopeless, they may believe that even nothingness would be better

**Q3. Have you ever wished to go to bed and not wake up in the morning?**
Passive thoughts of death are common in mental illness and can also occur in the elderly, especially after the loss of a spouse or peers

**Q4. Have you had thoughts about ending your life?**
If so, it is important to inquire about the frequency of these thoughts. Are they fleeting and easily dismissed, or do they persist for longer periods? Are they becoming more frequent?

**Q5. Have you had thoughts of ending your life?**
It is concerning if the patient has considered violent methods that are likely to be fatal, such as shooting, hanging, or jumping from a height

**Q6. Have you thought about how you would do it?**
Ask about the methods of suicide the patient has considered. Particularly worrying are violent methods that are likely to succeed (e.g., shooting, hanging, or jumping from a height)

**Q7. Have you made any preparations?**
Aim to establish how far the patient's plans have progressed from ideas to action. Have they considered a place, bought pills, carried out a final act (e.g., suicide note, or begun putting their affairs in order)?

**Q8. Have you tried to take your own life?**
Further assessment may be needed if there has been a recent concealed attempt (e.g., overdose)

If there was a recent suicide attempt, enquire about the following:

- *Preparatory acts:*
  - The extent of isolation at the time of the attempt.
  - The timing of the event and whether intervention and discovery were possible.
  - Measures taken to ensure they are not discovered, such as locking the door.
  - Making efforts to contact or notify family or friends regarding the suicidal attempt.
  - Actively planning and preparing for the suicidal act.
- *Intentionality and lethality of the attempt:*
  - Whether the purpose of the attempt was to seek attention, take revenge, or manipulate, or it was to end the pain and solve all problems.
  - The expectation of fatality with the type of method used for the suicidal act.
  - The seriousness of the attempt in terms of their desire to actually end life.
  - The desire and option that one could be rescued.
- Reaction to the attempt in the form of remorse toward it, and their attitude toward life in terms of wanting to live.

## RISK STRATIFICATION

With the information obtained above, a comprehensive risk level can be determined depending upon risk factors, protective factors, intentionality and lethality of suicidal thoughts or behaviors, and accessibility to lethal means[5] **(Table 1, Box 3)**.

**TABLE 1:** Risk stratification.

| *Risk level* | *Based on risk factors and warning signs* | *Based on suicidal behavior* |
|---|---|---|
| High | • Depression or other psychiatric illnesses<br>• Multiple risk factors and warning signs<br>• Few protective factors<br>• Triggering events<br>• Absence of protective factors | • Has made a lethal attempt<br>• Recent suicidal attempts<br>• Recurring suicidal thoughts |
| Moderate | • More risk factors and warning signs<br>• Few protective factors | • Ideation with a plan |
| Low | • A few risk factors<br>• Strong protective factors | • Thoughts of death<br>• No plan, intent, or behavior |

**BOX 3:** Modified SADPERSONS scale.

The score is calculated from ten yes/no questions, with points given for each affirmative answer as follows:
- S: Male sex → 1
- A: Age 15–25 or 59+ years → 1
- D: Depression or hopelessness → 2
- P: Previous suicidal attempts or psychiatric care → 1
- E: Excessive ethanol or drug use → 1
- R: Rational thinking loss (psychotic or organic illness) → 2
- S: Single, widowed, or divorced → 1
- O: Organized or serious attempt → 2
- N: No social support → 1
- S: Stated future intent (determined to repeat or ambivalent) → 2

This score is then mapped onto a risk assessment scale as follows:
- 0–5: May be safe to discharge (depending upon circumstances)
- 6–8: Probably requires psychiatric consultation
- >8: Probably requires hospital admission

## CONCLUSION

The process of suicide risk identification requires a comprehensive understanding of the patient's psychiatric history, assessment of suicidal ideation, evaluation of contributing and protective factors, and a collaborative approach to safety planning. By employing these basic components of psychiatry, history taking, healthcare professionals can better identify individuals at risk and provide timely intervention and support.

## REFERENCES

1. Amudhan S, Gururaj G, Varghese M, Benegal V, Rao GN, Sheehan DV, et al. A population-based analysis of suicidality and its correlates: findings from the National Mental Health Survey of India, 2015-16. Lancet Psychiatry. 2020;7(1):41-51.
2. Dandona R, Bertozzi-Villa A, Kumar GA, Dandona L. Lessons from a decade of suicide surveillance in India: who, why and how? Int J Epidemiol. 2017;46(3):983-93.
3. Vijayakumar L. Indian research on suicide. Indian J Psychiatry. 2010;52(Suppl1):S291-6.
4. Vijayakumar L, John S, Pirkis J, Whiteford H. Suicide in developing countries (2): risk factors. Crisis. 2005;26(3):112-9.
5. Isaac M, Elias B, Katz LY, Belik SL, Deane FP, Enns MW, et al. Gatekeeper training as a preventative intervention for suicide: a systematic review. Can J Psychiatry. 2009; 54(4):260-8.

CHAPTER 41

# Management of Suicidal Behavior

*Anju Kuruvilla*

## INTRODUCTION

The management of suicidal behavior includes assessing the individual's current risk of harm to self and formulating an individualized treatment plan in collaboration with the patient and available supports, with a goal of reducing death from suicide and the frequency and intensity of suicide attempts.

## STEPS IN THE MANAGEMENT OF SUICIDAL BEHAVIOR

- Stabilize and manage medical problems if present.
- *Establish a therapeutic relationship with the patient*, beginning with the first interaction. Conveying a nonjudgmental, empathetic attitude will help to elicit information and understand the context of the suicidal behavior. Acknowledge their distress and offer support.[1]
- *Ensure immediate safety of the patient* even while the initial evaluation is being carried out. Place the patient under constant supervision so that they are never alone and remove potentially hazardous items (medication, pesticides, firearms, sharp objects, rope, etc.) from the patient's vicinity, belongings, and person.
- *Assess the current risk of harm to self* by evaluating present suicidal ideation/intent, precipitating circumstances, predisposing and protective factors. ("How to Assess Suicidal Behavior?" Chapter 40).
- *Based on the risk assessment, determine the safest place to manage the patient.* In general, patients should be treated in the setting that is least restrictive, yet most likely to provide safe and effective care. While hospitalization does not eliminate the potential for suicide, it provides a treatment setting that facilitates detailed evaluation, implementation of constant observation, and physical or pharmacological restraint that may restrict an individual's ability to act on suicidal impulses[2] **(Table 1)**.
- *Involve existing support systems* of family and friends in the care of the patient.

**TABLE 1:** Risk assessment and treatment setting.[1]

| *Level of risk* | *Risk and protective factors* | *Suicidality* | *Treatment setting* |
|---|---|---|---|
| High | Presence of psychiatric diagnoses with severe symptoms, acute precipitating event, substance abuse/dependence, severe depression, and command hallucinations. Few/absent protective factors, poor support system | Potentially lethal suicide attempt; persistent ideation with strong intent; preparatory actions present | Admission indicated |
| Moderate | Multiple risk factors present with few protective factors; inconsistent support system | Suicidal ideation with plan, but no intent or behavior; no preparatory acts made | Admission indicated |
| Low | Modifiable risk factors present, along with strong protective factors; a good social support system is available at home | Ideation is limited in frequency, intensity, or duration. No plan, intent, or behavior | Outpatient management may be considered, with a well-documented safety plan. Monitor closely for any change in risk |

- Address underlying factors for suicide, including precipitating events, ongoing life difficulties, and mental disorders.
  - Identify and treat mental disorders with appropriate pharmacotherapeutic and psychological strategies. Disorders commonly associated with suicidal behavior include depressive episodes, bipolar disorder, schizophrenia, substance use disorders, anxiety disorders, borderline personality disorder, and adjustment disorders.

  *Pharmacotherapy: Antidepressants* in adequate doses are required for the treatment of suicidal patients suffering from depressive and anxiety disorders.
    - After the initiation of antidepressant medication, there is usually a delay before clinical improvement occurs, though energy to act on suicidal impulses may increase.
    - Nontricyclic, non-monoamine oxidase inhibitors (non-MAOI) antidepressants are relatively safe as they have a low risk of lethality in overdose.
    - Medication for suicidal patients should be dispensed for limited periods at a time to restrict the amount of drugs available for overdose.
    - Family members must be advised regarding the safe storage and supervised dispensing of medication.

  *Lithium* reduces the risk of suicide and suicide attempts in patients with bipolar disorder and major depressive disorder. The potential lethality of lithium in overdose should be kept in mind when deciding on the quantity to give with each prescription.

  *Antipsychotic agents* are required for suicidal patients with psychotic disorders. The use of clozapine has been shown to produce significant reductions in suicide attempts and hospitalization for suicidality.

  *Antianxiety agents:* Anxiety and insomnia are significant risk factors for suicide, which can be reduced by closely supervised short-term (1–4 weeks) benzodiazepines or sedating antidepressants.

  *Electroconvulsive therapy (ECT)* is effective in the short-term reduction of suicidal ideation in patients with severe depressive illness, manic and depressive episodes of bipolar disorder, and psychosis.

  *Psychological therapy and psychosocial interventions:* Cognitive behavior therapy, interpersonal psychotherapy, and problem-solving methods are effective in reducing suicidal ideation and behavior, while dialectical behavior therapy is especially useful for patients with personality disorders.
  - *Address precipitating events and ongoing life difficulties:* Suicidal behavior may be precipitated by acute stress (bereavement, loss of a job, financial difficulties, breakup of a marriage, or relationship) or chronic stress and intolerable life circumstances (abusive relationships, financial difficulties). Problem-solving techniques can help the patient look for possible solutions to some of these problems, while psychotherapy aimed at acceptance and changes in thinking and behavior are required for those adverse life situations that may be difficult to resolve.
  - *Suggest general stress reduction and coping strategies* such as yoga, meditation, regular physical exercise, involvement in hobbies, leisure, and religious activities.
  - *Alter high-risk behavioral and environmental factors.* Modify the patient's environment to restrict access to lethal means of suicide, and drugs and alcohol, which have disinhibiting effects. Increase social support by utilizing family, friends, and community resources.
- *Formulate and document a safety plan* in collaboration with the patient and their support system. This is a stepwise list of coping strategies and sources of support that can be used during or preceding a future suicidal crisis, to reduce the likelihood of engaging in suicidal behavior, tailored to the individual's needs and strengths, and modified as the patient's clinical status or circumstances change **(Box 1)**.

  A *"No Suicide Contract"* is a written commitment by the patient to not engage in suicidal behavior. It is not a legal document and will have benefit only if the treating doctor/team has a reasonably good therapeutic relationship with the patient. It is not routinely recommended as it could falsely lead the clinician to feel that the patient is safer than they actually are.
- *Help the patient identify and focus on sources of strength* that give a sense of purpose and can be a deterrent to self-harm, such as children in the home, family relationships, work, and cultural or religious beliefs. This will also help the patient focus on the

**BOX 1:** Components of a safety plan.[1]

- *Identify warning signs or triggers* that indicate suicidal ideation is likely to occur, including situations, thoughts, feelings, and behaviors such as anxiety, social withdrawal, and mood fluctuations
- *List personalized internal coping strategies* that the individual can carry out on their own to distract himself/herself when experiencing suicidal ideation, such as listening to music, watching sports, physical activity, and breathing exercises.
- *Identify social contacts* and social locations that may provide a distraction
- *List people that can be turned to for support and help*—family members, friends, religious leaders, other members of the community, with their contact information
- *Document contact details of mental health emergency resources*, including the treating doctor, hospital, and suicide helplines
- *Take steps to ensure the safety of the home environment* by restricting the patient's access to lethal means

**Flowchart 1:** Algorithm for management of patients with suicidal ideation.

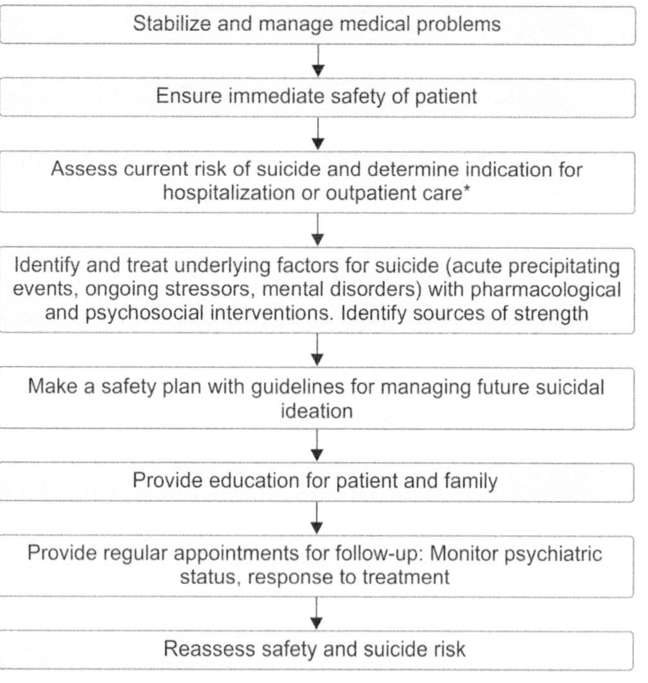


positive aspects of their life rather than just on the difficulties.

- *Provide support and psychoeducation to family members* regarding the nature, course, and management of the psychiatric/psychological problem. Help them identify symptoms that may herald suicidality, such as insomnia, hopelessness, anxiety, depression, command hallucinations, behaviors such as giving away possessions, arranging legal or financial affairs, or communicating suicidal intentions. Discuss about what to do in case of an emergency.[3]
- *Provide regular follow-up appointments:*
  - Schedule appointments at short intervals during the period of acute crisis; alter the frequency based on the clinical situation.
  - During each review, monitor the patient's psychiatric status, response to treatment, and current suicide risk.
  - Address modifiable factors that may interfere with adherence to treatment, such as inadequate understanding of the medication regimen and side effects.
  - Plan for methods to track and re-engage patients in case they fail to attend follow-up appointments with telephone calls, e-mails, or letters.
- *Reassess safety and suicide risk:*
  - Despite every effort at suicide assessment and treatment, suicides occur in clinical practice. No risk factor can be used exclusively to accurately predict suicidality. An ongoing process of assessment is required as the risk varies over time.
  - Repeat assessments are necessary, especially when there is a change in the treatment setting (from continuous supervision to routine inpatient care, after discharge from the hospital), worsening in the clinical condition, or the occurrence of an adverse life event.
  - Be alert to symptoms that may be associated with increased suicide risk.
  - The new emergence of suicidality should be responded to by a change in treatment setting, an increase in level of observation or frequency of outpatient visits, and a change of medication and/or psychotherapeutic approach.
  - In patients with chronic and repetitive self-injurious behavior, each act needs to be assessed in its context. Outpatient management may be appropriate at some times, while under other circumstances (e.g., brief psychotic episodes, following life-threatening suicide attempts), hospitalization may be indicated. In general, hospitalization should be used for short-term stabilization, as prolonged hospital stays can lead to regression and worsening of behavior[4] **(Flowcharts 1 and 2)**.

**Flowchart 2:** Assessment to determine treatment setting.[5]

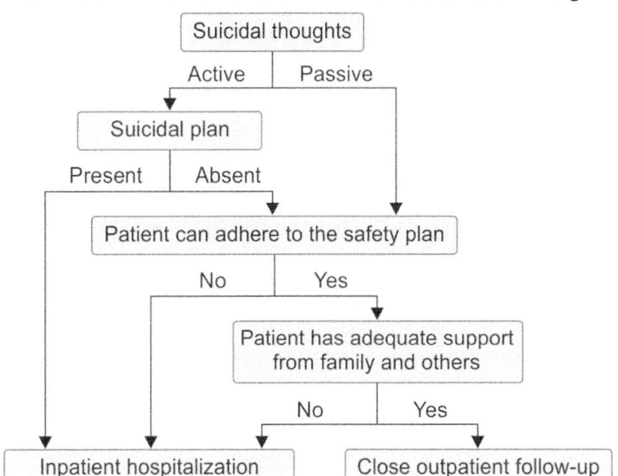


## REFERENCES

1. Sarkhel S, Vijayakumar V, Vijayakumar L. Clinical Practice Guidelines for Management of Suicidal Behaviour. Indian J Psychiatry. 2023;65(2):124-30.
2. Alabi AA. Management of self-harm, suicidal ideation and suicide attempts. S Afr Fam Pract (2004). 2022;64(1):e1-4.
3. Jacobs DG, Baldessarini RS, Conwell Y, Fawcett JA, Horton L, Meltzer H, et al. (2003). Practice Guideline for the Assessment and Treatment of patients with Suicidal Behaviors. [Online]. Available from: https://psychiatryonline.org/pb/assets/raw/sitewide/practice_guidelines/guidelines/suicide.pdf [Last accessed June, 2025].
4. Welton RS. The management of suicidality: assessment and intervention. Psychiatry (Edgmont). 2007;4(5):24-34.
5. Shreiber J, Culpepper L. Suicidal ideation and behavior in adults. [Online] Available from https://www.uptodate.com/contents/suicidal-ideation-and-behavior-in-adults [Last accessed June, 2025].

CHAPTER 42

# Management of Acute Gastrointestinal Side Effects of Antidepressants

*Arghya Pal, Arpit Parmar, Amit Singh*

## INTRODUCTION

- Major depressive disorder (MDD) and anxiety disorders are arguably the two most common groups of disorders encountered in nationwide psychiatric epidemiological studies.[1,2]
- Antidepressant drugs are among the most prescribed psychotropics for a range of psychiatric disorders.
- All recent guidelines recommend the personalization of pharmacotherapy in MDD based on various factors, including medical comorbidities, patient preferences, and predisposition to adverse effects from prescribed drugs.
- In the 1950s, the introduction of tricyclic antidepressants (TCA) and monoamine oxidase inhibitors (MAOI) revolutionized the management of MDD, but their popularity declined due to their adverse effect profiles. Over the last few decades, the search for safer and more tolerable alternatives has continued.

## PROBLEM STATEMENT

- The prevalence of adverse effects after initiating antidepressants has been estimated to be as high as 86%, with about 55% of these effects rated as troublesome. However, evidence shows that clinicians often tend to underestimate the prevalence of these adverse effects.[3]
- The prevalence of gastrointestinal side effects in a sample of patients attending a primary care setting was approximately 20%, including issues such as indigestion, diarrhea, constipation, and dry mouth.[4]
- Gastrointestinal adverse effects are also among the common reasons for discontinuation of antidepressant drugs.[5]

## NEUROBIOLOGICAL UNDERPINNING

- The gastrointestinal adverse effects of antidepressant drugs are largely mediated by the interrelationship between the central nervous system and the enteric nervous system. Serotonin is the most important neurotransmitter implicated in this mediation.
- The gut contains a very high concentration of the serotonergic (5HT) receptors, which play a critical role in the physiological functioning of the gut, including motility, endocrine/metabolic, immunological, and microbial signaling.
- The prescription of antidepressants, which often act by modulating serotonergic receptors, can lead to the emergence of gastrointestinal side effects due to their non-specific effects on the body.
- Studies on gut microbiota also show significant changes following the initiation of antidepressants, further substantiating the close interaction between the central nervous system and the enteric nervous system.

## COMMON GASTROINTESTINAL SIDE EFFECTS OF ANTIDEPRESSANT THERAPY

The onset of gastrointestinal side effects following antidepressant exposure can be both acute and chronic. For this chapter, our review will be limited solely to the acute effects, while symptoms involving the hepatobiliary system are out of the purview of this chapter. A hierarchy of the propensity of drugs to cause such side effects is provided in **Table 1**. A suggested management algorithm is depicted in **Flowchart 1**.

### Nausea

- Nausea is one of the most common adverse effects seen with antidepressant pharmacotherapy. The prevalence of it has been reported to be up to 17–26% in various studies.[3,6]
- The onset of nausea is usually acute, and up to 83% of the users reported its onset within the first 2 weeks of initiation.

**TABLE 1:** Summary of common gastrointestinal adverse effects of antidepressants and their management strategies.

| *Adverse effects* | *Drugs with higher propensity* | *Drugs with safer profile* | *Management strategies* |
|---|---|---|---|
| Nausea | • Duloxetine<br>• Vortioxetine<br>• Levomilnacipran<br>• Venlafaxine<br>• Reboxetine<br>• Desvenlafaxine<br>• Sertraline<br>• Fluvoxamine<br>• Escitalopram<br>• Paroxetine | Mirtazapine | • Divided dosing<br>• Taking drugs with food<br>• Ginger containing foods<br>• H2 antagonists (Ranitidine)<br>• Proton pump inhibitors (Pantoprazole)<br>• Promethazine<br>• Ondansetron |
| Diarrhea | • Sertraline<br>• Fluvoxamine<br>• Escitalopram<br>• Citalopram<br>• Duloxetine | • Agomelatine<br>• Bupropion<br>• Desvenlafaxine<br>• Fluoxetine<br>• Levomilnacipran<br>• Paroxetine<br>• Vortioxetine<br>• Venlafaxine | • Usually self-limiting<br>• Limited evidence for:<br>– Antidiarrheal agents such as loperamide, or diphenoxylate hydrochloride<br>– Cyproheptadine<br>– Lactobacillus acidophilus culture |
| Constipation | • Amitriptyline<br>• Levomilnacipran<br>• Desvenlafaxine<br>• Duloxetine<br>• Venlafaxine<br>• Sertraline<br>• Reboxetine<br>• Paroxetine<br>• Agomelatine<br>• Vortioxetine<br>• Bupropion | • Citalopram<br>• Escitalopram,<br>• Fluoxetine<br>• Fluvoxamine<br>• Mirtazapine | • Increase fiber intake<br>• Physical activity<br>• Increase water intake<br>• Bulk forming laxative<br>• Stool softeners<br>• Osmotic laxatives |
| Dyspepsia | • Sertraline<br>• Escitalopram | Fluoxetine | • Divided dosing<br>• Taking drugs with food<br>• H2 antagonists (ranitidine)<br>• Proton pump inhibitors (pantoprazole) |
| Anorexia | • Fluvoxamine<br>• Desvenlafaxine<br>• Venlafaxine<br>• Paroxetine<br>• Duloxetine<br>• Fluoxetine<br>• Escitalopram<br>• Sertraline<br>• Vortioxetine | • Agomelatine<br>• Bupropion<br>• Citalopram | • Change of drug<br>• Off-label trial of cyproheptadine (but increased depressive symptoms) |
| Increased appetite | • Mirtazapine | • Fluvoxamine<br>• Venlafaxine | Change of drug |
| Dry mouth | • Amitriptyline<br>• Duloxetine<br>• Desvenlafaxine<br>• Venlafaxine<br>• Sertraline<br>• Bupropion<br>• Paroxetine<br>• Escitalopram<br>• Levomilnacipran<br>• Fluvoxamine | • Agomelatine<br>• Citalopram<br>• Fluoxetine<br>• Mirtazapine<br>• Vortioxetine | • Increase water intake<br>• Gustatory sialogs:<br>• Acid-tasting substances (e.g., citrus fruits)<br>• Sugar-free chewing gums or candies<br>• Pilocarpine, bethanechol, benzopyrone, or carbachol |

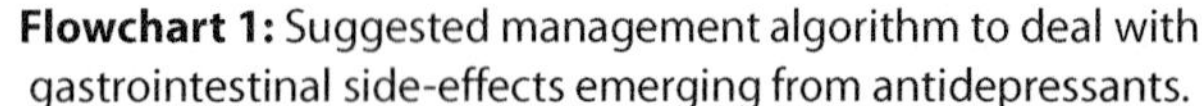
**Flowchart 1:** Suggested management algorithm to deal with gastrointestinal side-effects emerging from antidepressants.

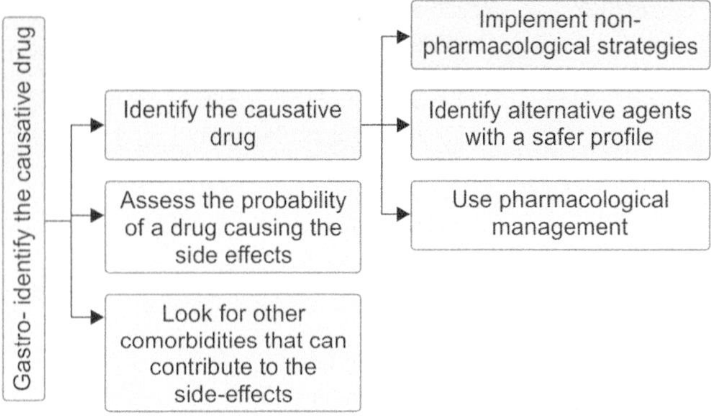


- The Serotonin and norepinephrine reuptake inhibitors (SNRIs) and Selective serotonin reuptake inhibitors (SSRIs) seem to be the most notorious group in causing these side effects. Paroxetine appears to be the most predisposing among the SSRIs, though its extended-release formulation appears to be a bit safer.
- In order to deal with nausea, strategies like dividing the doses and taking drugs with food can be helpful.
- Pharmacologically, nausea can be managed using drugs, such as ondansetron, proton pump inhibitors, and H2 antagonists.

## Diarrhea

- The prevalence of diarrhea has been estimated to be around 15%, and in about 75% of the cases, the onset of these symptoms has been within the first 2 weeks.[6]
- The use of SSRIs has been most commonly linked with the incidence of diarrhea.
- In most cases, diarrhea is self-limiting. Pharmacological management, if required, can be done using antidiarrheal drugs such as loperamide and diphenoxylate hydrochloride.

## Constipation

- The rates of constipation as an adverse effect of antidepressant exposure have been found to be around 11–12.5% in various studies.[3,6]
- Among the various antidepressants, TCA has a high propensity to develop constipation, and this has been one of the major reasons for their limited tolerability.[7]
- Most of the SSRI has a beneficial profile in terms of constipation, other than Paroxetine.
- The management of constipation mostly deals with dietary modifications (increase in dietary fiber and water intake) and an increase in physical activities.
- Pharmacological management consists of the use of appropriate laxatives.[8]

## Changes in Appetite

- Antidepressant drugs can be associated with both an increase and a decrease in appetite.
- The number of drugs known to be associated with a decrease in appetite is significantly higher. Most of the serotonergic antidepressants can be associated with a decrease in appetite.
- Mirtazapine is the most prominent drug that has been linked to an increase in appetite.
- The management of these dietary changes mostly involves tactful switching of the drugs.
- There is minimal pharmacological management to suggest for such adverse effects.

## Dry Mouth

- The most implicated group of antidepressants causing dry mouth is the TCAs.
- However, in the meta-analysis by Oliva et al.,[9] a substantial number of other antidepressants also presented with significant dryness of the mouth. This included SNRI, such as duloxetine, desvenlafaxine, and venlafaxine; SSRIs like sertraline, paroxetine, escitalopram, and fluvoxamine.
- The management of dryness of the mouth can be done by increasing the water intake and use of gustatory sialogs like citrus fruits.
- Pharmacologically, it can be managed using drugs, such as pilocarpine, bethanechol, benzopyrone, and carbachol, but they are rarely required.

# CONCLUSION

- Gastrointestinal side effects are quite frequently seen with the administration of antidepressants.
- The various commonly encountered adverse effects include nausea, diarrhea, constipation, changes in appetite, and dry mouth.
- Though classes of antidepressants such as SSRIs and SNRIs are more tolerable as compared to TCAs and MAOIs, the prevalence of gastrointestinal side effects is seen quite frequently in these groups as well.

- The management of these adverse effects is usually not very challenging and can be done using a simple modification of lifestyle and diet, and rarely requires a change of the prescribed drug.
- Pharmacological management of these adverse effects is usually not required, though options are available.

## REFERENCES


1. GBD 2019 Diseases and Injuries Collaborators. Global burden of 369 diseases and injuries in 204 countries and territories, 1990-2019: a systematic analysis for the Global Burden of Disease Study 2019. Lancet (London, England). 2020;396(10258):1204-22.
2. GBD 2016 Causes of Death Collaborators. Global, regional, and national age-sex specific mortality for 264 causes of death, 1980-2016: a systematic analysis for the Global Burden of Disease Study 2016. Lancet (London, England). 2017;390(10100):1151-210.
3. Hu XH, Bull SA, Hunkeler EM, Ming E, Lee JY, Fireman B, Markson LE. Incidence and duration of side effects and those rated as bothersome with selective serotonin reuptake inhibitor treatment for depression: patient report versus physician estimate. J Clin Psychiatry. 2004;65(7):959-65.
4. Ramic E, Prasko S, Gavran L, Spahic E. Assessment of the Antidepressant Side Effects Occurrence in Patients Treated in Primary Care. Mater Sociomed. 2020;32(2):131-4.
5. Lin EHB, Von Korff M, Katon W, Bush T, Simon GE, Walker E, Robinson P. The role of the primary care physician in patients' adherence to antidepressant therapy. Med Care. 1995;33(1):67-74.
6. Trindade E, Menon D, Topfer LA, Coloma C. Adverse effects associated with selective serotonin reuptake inhibitors and tricyclic antidepressants: a meta-analysis. C Can Med Assoc J. 1998;159(10):1245-52.
7. Steffens DC, Krishnan KR, Helms MJ. Are SSRIs better than TCAs? Comparison of SSRIs and TCAs: a meta-analysis. Depress Anxiety. 1997;6(1):10-8.
8. Kelly K, Posternak M, Alpert JE. Toward achieving optimal response: understanding and managing antidepressant side effects. Dialogues Clin Neurosci. 2008;10(4):409-18.
9. Oliva V, Lippi M, Paci R, Del Fabro L, Delvecchio G, Brambilla P, et al. Gastrointestinal side effects associated with antidepressant treatments in patients with major depressive disorder: A systematic review and meta-analysis. Prog Neuropsychopharmacol Biol Psychiatry. 2021;109:110266.

CHAPTER 43

# Management of Treatment-Emergent Sexual Dysfunction due to Antidepressants

*Adarsh Tripathi, Aditya Agarwal*

## INTRODUCTION

- Antidepressants (ADs) are a group of medications used for a wide range of clinical conditions, including depression, anxiety disorders, obsessive-compulsive disorder (OCD), trauma, and stress-related disorders, among others.[1,2]
- Treatment emergent sexual dysfunctions (TESD) are common side effects of ADs and are among the most frequent reasons for noncompliance and poor treatment response. However, TESD is often underreported in clinical practice.[3,4]
- Studies have reported that TESD often goes unreported when relying solely on spontaneous reporting by patients. The routine use of questions and rating scales significantly increases the rates of TESD reported by patients using ADs.[5]
- Most ADs, especially those acting on serotonergic system, negatively affect sexual functioning. The rates of TESD vary greatly among various AD medications, with studies reporting a range of 20–80% patients using ADs experiencing TESD.[6]
- ADs can influence any or all phases of sexual functioning, including sexual desire, arousal, ejaculation, and orgasm.[7]

## ASSESSMENT

- When assessing sexual dysfunctions associated with ADs, clinicians must consider that sexual disorders and psychiatric disorders may occur due to several reasons. Factors that may have a common causative influence on both sexual and psychiatric disorders include:[5,8,9]
  - Common etiological factors such as genetic factors, endocrine dysfunctions, metabolic syndrome, and immunological disorders
  - Comorbid medical and substance use disorders
  - Interpersonal factors such as interpersonal conflicts and divorce
  - Poor educational attainment, occupational functioning, and social factors may indirectly influence the risk of causation.
  - Personality factors such as poor self-esteem, unstable interpersonal relationships, and poor emotional management
  - Economic conditions and living situations
  - Medications used to treat various medical disorders such as hypertension, endocrine disorders, and steroids
  - Stigma and discrimination resulting from illnesses
- The assessment necessary for the management of TESD due to ADs includes:[5,10]
  - Reviewing current illness severity, functioning, and improvement with the current treatments
  - Considering past episodes, risk of relapse, and potential consequences of relapse
  - Assessing previous, current, and future sexual activity, as well as relationship status

## MANAGEMENT

- The aim of management is to eliminate TESD. If complete reversal of TESD is not possible, partial improvement is targeted. As several strategies targeted at improving TESD caused by ADs may have a variable risk of destabilizing the patients' clinical condition or risk of relapse or worsening of symptoms, the risk-benefit ratio must be clearly assessed in consultation with the patient for potential management strategies **(Flowchart 1)**.
- The strategies for managing TESD include:
  - *Reassurance:* If the treatment has recently started, improvement is unsatisfactory, or the risk of relapse is very high, along with the patient's personal situation suggesting that sexual activity may delayed or postponed for the time being, the patient may be reassured about the temporary nature of the

**Flowchart 1:** Deciding management options for antidepressant (AD)-emergent sexual dysfunction (SD).

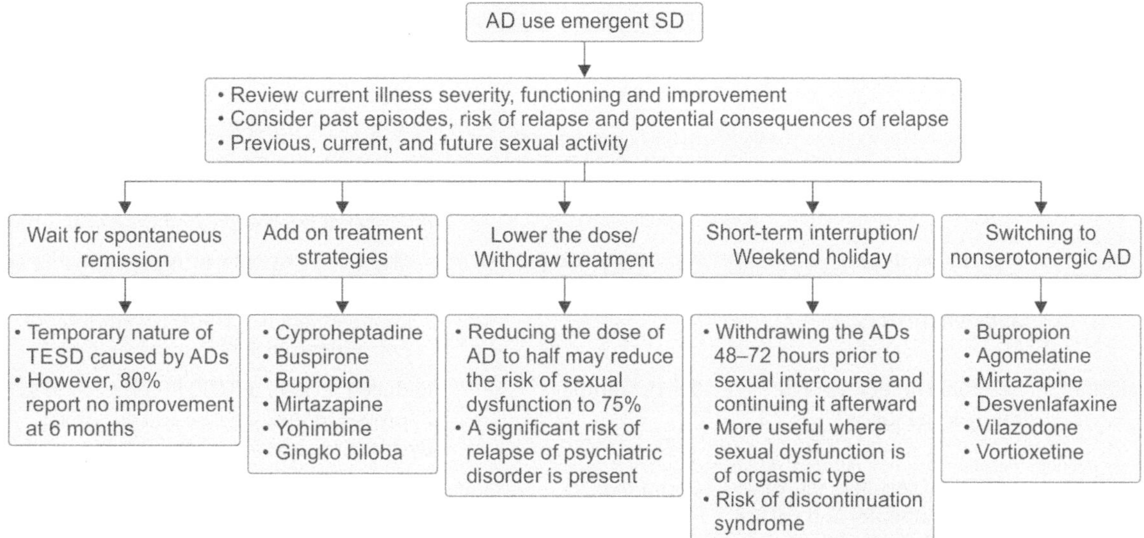


**TABLE 1:** Add-on treatment strategies for TESD caused by AD medications.

| *Drug* | *Mechanism of action* | *Dosages and use pattern* | *Comments* |
|---|---|---|---|
| Cyproheptadine[14] | 5HT antagonism | 4–16 mg/day, usually in evening | May cause sedation and weight gain |
| Buspirone[15] | $5HT_{1A}$ partial agonism | 15–30 mg/day, three divided doses | Usually well tolerated |
| Bupropion[16] | Dopaminergic, adrenergic effect | 150–300 mg in the morning | May increase anxiety |
| Mirtazapine[17] | $5HT_2$ antagonism | 7.5–30 mg at night | May cause sedation, increased appetite and weight gain |
| Yohimbine[18] | $\alpha_2$ adrenergic antagonism | Up to 30 mg/day in three divided dosages | Efficacy is doubtful |
| Gingko biloba extract[19,20] | Heterogenous | 120–360 mg in two to three divided dosages | Efficacy is doubtful |

(AD: antidepressant; TESD: treatment emergent sexual dysfunction)

TESD caused by ADs. It may be prudent to wait and watch for spontaneous recovery. As the symptoms of psychiatric disorders and overall wellbeing of the patient improve, sexual functioning of the individual may also improve. However, this strategy is not often successful, and it is reported that most patients (up to 80%) may not report any improvement after 6 months of treatment.[11,12]

- *Lowering the dose* or *withdrawing the treatment:* TESDs are almost always reversible after withdrawal of the offending agent. Hence, if the patient's clinical condition, past history, and other factors permit, this strategy may be attempted after informed decision-making with the patient. Reducing the dose of AD to half may reduce the risk of sexual dysfunction to 75%. Gradually, reducing the dosages reduces the withdrawal syndrome caused by ADs. However, a significant risk of relapse of psychiatric disorder is present.[12]
- *Add-on treatment:* This strategy is also commonly used for the treatment of TESD. Another medication with a different mechanism of action and potential to reverse TESD is added to the ongoing treatment.[13] Medications used for this purpose are described in **Table 1**.
- *Short-term interruption of treatment* or *weekend holidays:* This strategy involves withdrawing the AD 48–72 hours prior to sexual intercourse and resuming it afterward. It may be attempted in patients where treatment cannot be stopped or

**TABLE 2:** Alternative medications to SSRI for avoiding or managing TESD.

| *Drug* | *Mechanism of action* | *Dosages and use pattern* | *Comments* |
|---|---|---|---|
| Bupropion[23] | Dopaminergic, adrenergic effect | 150–300 mg in the morning | Incidence of treatment emergent sexual dysfunction is almost similar to placebo, may exacerbate symptoms of anxiety |
| Agomelatine[24] | Agonist at $MT_1$ and $MT_2$ receptors; antagonizes $5HT_{2C}$ | 25–50 mg at bed time | Comparable antidepressants efficacy has been reported in trials. However, concerns related to efficacy has been expressed in clinical settings |
| Mirtazapine[25] | Noradrenergic and specific serotonergic receptor antagonism (NaSSA) | 7.5–30 mg in night | • May cause sedation, increased appetite and weight gain<br>• Improvement in 70–90% is reported of TESD after switching from SSRI to mirtazapine |
| Desvenlafaxine[26] | Serotonin norepinephrine reuptake inhibitor | 50–150 mg/day | Reduced severity of TESD in comparison to SSRIs. Improved in sexual desire and orgasmic dysfunction, sexual arousal my/or may not improve |
| Vilazodone[26] | Combined selective serotonin reuptake inhibitor and partial $5\text{-}HT_{1A}$ receptor agonist | 40 mg/day | • Gradual dose increment is needed to avoid GI intolerability. Need to be taken with food<br>• Low rates of TESD |
| Vortioxetine[27] | $5\text{-}HT_3$ and $5\text{-}HT_7$ receptor antagonism, $5\text{-}HT_{1B}$ receptor partial agonism, $5\text{-}HT_{1A}$ receptor agonism, and serotonin transporter inhibition | 10–20 mg/day | • There may be improvement in all three phases of sexual functioning (desire, arousal and orgasm)<br>• Incidence of TESD is low<br>• Tolerability is good<br>• Comparable efficacy to SSRIs but SNRIs may show greater efficacy |

(SNRI: serotonin-norepinephrine reuptake inhibitor; SSRI: selective serotonin reuptake inhibitor; TESD: treatment emergent sexual dysfunction)

changed. This approach may be more useful when primary sexual dysfunction is orgasmic dysfunction and an selective serotonin reuptake inhibitor (SSRI) other than fluoxetine is being used.[13] However, there is a risk of withdrawal symptoms and discontinuation syndrome. Additionally, there are increased chances of irregular compliance and relapse with this treatment strategy. Another approach involves reducing the dosage to half for 2 consecutive days before planned sexual intercourse, followed by resuming the usual dose. While reducing the plasma level of AD may improve erection/lubrication during sexual intercourse, lack of desire frequently does not change with this treatment strategy.[21]

- *Switching to a nonserotonergic AD:* Switching treatment from an SSRI to a medication that acts via a nonserotonergic mechanism may be helpful in alleviating TESD **(Table 2)**. Careful alteration in treatment is required to avoid any discontinuation syndrome or emergence of the symptoms of the psychiatric disorder. However, this approach may not be feasible for clinical conditions where SSRIs are the preferred treatment options, such as OCD and related disorders, and impulse control disorders.[13,22]
- *Psychoeducation:* Psychoeducation is necessary for preparing the patient for possible TESD. Prior information and education can prevent panic if TESD occurs and help patients cooperate in the evaluation and management of these side effects. Maintaining a healthy diet, engaging in physical exercise, and fostering good interpersonal relationships are very helpful in having a mutually satisfying sexual life.[7]

## REFERENCES

1. Chu A, Wadhwa R. Selective Serotonin Reuptake Inhibitors [Internet]. In: StatPearls. Treasure Island (FL): StatPearls Publishing; 2021.
2. Stahl SM. Stahl's essential psychopharmacology: Prescriber's guide, 5th edition. New York, NY, US: Cambridge University Press; 2014.

3. Serretti A, Chiesa A. Treatment-Emergent Sexual Dysfunction Related to Antidepressants: A Meta-Analysis. J Clin Psychopharmacol. 2009;29(3):259-66.
4. Kennedy SH, Rizvi S. Sexual Dysfunction, Depression, and the Impact of Antidepressants. J Clin Psychopharmacol. 2009;29(2):157-64.
5. Jespersen S. Antidepressant induced sexual dysfunction Part 2: assessment and management. S Afr Psychiatry Rev. 2006;9:79-83.
6. SALSEX Working Study Group; Montejo AL, Calama J, Rico-Villademoros F, Montejo L, González-García N, Pérez J. A Real-World Study on Antidepressant-Associated Sexual Dysfunction in 2144 Outpatients: The SALSEX I Study. Arch Sex Behav. 2019;48(3):923-33.
7. Montejo AL, Prieto N, de Alarcón R, Casado-Espada N, de la Iglesia J, Montejo L. Management Strategies for Antidepressant-Related Sexual Dysfunction: A Clinical Approach. J Clin Med. 2019;8(10):1640.
8. Bartlik BD, Rosenfeld S, Beaton C. Assessment of sexual functioning: Sexual history taking for health care practitioners. Epilepsy Behav. 2005;7:15-21.
9. Avasthi A, Grover S, Sathyanarayana Rao T. Clinical Practice Guidelines for Management of Sexual Dysfunction. Indian J Psychiatry. 2017;59(5):91.
10. Vaishnav M, Rao TSS, Adarsh T, Nebhinani N. IPS Textbook of Sexuality and Sexual Medicine. Delhi: Jaypee Brothers Medical Publishers Pvt Limited; 2022.
11. Montejo AL, Llorca G, Izquierdo JA, Rico-Villademoros F. Incidence of sexual dysfunction associated with antidepressant agents: a prospective multicenter study of 1022 outpatients. Spanish Working Group for the Study of Psychotropic-Related Sexual Dysfunction. J Clin Psychiatry. 2001;62 Suppl 3:10-21.
12. Montejo-González AL, Llorca G, Izquierdo JA, Ledesma A, Bousoño M, Calcedo A, et al. SSRI-induced sexual dysfunction: fluoxetine, paroxetine, sertraline, and fluvoxamine in a prospective, multicenter, and descriptive clinical study of 344 patients. J Sex Marital Ther. 1997;23(3):176-94.
13. Clayton AH, Alkis AR, Parikh NB, Votta JG. Sexual Dysfunction Due to Psychotropic Medications. Psychiatric Clinics of North America. 2016;39(3):427-63.
14. Gutierrez MA, Stimmel GL. Management of and Counseling for Psychotropic Drug-Induced Sexual Dysfunction. Pharmacotherapy. 1999;19(7):823-31.
15. Norden MJ. Buspirone treatment of sexual dysfunction associated with selective serotonin re-uptake inhibitors. Depression. 1994;2(2):109-12.
16. Taylor MJ, Rudkin L, Bullemor-Day P, Lubin J, Chukwujekwu C, Hawton K. Strategies for managing sexual dysfunction induced by antidepressant medication. Cochrane Database of Systematic Reviews. 2013;2013(5):CD003382.
17. Ozmenler NK, Karlidere T, Bozkurt A, Yetkin S, Doruk A, Sutcigil L, et al. Mirtazapine augmentation in depressed patients with sexual dysfunction due to selective serotonin reuptake inhibitors. Hum Psychopharmacol Clin Exp. 2008;23(4):321-6.
18. Hollander E, McCarley A. Yohimbine treatment of sexual side effects induced by serotonin reuptake blockers. J Clin Psychiatry. 1992;53(6):207-9.
19. Cohen AJ, Bartlik B. Ginkgo biloba for antidepressant-induced sexual dysfunction. J Sex Marital Ther. 1998;24(2):139-43.
20. Kang BJ, Lee SJ, Kim MD, Cho MJ. A placebo-controlled, double-blind trial of Ginkgo biloba for antidepressant-induced sexual dysfunction. Hum Psychopharmacol Clin Exp. 2002;17(6):279-84.
21. Rothschild AJ. Selective serotonin reuptake inhibitor-induced sexual dysfunction: efficacy of a drug holiday. Am J Psychiatry. 1995;152(10):1514-6.
22. Gregorian RS, Golden KA, Bahce A, Goodman C, Kwong WJ, Khan ZM. Antidepressant-Induced Sexual Dysfunction. Ann Pharmacother. 2002;36(10):1577-89.
23. Clayton AH, Warnock JK, Kornstein SG, Pinkerton R, Sheldon-Keller A, McGarvey EL. A Placebo-Controlled Trial of Bupropion SR as an Antidote for Selective Serotonin Reuptake Inhibitor–Induced Sexual Dysfunction. J Clin Psychiatry. 2004;65(1):62-7.
24. Montejo AL, Perez Urdaniz A, Mosqueira I, Prieto N, De La Rica A, Gallego MT, et al. EPA-1719 – Effectiveness of switching to agomelatine in antidepressant-related sexual dysfunction. Eur Psychiatry. 2014;29:1.
25. Koutouvidis N, Pratikakis M, Fotiadou A. The use of mirtazapine in a group of 11 patients following poor compliance to selective serotonin reuptake inhibitor treatment due to sexual dysfunction. Int Clin Psychopharmacol. 1999;14(4):253-5.
26. Carvalho AF, Sharma MS, Brunoni AR, Vieta E, Fava GA. The Safety, Tolerability and Risks Associated with the Use of Newer Generation Antidepressant Drugs: A Critical Review of the Literature. Psychother Psychosom. 2016;85(5):270-88.
27. Jacobsen PL, Mahableshwarkar AR, Chen Y, Chrones L, Clayton AH. Effect of Vortioxetine vs. Escitalopram on Sexual Functioning in Adults with Well-Treated Major Depressive Disorder Experiencing SSRI-Induced Sexual Dysfunction. J Sexual Med. 2015;12(10):2036-48.

CHAPTER 44

# Management of Antipsychotic-induced Sexual Dysfunction

*Sujita Kumar Kar, Babita Sharma*

## INTRODUCTION

The class of pharmaceuticals known as antipsychotic drugs, commonly referred to as neuroleptics, is largely used to treat various psychiatric diseases such as schizophrenia, bipolar disorder, and severe depression with psychotic symptoms. These drugs are also recommended for the management of behavioral symptoms of dementia, disruptive disorders in children and adolescents, control of aggression, and as an adjuvant for a number of psychiatric issues. The key neurotransmitters that these drugs target and alter to function are dopamine and serotonin, two of the most crucial neurotransmitters for regulating mood, perception, and cognition.[1,2] The primary purpose of antipsychotic medications is to manage psychotic symptoms, such as hallucinations, delusions, and disorganized thinking. They help in reducing the severity and frequency of these symptoms. Antipsychotics can help patients maintain long-term stability by reducing or eliminating the occurrence of psychotic episodes.

Antipsychotic medications produce a spectrum of side effects including constipation, excessive sedation, postural hypotension, extrapyramidal side effects, galactorrhea, falls, metabolic side effects, along with sexual dysfunction. The older (typical) antipsychotics have higher propensity to cause extrapyramidal side effects, while the newer (atypical) antipsychotics are more likely to cause metabolic side effects.[1,2]

## ANTIPSYCHOTICS CAUSING SEXUAL DYSFUNCTION

Although antipsychotic medications are highly beneficial in treating several mental health issues, they can have the side effect of causing sexual dysfunction. These dysfunctions can vary in nature and severity depending on the specific medication and individual factors. Some common sexual dysfunctions associated with antipsychotic drugs include erectile dysfunction (impotence), reduced libido, anorgasmia, delayed ejaculation, and irregular menstruation in some women. The degree of these sexual dysfunctions might vary from person to person, and it is important to note that not everyone who takes antipsychotic medications will experience these issues. **Table 1** lists the antipsychotic medications and their associated sexual side effects. The mechanism of sexual dysfunction linked to antipsychotic drug usage are described in **Table 2**. **Flowchart 1** represents the effects of neurotransmitters on various stages of human sexual response.

## MANAGEMENT OF SEXUAL DYSFUNCTION CAUSED BY ANTIPSYCHOTIC MEDICATIONS

Sexual dysfunctions need to be identified accurately, and prompt intervention should be done to minimize patient distress. It is important to obtain a detailed history of sexual life and assess for any possibility of sexual dysfunction in patients receiving antipsychotic medications. Patients on antipsychotic medications may also be receiving other medications concomitantly, which can also adversely affect sexual functioning. Additionally, patients with psychiatric illnesses receiving antipsychotic medications may have sexual dysfunction that was present before the initiation of medication, or the dysfunction may be a direct effect of mental illness itself. Hence, it is important to exclude all these possibilities before diagnosing antipsychotic medication-induced sexual dysfunction. Before attributing the sexual dysfunction to the medication, it is important to evaluate the following:[3]

- Baseline sexual functioning
- Psychological issues
- Impact of the acute illness on the sexual functioning
- Comorbid physical disorders
- Comorbid substance use

**TABLE 1:** Types of antipsychotics drugs causing sexual dysfunction with the rate of dysfunction and underlying mechanism.[4-7]

| *Antipsychotic drugs* | *Sexual side effects* | | *Mechanism* | *Rate of sexual dysfunction* |
|---|---|---|---|---|
| | *Men* | *Women* | | |
| Haloperidol | • Decreased libido<br>• Erectile dysfunction<br>• Ejaculatory disorder<br>• Higher arousal and orgasm dysfunction | • Decreased libido<br>• Arousal disorder | • Strong D2 antagonism and decrease of dopamine function<br>• Elevated prolactin levels | High |
| Trifluoperazine | Impairs erection and ejaculation | • Decreased libido<br>• Orgasmic dysfunction | | High |
| Iloperidone | Erectile or ejaculatory dysfunction gynecomastia decreased libido | – | Blockade of alpha 1-adrenergic receptor | High |
| Chlorpromazine (Thorazine) | • Impairs erection and ejaculation<br>• Painful erection/priapism | – | – | High |
| Thioridazine | • Desire, arousal and orgasm dysfunction<br>• Painful erection | • Decreased libido<br>• Orgasmic dysfunction | – | High |
| Fluphenazine | • Decreased libido<br>• Erectile dysfunction<br>• Orgasmic problems | • Decreased libido<br>• Orgasmic dysfunction | – | High |
| Amisulpride | • Gynecomastia<br>• Reduced libido | Amenorrhea | • Strong D2 antagonism and decrease of dopamine function<br>• Increase prolactin levels | High |
| Risperidone | • Erectile or ejaculatory dysfunction Azoospermia, gynecomastia<br>• Decreased libido<br>• Higher arousal and orgasm dysfunction | • Infertility<br>• Decreased libido<br>• Vaginal dryness<br>• Arousal and orgasmic difficulty | • Strong D2 antagonism and decrease of dopamine function, weak 5HT2C antagonism | High |
| Paliperidone | • Decreased libido<br>• Erectile dysfunction<br>• Ejaculatory problems<br>• Impaired orgasm | • Decreased libido<br>• Impaired orgasm<br>• Vaginal dryness<br>• Menstrual irregularities | Elevate prolactin levels | High |
| Olanzapine | • Reduced libido<br>• Erectile or ejaculatory dysfunction | • Reduced libido<br>• Decreased lubrication | • Strong 5HT2A antagonism and moderate D2 antagonism and 5HT2C antagonism<br>• Causes transient increase in prolactin levels | Contrasting evidence exists |
| Clozapine | • Retrograde ejaculation<br>• Gynecomastia<br>• Decreased libido<br>• Priapism | • Decreased libido<br>• Impaired arousal | Weak D2 antagonism, mild 5HT2A antagonism, H1 and M1 antagonism | High |
| Quetiapine | • Decreased libido<br>• Impaired arousal | • Decreased libido<br>• Impaired arousal | Weak D2 antagonism, mild 5HT2A and 5HT2C antagonism | High |
| Aripiprazole | • Decreased libido<br>• Ejaculatory dysfunction | • Arousal difficulty<br>• Delayed orgasm | – | Low |
| Ziprasidone | Desire, arousal and orgasm dysfunction | Desire, arousal and orgasm dysfunction | Strong 5HT2A antagonism and moderate D2 antagonism and 5HT2C antagonism | No significant difference |

**TABLE 2:** Mechanism of action and sexual effects of antipsychotic drugs.[8-10]

| Drug effects | Physiological effects | Mechanism of sexual effects |
|---|---|---|
| Cholinergic receptor antagonism | Reduced peripheral vasodilatation | Induce erectile dysfunction (men) and decreased lubrication (women) by reducing peripheral vasodilation |
| Alpha-adrenergic alpha receptor antagonism | Reduced peripheral vasodilatation | • Induce erectile dysfunction in men<br>• Decreased lubrication in women by reducing peripheral vasodilation<br>• May cause abnormal ejaculation associated with priapism |
| Histamine receptor antagonism | Sedation | Impair arousal by directly increasing sedation |
| Dopamine receptor antagonism | Inhibition of motivation and reward | Decrease the libido by inhibiting motivation and reward |
| Dopamine D2 receptor antagonism | Hyperprolactinemia | Decrease the libido, impair arousal, impair orgasm indirectly by increasing prolactin levels |

**Flowchart 1:** Effects of neurotransmitters on various stages of human sexual response.[11-12]

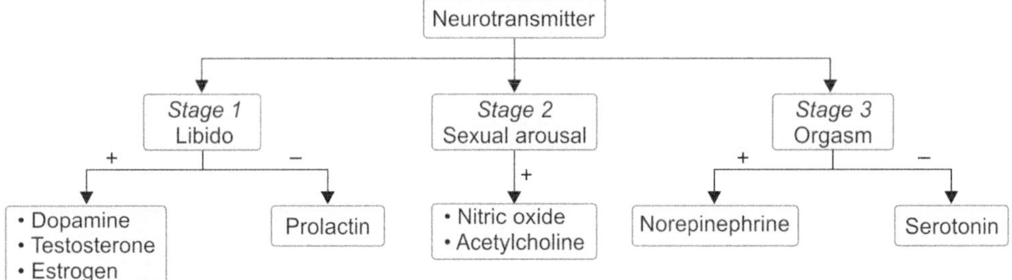


- Concomitant medications
- Age-related changes
- Relationship Issues

## Examining Historical Records to find Associations and Impacts of Sexual Dysfunction

To fully comprehend the onset of the initial signs of sexual dysfunction, obtaining a complete sexual medical history is helpful. Understanding the following domains is important from the management point of view.[5]

- Onset and severity of sexual dysfunction
- Effects of sexual dysfunction on the patient's and their partner's sexual lives
- Sexual dysfunction's impact on the patient's quality of life

This comprehensive assessment would also aid in determining whether sexual dysfunction is indeed a side effect of treatment or whether it is caused by other variables, including comorbidities, substance addiction, or other prescription medications.

Various strategies have been adopted to manage sexual dysfunction caused by antipsychotic medications, which are as follows:

- Sometimes the sexual dysfunctions are self-limiting; hence, a wait-and-watch strategy may be followed initially.[5]
- Dose reduction of antipsychotic drugs is an important strategy to deal with antipsychotic treatment-emergent sexual dysfunction.[5,13] If the psychotic symptoms are well controlled, dose reduction may be actively considered. If the patient is receiving a combination of antipsychotic drugs, dose reduction strategy may be adopted. However, clinicians need to be cautious and vigilant to look for any signs of relapse of psychotic symptoms.
- Prescribing antipsychotics with fewer sexual side effects (e.g., aripiprazole, cariprazine, and brexpiprazole) as the primary treatment option.[5,10]
- Switching to antipsychotic medications with a relatively better safety profile, such as olanzapine, quetiapine, ziprasidone, and aripiprazole.[5,10,13]

- Use of phosphodiesterase-5 inhibitors such sildenafil and tadalafil for erectile dysfunction caused by antipsychotic medications.[5,10,13]
- There is some evidence supporting the use of dopamine agonistic agents such as cabergoline, bromocriptine, and amantadine in the management of antipsychotic medication-induced sexual dysfunction;[10] however, there is a concern about the potential for relapse and worsening of psychotic symptoms.
- Drug holiday (discontinuing the antipsychotic medication for 2–3 days prior to sexual intercourse) is another strategy found to be beneficial in some patients.[13]
- Considering nonpharmacological strategies such as relaxation technique, psychoeducation, supportive psychotherapy, and couple therapy, wherever possible.

Antipsychotic medication-related sexual dysfunction can be treated with nonpharmacological therapies such as psychoeducation, counseling, and psychotherapy. These interventions are designed to inform patients about the possible negative effects of antipsychotic drugs, offer coping mechanisms, and deal with any underlying psychological or interpersonal difficulties that might be contributing to the problem.

Involving the patient's partner in the treatment can also be advantageous, as it encourages honest dialogue and understanding between the partners. Couples or sex therapy may occasionally be advised to help increase sexual functioning and improve the overall sexual experience. It is crucial to stress that treatment for sexual dysfunction caused by antipsychotic drugs should be individualized and tailored to each patient's unique requirements and preferences.

## CONCLUSION

Managing sexual dysfunction caused by antipsychotic medications necessitates a thorough and comprehensive strategy that involves medication management, psychoeducation, counseling, and possibly supplementary pharmacotherapy. Healthcare practitioners can improve the overall well-being and treatment outcomes of individuals with psychiatric disorders by addressing this important side effect.

## REFERENCES

1. Hudepohl NS, Nasrallah HA. Antipsychotic drugs. Handb Clin Neurol. 2012;106:657-67.
2. Meltzer HY. Update on typical and atypical antipsychotic drugs. Annu Rev Med. 2013;64:393-406.
3. Kandeel FR, Koussa VK, Swerdloff RS. Male sexual function and its disorders: physiology, pathophysiology, clinical investigation, and treatment. Endocr Rev. 2001;22(3):342-88.
4. Gowda SM, Kg VK, Venkatasubramanian G. Retrograde Ejaculation With Second-Generation Antipsychotics in Schizophrenia: A Case Series and Literature Review. Prim Care Companion CNS Disord. 2021;23(2):20l02654.
5. Montejo AL, de Alarcón R, Prieto N, Acosta JM, Buch B, Montejo L. Management Strategies for Antipsychotic-Related Sexual Dysfunction: A Clinical Approach. J Clin Med. 2021;10(2):308.
6. Roughley M, Lyall M. Retrograde ejaculation associated with quetiapine and treatment with low-dose imipramine. BMJ Case Rep. 2019;12(8):e228539.
7. Serretti A, Chiesa A. A meta-analysis of sexual dysfunction in psychiatric patients taking antipsychotics. Int Clin Psychopharmacol. 2011;26(3):130-40.
8. Just MJ. The influence of atypical antipsychotic drugs on sexual function. Neuropsychiatr Dis Treat. 2015;11:1655-61.
9. La Torre A, Conca A, Duffy D, Giupponi G, Pompili M, Grözinger M. Sexual dysfunction related to psychotropic drugs: a critical review part II: antipsychotics. Pharmacopsychiatry. 2013;46(6):201-8.
10. Park YW, Kim Y, Lee JH. Antipsychotic-Induced Sexual Dysfunction and Its Management. World J Mens Health. 2012;30(3):153-9.
11. Gutierrez MA, Stimmel GL. Management of and counseling for psychotropic drug-induced sexual dysfunction. Pharmacotherapy. 1999;19(7):823-31.
12. Stahl SM. The psychopharmacology of sex, part 2: effects of drugs and disease on the 3 phases of human sexual response. J Clin Psychiatry. 2001;62(3):147-8.
13. Schmidt HM, Hagen M, Kriston L, Soares-Weiser K, Maayan N, Berner MM. Management of sexual dysfunction due to antipsychotic drug therapy. Cochrane Database Syst Rev. 2012;2012(11):CD003546.

CHAPTER 45

# Managing Renal Effects of Lithium Treatment

*Naresh Nebhinani, Aanushka Suklabaidya*

## INTRODUCTION

- Lithium is one of the first drugs approved for use in bipolar disorder that is still used to this date.
- Lithium is widely known to be associated with renal side effects. However, there is wide variability in the risk associated with the same among various studies.
- Lithium is not contraindicated in all cases of kidney disease, especially if the patient has had multiple relapses in the past and lithium has been most efficacious for the patient.
- Active liaison between psychiatrists and nephrologists is required along with careful monitoring.
- *Factors influencing renal side effects:*
    - *Lithium-related risk factors:* Cumulative dose of lithium, total treatment duration, multiple dosing, maintaining higher serum levels, acute lithium toxicity.
    - *Simultaneous use of nephrotoxic medications:* Nonsteroidal anti-inflammatory drugs, angiotensin converting enzyme inhibitors, angiotensin receptor blockers, and thiazide diuretics
    - *Comorbid physical illness:* Diabetes, hypertension, obesity, cardiovascular disease, hyperparathyroidism, systemic lupus erythematosus, and recurrent renal calculi
- Lithium nephrotoxicity can be divided into the following types broadly:
    - Nephrogenic diabetes insipidus
    - Chronic kidney disease (CKD) and end-stage renal disease (ESRD)
    - Acute renal failure
    - Nephrotic syndrome
    - *Other conditions:* Renal tubular acidosis, hypercalcemia, and hyperparathyroidism

## LITHIUM-INDUCED NEPHROGENIC DIABETES INSIPIDUS

- Impairment in concentrating urine is one of the most common adverse effects affecting up to 40% of patients.[1]
- Symptoms include polyuria (>3 liters of urine production per day), thirst, and compensatory polydipsia.
- Symptoms usually start by 6–8 weeks. It mostly remains reversible during the first 6 years of treatment, following which it may be irreversible.[2]
- The mechanisms of the side effect include decreased effectiveness of the antidiuretic hormone on the kidney, reduction in the number of aquaporin 2 water channels in the collecting ducts, and increase in renal prostaglandin E2, which increases diuresis.
- It increases the risk of severe dehydration, electrolyte imbalances, and increases the risk of lithium intoxication.
- Following is the treatment approach for lithium-induced nephrogenic diabetes insipidus (Li-NDI) **(Flowchart 1)**.

## CHRONIC KIDNEY DISEASE AND END-STAGE RENAL DISEASE

- The most common form of CKD associated with lithium treatment is chronic tubulointerstitial nephritis (CTIN). The biopsy usually reveals cortical and medullary tubular atrophy and interstitial fibrosis.
- It can also cause glomerular impairment, which ultimately leads to renal insufficiency.
- NICE guidelines describe five stages of CKD based on estimated glomerular filtration rate (eGFR), and stage 5 CKD is known as ESRD, which requires hemodialysis.

- eGFR declines at the rate of around 0.92 mL/min/1.73 $m^2$ with each year of being on lithium treatment.[4]
- Renal dysfunction may persist or worsen even after stopping lithium if the eGFR at the cessation time is ≤40–45 mL/min/1.73 $m^2$ at cessation.[5]

**Flowchart 1:** Treatment approach for lithium-induced nephrogenic diabetes insipidus.

Lithium-treated patient if present with symptoms of polydipsia, polyuria, and excessive thirst causing significant impairment

↓

As side effects are considered dose-related, *reducing the dose* to maintain serum lithium levels towards the lower end of the therapeutic level and *once-daily dosing* may help

↓

The following assessments should be done:
- 24-hour urinary collection to look for the volume of urine
- Both serum and urine sodium levels and osmolality are to be checked
- Water deprivation test (for 12 hours), following which desmopressin is administered to demonstrate renal unresponsiveness

↓

If symptoms persist, weighing of risks vs. benefits should be done
- Alternative options may be considered
- *Amiloride* is recommended and can be added (5–10 mg twice daily) It increases the production of urea transporters in medullary collecting ducts and restores the concentrating power of the kidney. Most useful in mild-to-moderate cases[3]
- *Other medications were tried but with less evidence:* Thiazide or indomethacin

- Until the eGFR falls below 60 mL/min/1.73 $m^2$ and there are no clinical symptoms of renal disease, Lithium can be safely prescribed with adequate monitoring[6] **(Table 1)**.
- In case of symptoms of CKD or other red flag symptoms, nephrology referral would be required as highlighted in **Box 1**.

## ACUTE RENAL FAILURE

- Intoxication with lithium (both acute and chronic) can cause acute kidney injury due to intravascular volume loss and hypotension.
- It can be a result of direct tubular epithelial damage.
- It usually responds to the correction of dehydration by proper fluid and electrolyte management. Hemodialysis is required for severe lithium intoxication.
- There is usually a reversal of the acute injury in most cases.
- Monitoring of urea and creatinine levels, eGFR would be required to look for the return of levels to the baseline and to consider restarting lithium.

## NEPHROTIC SYNDROME

- The nephrotic syndrome usually presents with marked edema, proteinuria, and hypoalbuminemia.

**TABLE 1:** Renal monitoring in patients on lithium treatment (based on NICE guidelines for chronic kidney disease).[7]

| *Stage of CKD* | *eGFR (mL/min/1.73 $m^2$ body surface)* | *Steps to be taken* |
|---|---|---|
| Normal mildly reduced eGFR (CKD stages 1 and 2) | >60 | • To check the estimated glomerular filtration rate (eGFR) annually<br>• To monitor BP regularly<br>• In the case of mild proteinuria, monitor the albumin: creatinine ratio annually<br>• In case of moderate to heavy proteinuria, refer to nephrologist |
| Moderately reduced eGFR (CKD stages 3a and 3b) | >30 | • To monitor eGFR, urinalysis (for proteinuria and hematuria) 3-monthly<br>• *To monitor albumin:* Creatinine ratio annually, in case of an abnormal result, to confirm with early morning sample<br>• To look for cardiovascular risks, including hypertension and management with antihypertensives, antiplatelets, and statins<br>• In case of heavy proteinuria, or proteinuria along with hematuria, nephrology referral, and discontinuation of lithium can be considered |
| Severely reduced eGFR (CKD stages 4 and 5) | <30 | • Active liaison with nephrology<br>• Lithium is usually contraindicated |

(CKD: chronic kidney disease; eGFR: estimated glomerular filtration rate)

**BOX 1:** Nephrology referral to be considered under the following circumstances.[8]

- If the patient has stage 4 or 5 chronic kidney disease (eGFR <30 (mL/min/1.73 $m^2$ body surface)
- Rapid fall in eGFR (>5 mL/min/1.73 $m^2$ over one year, or >10 mL/min/1.73 $m^2$ over 5 years) and persistently low eGFR, especially in a younger patient
- If there is proteinuria (ACR ≥30 mg/mmol, or urinary protein excretion ≥0.5 g/24 h) together with hematuria
- Complications of CKD (such as anemia, edema, electrolyte imbalances, and hypertension)

(ACR: albumin-to-creatinine ratio; CKD: chronic kidney disease; eGFR: estimated glomerular filtration rate)

- Lithium is to be stopped immediately if nephrotic syndrome is suspected and immediately refer to a nephrologist.
- After the resolution of the same, a risk-benefit analysis has to be performed if lithium should be reintroduced based on previous response to medications.

## OTHER ASSOCIATED CONDITIONS

### Hypercalcemia and Hyperparathyroidism

- Develops in about 15–60% of patients on lithium treatment[9]
- Hyperparathyroidism presents with either single or multiple adenomas or diffuse hyperplasia, which usually leads to hypercalcemia.
- Hypercalcemia presents as dyspepsia, nephrolithiasis, nephrocalcinosis, osteoporosis, and cognitive impairment symptoms.
- In case of moderate-to-severe hypercalcemia or with symptomatic patient, following approach is generally recommended:
  - Endocrinologist opinion should be sought.
  - If lithium is considered to be the cause of hypercalcemia after evaluation, then it should be *withdrawn gradually*, and other psychotropics can be considered after risk-benefit analysis
  - Cinacalcet, calcimimetic drug, has been used to treat patients with lithium-induced hyperparathyroidism
  - Surgical intervention may also be required to treat hyperparathyroidism, for which liaison with endocrinology and ear, nose, and throat (ENT)/ general surgery may be required.

Clinician should be aware about lithium-related concern, dosing, prelithium work-up and subsequent monitoring, and appropriate liaison. General approach to prevent renal side effects is depicted in **Box 2**.

**BOX 2:** Guidelines for prescribing lithium to patients to prevent renal side effects.

- *Before starting medications:*
  - To look for comorbid physical illness, substance use history, and concomitant nephrotoxic medications
  - Baseline investigations: Kidney function test, estimated glomerular filtration rate (eGFR) (NICE guidelines suggest using the Chronic Kidney Disease Epidemiology Collaboration (CKD-EPI) creatinine equation for the same)
- Educate patients and family about risk associated, caution, potential side effects, and monitoring
- To target the lowest therapeutic serum lithium level[3]
- Once daily dosing is preferable[3]
- Prevention of lithium intoxication
- To monitor serum lithium levels every 3–6 months and after dose adjustments, monitoring of serum urea and creatinine (biannually according to NICE guidelines), eGFR, serum calcium levels, urinalysis, and urine/albumin creatinine ration once per year
- Monitor blood pressure levels (as the decline in renal function has an impact on cardiovascular health)

## CONCLUSION

Lithium use has declined over the years due to concerns about its long-term effects. However, the absolute risk of lithium-induced ESRD is low. Hence, for patients in whom lithium has been helpful in stabilizing the course of illness, as well as those at high risk of suicide for whom alternative treatments have not been effective, the use of lithium should be considered, after discussion with the patient and their family. Additionally, if necessary, collaboration with other clinicians, including nephrologists, is recommended. Strict monitoring and adherence to treatment algorithms and guidelines are essential components of lithium therapy.

## REFERENCES

1. Stone KA. Lithium-induced nephrogenic diabetes insipidus. J Am Board Fam Pract. 1999;12(1):43-7.
2. Grandjean EM, Aubry JM. Lithium: updated human knowledge using an evidence-based approach: part III: clinical safety. CNS drugs. 2009;23:397-418.
3. Schoot TS, Molmans TH, Grootens KP, Kerckhoffs AP. Systematic review and practical guideline for the prevention and management of the renal side effects of lithium therapy. European Neuropsychopharmacology. 2020; 31:16-32.

4. Tondo L, Abramowicz M, Alda M, Bauer M, Bocchetta A, Bolzani L, et al. Long-term lithium treatment in bipolar disorder: effects on glomerular filtration rate and other metabolic parameters. Int J Bipolar Disord 2017;5(1):1-2.
5. Bocchetta A, Ardau R, Fanni T, Sardu C, Piras D, Pani A, et al. Renal function during long-term lithium treatment: a cross-sectional and longitudinal study. BMC Med. 2015;13(1):1-7.
6. Kripalani M, Shawcross J, Reilly J, Main J. Lithium and chronic kidney disease. BMJ. 2009;3:339.
7. National Institute for Health and Clinical Excellence. (2008). Early identification and management of chronic kidney disease in adults in primary and secondary care (Clinical guideline 73). [online] Available from www.nice.org.uk/Guidance/CG73 [Last accessed June, 2025].
8. Davis J, Desmond M, Berk M. Lithium and nephrotoxicity: a literature review of approaches to clinical management and risk stratification. BMC Nephrol. 2018;19:1-7.
9. Khandwala HM, Van Uum S. Reversible hypercalcemia and hyperparathyroidism associated with lithium therapy: case report and review of literature. Endocr Pract. 2006;12(1):54-8.

CHAPTER 46

# Management of Lithium-induced Cognitive Dysfunction

*Biswa Ranjan Mishra, Dibyendu Mohanty*

## INTRODUCTION

Lithium is a naturally occurring metal first discovered as early as 1800 AD. Its use in psychiatry has been documented since the nineteenth century and gained momentum in the latter half of the twentieth century for its mood-stabilizing effects.[1]

Lithium is readily available, low-cost, and has good mood-stabilizing properties. Lithium carbonate is the most common salt of lithium used in tablet form as an oral prescription. In addition to bipolar disorder (BD), lithium has shown efficacy in depression, where it is recommended as an augmenting agent and as a prophylactic agent to prevent further episodes. In schizoaffective disorder, it can be used as a mood stabilizer for acute management and prophylactically to prevent future episodes. Lithium has also been found to be effective in reducing self-harming behavior in patients with personality disorders. Furthermore, it has been shown to reduce the risk of suicidality in both unipolar depression and BD, independent of its therapeutic effects. Additionally, lithium is sometimes used to reverse clozapine-induced neutropenia.[2]

However, lithium has its limitations, including its narrow therapeutic range and a side-effect profile that ranges from mild acne to severe hypothyroidism, renal dysfunction, cerebellar involvement, and cardiac conduction defects. In addition to these established side effects, recent studies have shown a negative impact on cognition, contradicting earlier reports of cognitive improvements. Hence, there is a need for closer inspection of the role of lithium in cognition and its implication in patient care.

## LITHIUM AND COGNITION: AN OVERVIEW

Lithium's protective effect on cognition in BD by its direct effect on the course of the illness is well established. Other mechanisms have been proposed, such as increasing the brain-derived natriuretic factor (BDNF), enhancing the number of neurons and synapses in the hippocampal area and the overall brain volume, and reducing the production of reactive oxygen species secondary to brain hyperactivity.[3]

However, recent studies have started showing some specific undesirable effects of lithium on cognition.[4] The general perception of lithium's predominantly positive effects on cognition, independent of its therapeutic action, is now being debated. The reasons for this debate are multifactorial.[5]

Firstly, the effect of lithium on cognition is mainly studied in BD, where it is most commonly used. Cognitive decline in BD can occur secondary to disease progression and increased episode frequency. Lithium tends to reduce episodes and halts the disease progression, thereby potentially improving cognition as a secondary effect of treating the illness rather than through primary effects on cognition. Secondly, more controlled trials with healthy controls are needed to better understand the complex mechanisms at play. Thirdly, the negative effect of lithium on cognition might be subtle, making it challenging to assess using standard tools in everyday clinical practice.

## ADVERSE EFFECTS OF LITHIUM ON COGNITION

Patients on lithium who report cognitive difficulties often describe symptoms such as "mental fogging," "feeling blurry" or slow, experiencing word-finding issues, memory difficulties, and a "dampening in creativity."[4] Various studies have shown impaired performance across multiple cognitive domains, including executive functioning, verbal memory, psychomotor speed, verbal fluency, visual memory, and social cognition (reading emotions).[4,5] Magnetic resonance imaging (MRI) studies in patients on long-term lithium therapy suggest that as patients age, there is an increase in brain lithium levels that do not correlate with serum lithium levels, leading to increased cognitive side effects, particularly involving the frontal lobes.[6]

Lithium-induced cognitive dysfunction tends to remain static and usually improves within 2 weeks of discontinuation.[4,7,8] In contrast to the cognitive dysfunction secondary to BD, which is typically progressive, cumulative, and permanent, cognitive dysfunction resulting from lithium use is temporary, non-progressive, and reversible. Therefore, accurate diagnosis is crucial, as lithium-induced cognitive dysfunction generally carries a better outcome.

## MANAGEMENT OF LITHIUM-INDUCED COGNITIVE DYSFUNCTION

### Cognitive Assessment Tools

Based on the findings mentioned above, Malhi et al. proposed a lithium battery for clinical purposes to assess for lithium-induced cognitive dysfunction. This battery includes the Trail Making Test A and B (TMT A and B) for assessing psychomotor and processing speed, the Controlled Oral Word Association Test (COWAT) for verbal fluency, and the Rey Auditory Learning Verbal Test (RAVLT) for evaluating verbal learning and memory. These tests require 10–15 minutes to administer, making them feasible in a clinical setting.[5]

Other than these specific tests, standard scales like the Mini Mental Score Examination (MMSE) or the Montreal Cognitive Assessment (MoCA) can be used adjunctively to cover other cognitive domains and obtain a more detailed picture of a patient's baseline functioning.

A baseline cognitive assessment should be done in patients on lithium or those with BD when they present with complaints of cognitive dysfunction. Subsequently, monthly assessments should be performed following any relevant intervention, as outlined in the flowchart below. If lithium is discontinued, reassessments should be done after two weeks **(Flowchart 1)**. The reason is twofold: firstly, lithium-induced cognitive dysfunction starts improving within two weeks of cessation, and secondly, it is unwise to keep a patient with BD off mood stabilizers for extended periods, as this may increase the risk of relapse. Hence, the diagnosis of "lithium-induced cognitive dysfunction" should be promptly made after discontinuing lithium, and a subsequent plan should be implemented accordingly.

### Ruling Out Confounding Factors

Since several confounding factors complicate the diagnosis and considering the catastrophic effect of lithium discontinuation on the course of illness, lithium induced cognitive dysfunction should be a diagnosis of exclusion, only made after ruling out all other potential contributors.[9]

- *Acute mood episodes:* Before concluding drug-induced cognitive dysfunction, it is crucial to rule out acute manic or depressive episodes, as these invariably affect a patient's cognitive capabilities. A Young Mania Rating Scale (YMRS) score of <6 and a Hamilton Depression Rating Scale (HDRS) score of <8 are generally considered indicative of the absence of manic or depressive episodes. Clinicians should also be mindful of subsyndromal symptoms.
- *Metabolic syndrome:* Psychiatric patients are at a higher risk of metabolic syndrome due to genetic burden, psychotropic side effects, and sedentary lifestyle. Hence, ruling out metabolic syndrome and its associated effects on cognitive abilities is imperative.
- *Comorbid psychiatric or medical illnesses:* Patients with BD often have concurrent psychiatric disorders, such as anxiety disorders, substance use disorders, ADHD, and PTSD, which can negatively influence cognitive functioning.
- *Concurrent use of psychotropics:* Atypical antipsychotics and benzodiazepines are commonly used for their rapid tranquillizing and mood-stabilizing effects. However, their concomitant use can cause sedation and extrapyramidal side effects, negatively affecting cognition. Rationalizing the dose of these drugs (maintaining on minimum effective doses) and minimizing polypharmacy is essential in preserving cognitive function.
- *Serum lithium levels:* Lithium has a narrow therapeutic range in blood levels. Typically, a level of 0.8–1.2 mmol/L is considered adequate during acute episodes, and 0.6–0.8 mmol/L is appropriate during the maintenance phase of treatment as a mood stabilizer. Higher levels can lead to side effects, while levels below this range may result in inadequate control of illness and further

**Flowchart 1:** Approach to a case of lithium-induced cognitive dysfunction.

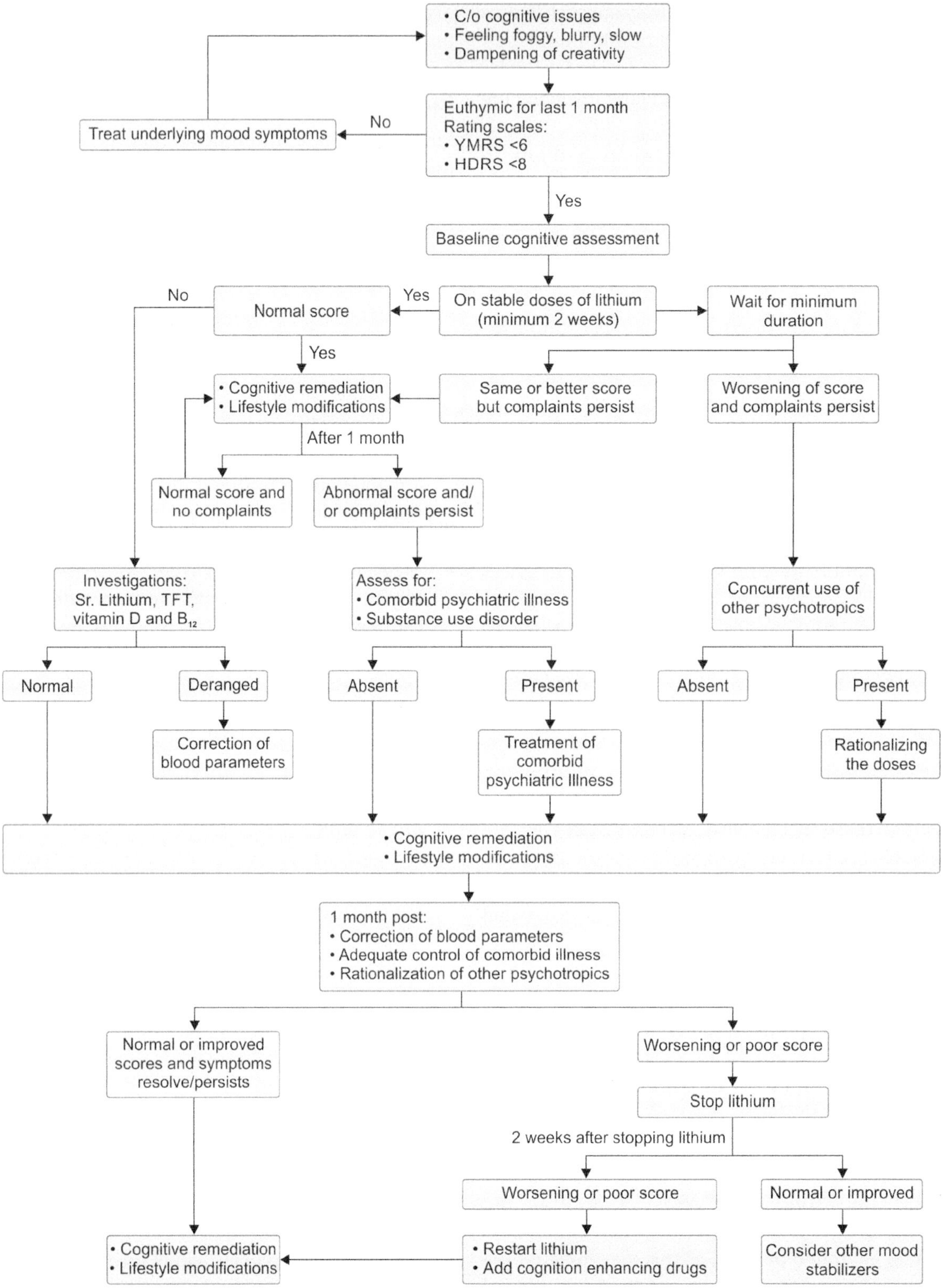

- C/o cognitive issues
- Feeling foggy, blurry, slow
- Dampening of creativity

Euthymic for last 1 month
Rating scales:
- YMRS <6
- HDRS <8

No → Treat underlying mood symptoms

Yes → Baseline cognitive assessment

On stable doses of lithium (minimum 2 weeks)

Wait for minimum duration

Normal score

No / Yes

- Cognitive remediation
- Lifestyle modifications

Same or better score but complaints persist

Worsening of score and complaints persist

After 1 month

Normal score and no complaints

Abnormal score and/ or complaints persist

Investigations: Sr. Lithium, TFT, vitamin D and $B_{12}$

Assess for:
- Comorbid psychiatric illness
- Substance use disorder

Concurrent use of other psychotropics

Normal | Deranged | Absent | Present | Absent | Present

Correction of blood parameters

Treatment of comorbid psychiatric Illness

Rationalizing the doses

- Cognitive remediation
- Lifestyle modifications

1 month post:
- Correction of blood parameters
- Adequate control of comorbid illness
- Rationalization of other psychotropics

Normal or improved scores and symptoms resolve/persists

Worsening or poor score

Stop lithium

2 weeks after stopping lithium

Worsening or poor score

Normal or improved

- Cognitive remediation
- Lifestyle modifications

- Restart lithium
- Add cognition enhancing drugs

Consider other mood stabilizers

(YMRS: Young Mania Rating Scale, HDRS: Hamilton Depression Rating Scale, c/o: complaints of, vit: vitamin; TFT: thyroid function test)

cognitive decline. Hence, regular monitoring of blood levels is necessary for optimal dosing.

- *Deficiencies:* Hypothyroidism is a common side effect of long-term lithium use, with the risk increasing over time, reaching up to 20%. Hypothyroidism can directly affect cognition or indirectly contribute to cognitive decline through metabolic side effects and inadequate control of the illness. Additionally, deficiencies in vitamin D and vitamin $B_{12}$ can mimic depressive symptoms and cause cognitive dysfunction.[10,11]
- *Lifestyle factors:* Major psychiatric illnesses are often associated with a sedentary lifestyle and a lack of physical activity, which can lead to long-term medical issues and impaired overall well-being.

## DECISION REGARDING DISCONTINUING LITHIUM

The decision to discontinue lithium should be carefully considered and based on the persistence or worsening of cognitive dysfunction, even after adequately treating confounding factors. If cognitive dysfunction persists or worsens despite addressing these factors, a trial discontinuation of lithium may be initiated, followed by reassessment of cognitive performance. If cognitive function improves after discontinuation, it can be inferred that lithium was the likely cause of cognitive decline, and alternative mood stabilizers can be considered. However, if cognitive dysfunction persists or worsens after discontinuation of lithium, factors other than lithium may be responsible and should be further explored. In such cases, restarting lithium and addressing the underlying factors is prudent.

In situations where discontinuing lithium is not feasible due to illness or patient-related factors, pharmacological and nonpharmacological interventions can be used to mitigate cognitive dysfunction. Nonpharmacological strategies such as exercise and cognitive remediation techniques, including mindfulness, have shown effectiveness in improving cognition. Exercise releases endorphins and improves overall mood and cognitive functioning, especially in depressive episodes. Additionally, certain pharmacological agents, including mifepristone, pramipexole, galantamine, and lurasidone, have shown promise in addressing cognitive dysfunction. Although evidence is inconclusive, intranasal insulin and erythropoietin can also be considered. Extracts of *Withania somnifera* have demonstrated benefits in auditory-verbal working memory and may be considered as well.[9]

## CONCLUSION

Even after nearly 70 years since its first use in BD, lithium remains an effective treatment. However, it is not without its side effects. Recent studies provide evidence of its negative impact on cognition, which can lead to poor socio-occupational functioning and increased dropout rates with significant consequences.

Diagnosing lithium-induced cognitive dysfunction should be approached cautiously, with a high threshold to improve specificity. It should only be diagnosed after excluding all other confounding factors. If the diagnosis is confirmed, discontinuing lithium and considering alternative mood stabilizers is advisable. If discontinuation of lithium is not feasible, other pharmacological and nonpharmacological treatment options should be explored to mitigate cognitive dysfunction. If cognitive dysfunction persists or worsens after discontinuing lithium, then the diagnosis of lithium-induced cognitive dysfunction should be revised, and lithium should be restarted. Our understanding of the effect of lithium on cognition is still evolving, and further research is needed to elucidate this complex relationship.

## REFERENCES


1. Shorter E. The history of lithium therapy. Bipolar Disord. 2009;11(Suppl 2):4-9.
2. In: Taylor DM, Barnes TRE, Young AH (Eds). The Maudsley prescribing guidelines in psychiatry, 14th edition. New Jersey: John Wiley & Sons; 2018.
3. De-Paula VJ, Gattaz WF, Forlenza OV. Long-term lithium treatment increases intracellular and extracellular brain-derived neurotrophic factor (BDNF) in cortical and hippocampal neurons at subtherapeutic concentrations. Bipolar Disord. 2016;18(8):692-5.
4. Pachet AK, Wisniewski AM. The effects of lithium on cognition: an updated review. Psychopharmacology (Berl). 2003;170(3):225-34.
5. Malhi GS, McAulay C, Gershon S, Gessler D, Fritz K, Das P, Outhred T. The Lithium Battery: assessing the neurocognitive profile of lithium in bipolar disorder. Bipolar Disord. 2016;18(2):102-15.
6. Forester BP, Streeter CC, Berlow YA, Tian H, Wardrop M, Finn CT, et al. Brain Lithium Levels and Effects on Cognition and Mood in Geriatric Bipolar Disorder: A Lithium-7 Magnetic Resonance Spectroscopy Study. Am J Geriatr Psychiatry. 2009;17(1):13-23.

7. Shaw E, Stokes P, Mann J, Manevitz Z. Effects of lithium carbonate on the memory and motor speed of bipolar outpatients. J Abnorm Psychol. 1987;96(1): 64-69.
8. Kocsis J, Shaw E, Stokes P, Wilner P, Elliot A, Sikes C, et al. Neuropsychologic effects of lithium discontinuation. J Clin Psychopharmacol. 1993;13(4):268-76.
9. Solé B, Jiménez E, Torrent C, Reinares M, Bonnin CDM, Torres I, et al. Cognitive Impairment in Bipolar Disorder: Treatment and Prevention Strategies. Int J Neuropsychopharmacol. 2017;20(8):670-80.
10. Marazziti D, Mangiapane P, Carbone MG, Morana F, Arone A, Massa L, et al. Decreased Levels of Vitamin D in Bipolar Patients. Life. 2023;13(4):883.
11. Jayaram N, Rao MG, Narasimha A, Raveendranathan D, Varambally S, Venkatasubramanian G, et al. Vitamin $B_{12}$ levels and psychiatric symptomatology: a case series. J Neuropsychiatry Clin Neurosci. 2013 Spring;25(2):150-2.

CHAPTER 47

# Management of Endocrine Effects of Lithium

*Deepak Kumar, Aparna Goyal*

## INTRODUCTION

Lithium is commonly used as a mood stabilizer for bipolar disorder (BD). Lithium has a narrow therapeutic index. Its precise mechanism of action in mood disorders is not entirely clear, but it is believed to reduce intracellular sodium and calcium levels, which are elevated in individuals with BD. Additionally, it may exert its effects through modulation of glycogen synthase kinase 3 (GSK 3), cAMP response element-binding protein (CREB), and $Na^+/K^+$ ATPase-related mechanisms. Moreover, lithium has been reported to have neuroprotective effects and may promote neurogenesis.[1]

Most of the side effects associated with lithium are dose and plasma concentration-dependent. Common adverse effects include gastrointestinal side effects like nausea and diarrhea. These are prominent in the early treatment course and are less common in long-term therapy. Weight gain, tremor, and cutaneous side effects such as acne and psoriasis are other common side effects. Nystagmus, myasthenia gravis, papilledema, photophobia, and dry eye are other reported side effects. Albuminuria, hypotension, cardiac arrhythmias, QT prolongation, and ECG changes like ST-segment and T-wave changes are uncommon. Lithium also exerts endocrine influences, affecting thyroid, parathyroid, kidney, and calcium levels **(Table 1)**. In predisposed individuals, endocrine abnormalities may manifest even within the reference range of lithium levels.

While there are no absolute contraindications for lithium use, it is strongly recommended that all patients prescribed lithium undergo thorough investigation and regular monitoring.

## THYROID

Hyperthyroidism is an uncommon complication of lithium use, with a reported incidence of 0.1–1.7%. The rate of hyperthyroidism is two to three times higher in lithium-treated individuals in comparison to the general population. One proposed mechanism suggests that lithium-induced thyroiditis results from maladaptation to disturbed iodine kinetics, leading to an escape phenomenon after the expansion of the intrathyroidal iodine pool.[2]

**TABLE 1:** Adverse impact of lithium on the endocrine system.[2-5]

| *Organ affected* | *Thyroid* | *Parathyroid* | *Kidney* |
|---|---|---|---|
| Endocrine abnormality | Goiter/Hypothyroidism<br>Hyperthyroidism | Hyperparathyroidism<br>Hypercalcemia | Nephrogenic Diabetes Insipidus (NDI) |
| Prevalence | 10–50% may develop[6] | 6.3–50%[7] | Approx 20–40%[8] |
| Risk factors | • Long-term treatment of lithium<br>• Iodine-deficient areas<br>• More common in women<br>• Those with preexisting thyroid antibodies.<br>• family history of thyroid disease<br>• Usually occurs more frequently within the first 2 years | • More prevalent in women (4:1). Both parathyroid adenomas and hyperplasia are observed.<br>• Can occur even after just 4 weeks of lithium treatment | • Those on any comorbid drugs like ACE inhibitors<br>• Gradual changes and manifested as polyuria, polydipsia, and low urinary osmolarity |

*Contd...*

*Contd...*

| *Organ affected* | *Thyroid* | *Parathyroid* | *Kidney* |
|---|---|---|---|
| Mechanism of action | • Inhibition of the release of thyroid hormones<br>• Increases secretion of immunoglobulins by lymphocytes, triggering a preexisting immune response or interfering with the function of CD8 suppressor cells<br>• Reduce iodine uptake, interferes with tyrosine iodination, changing thyroglobulin structure and colloid formation, causing interference in iodotyrosinase synthesis<br>• Increase nuclear triiodothyronine binding<br>• Inhibits the activity of ATP, inhibits cAMP, and the activity of adenylyl cyclase induced by stimulation of the TSH receptor | • Lithium increases the setpoint of the parathyroid calcium-sensing receptor<br>• Higher levels of serum calcium are required to inhibit PTH secretion<br>• Reduced urinary excretion of calcium due to increased renal resorption secondary to PTH increase<br>• May stimulate the growth of preexisting parathyroid tumors | • Kidney's inability to concentrate urine, even with normal levels of ADH<br>• Inhibition of adenylate cyclase activity<br>• Reduction of AQP2 mRNA synthesis, inhibition of adenosine triphosphatases, and interference with prostaglandin production<br>• Lithium inhibits the expression of aquaporins (mainly aquaporin 2, AQP2) (stimulated by binding of ADH with V2 receptors) in the renal collecting duct, yet unknown mechanisms |

(AQP2: aquaporin-2; ATP: adenosine triphosphate; cAMP: cyclic adenosine monophosphate)

**Flowchart 1:** Management of endocrine effects of lithium.

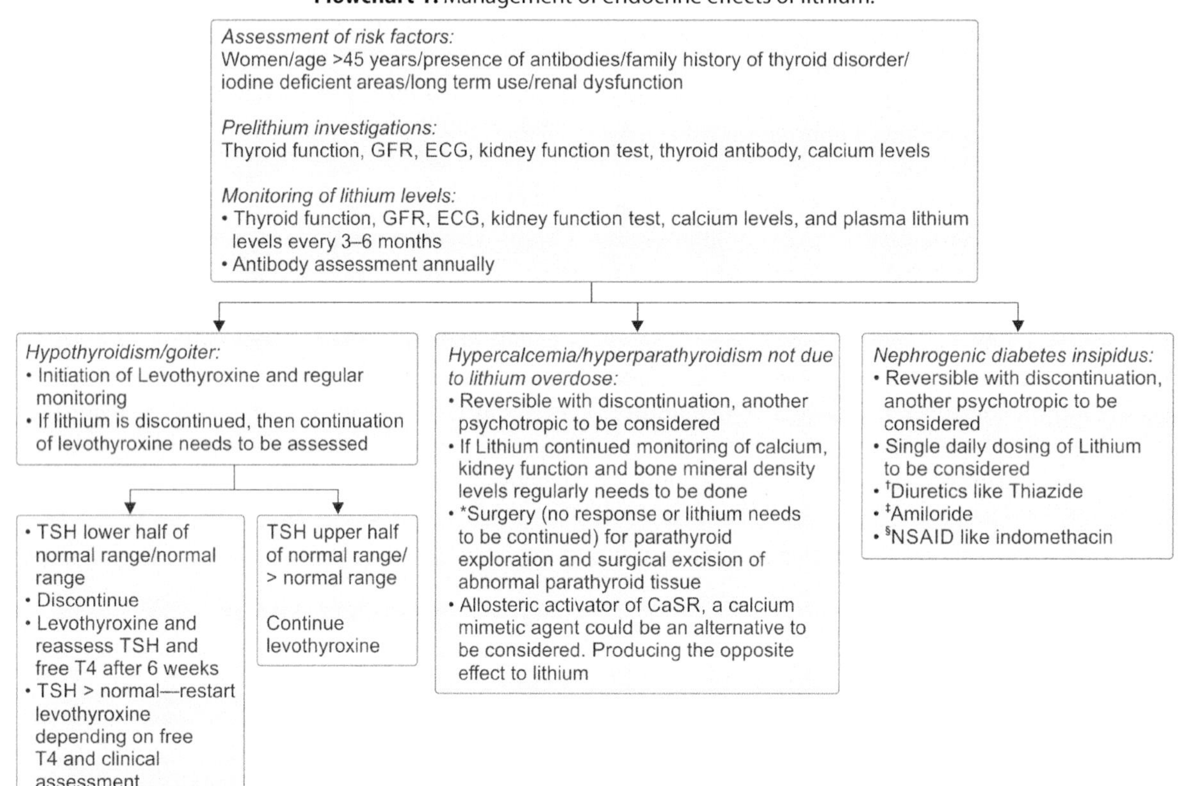


(CaSR: calcium sensing receptor; ECG: electrocardiogram; GFR: glomerular filtration rate; NSAID: nonsteroidal anti-inflammatory drug)

*The approach is disputed, as about 25–75% of people have multiglandular pathology. If preoperative localization of the lesion is possible and intraoperative PTH measurement is feasible, unilateral parathyroidectomy is preferred. If not, then bilateral exploration with removal only of the abnormal glands or subtotal parathyroidectomy (three- and one-half glands) is recommended wherever possible.

†Not hydrochlorothiazide as it can cause lithium toxicity.

‡Due to its natriuretic action (causing contraction of extracellular volume, consequent decrease in glomerular filtration, and ultimately leading to decreased urine volume), and reduces the entry of lithium in distal tubule cells.

§Should not be carried out on a long-term basis due to its side effects.

*Note:* NDI and hypercalcemia related to lithium can occur together, as dehydration can exacerbate hypercalcemia.

Silent thyroiditis and thyrotoxicosis are also reported, although less frequently reported after long-term lithium use, probably as a direct effect of the lithium on follicular cells. Paradoxically, lithium has been shown to be useful in low doses for controlling thyrotoxicosis in patients who do not respond to thionamides.

## PARATHYROID

In lithium-induced hyperparathyroidism, there are normal phosphate levels, increased circulating magnesium, and hypocalciuria compared to hyperparathyroidism, where plasma phosphates and urine calcium loss are increased. Additionally, some patients may remain hypercalcemic even after discontinuation of lithium therapy.

## NEPHROGENIC DIABETES INSIPIDUS

Recovery of renal concentrating ability may take several months or years after discontinuation of lithium therapy. However, occasionally, chronic interstitial nephropathy may cause irreversible kidney damage, leading to eventually end-stage renal failure (ESRF). The absolute risk of ESRF appears to be small, i.e., estimated at 0.5% in comparison to 0.2% in the general population.

## CONCLUSION

Key points to remember in the management of adverse endocrine effects due to lithium therapy include **(Flowchart 1)**:

- Individualized case-based analysis.
- Risk factors to be kept in mind.
- Prelithium investigations to be done before lithium initiation.
- Regular monitoring of lithium levels and various other investigations.
- There are no absolute contraindications in patients with preexisting thyroid disorders.
- Interactions with other drugs like angiotensin-converting enzyme inhibitors and calcium channel blockers can cause lithium toxicity should be forewarned.
- Cautious use in vulnerable populations like the elderly and preference for alternative drugs.
- Regular monitoring of the adverse effects if lithium is continued.

## REFERENCES

1. In: Taylor DM, Barnes TR, Young AH (Eds). The Maudsley prescribing guidelines in psychiatry. New Jersey: John Wiley & Sons; 2021.
2. Lerena VS, León NS, Sosa S, Deligiannis NG, Danilowicz K, Rizzo LF. Lithium and endocrine dysfunction. MEDICINA (Buenos Aires). 2022;82(1).
3. Krysiak R, Okopien B. Potentiation of Endocrine Adverse Effects of Lithium by Enalapril and Verapamil. The West Indian Medical Journal. 2014;63(7):803.
4. Giusti CF, Amorim SR, Guerra RA, Portes ES. Endocrine disturbances related to the use of lithium. Arq Bras Endocrinol Metabol. 2012;56(3):153-8.
5. García-Maldonado G, de Jesús Castro-García R. Endocrinological disorders related to the medical use of lithium. A narrative review. Revista Colombiana de Psiquiatría (English ed.). 2019;48(1):35-43.
6. McKnight RF, Adida M, Budge K, Stockton S, Goodwin GM, Geddes JR. Lithium toxicity profile: a systematic review and meta-analysis. Lancet. 2012;379(9817):721-8.
7. Livingstone C, Rampes H. Lithium: a review of its metabolic adverse effects. J Psychopharmacol. 2006;20(3):347-55.
8. Jackson BA, Edwards RM, Dousa TP. Lithium-induced polyuria: effect of lithium on adenylate cyclase and adenosine 3′,5′-monophosphate phosphodiesterase in medullary ascending limb of Henle's loop and in medullary collecting tubules. Endocrinology. 1980;107(6):1693-8.

# Managing Weight Gain with Lithium Treatment

*Shalini Kumari, Santanu Nath, Venkata Lakshmi Narasimha*

## INTRODUCTION

Lithium is a first-line pharmacological agent for managing bipolar disorder and is also utilized in treating various other psychiatric disorders. The use of lithium is associated with a 1.89 odds of experiencing weight gain compared to the use of a placebo.[1] While weight gain is a common side effect, it is also multifactorial, including factors such as concurrent use of multiple agents and inactivity. Weight gain can be distressing, leading to noncompliance and relapses. This chapter deals with possible mechanisms of weight gain with lithium and its management options.

## MECHANISM OF WEIGHT GAIN WITH LITHIUM

The potential risk factors for lithium-induced weight gain are outlined in **Box 1**. While the exact biological mechanisms underlying lithium-induced weight gain are not fully understood, researchers have proposed that multiple processes are likely involved **(Fig. 1)**, and various hypotheses have been put forward. One such hypothesis suggests that initial weight gain after lithium therapy is because patients regain previously lost weight during the illness.[2] Storlien and Smythe proposed four potential mechanisms of lithium-induced weight gain[3] **(Fig. 1)**.

**BOX 1:** Risk factors related to weight gain with lithium.

*Risk factors:*
- Female gender.
- History of overweight prior to lithium treatment.
- Higher serum lithium levels
- Increased calorie and fluid intake
- Other medications (e.g., concomitant use of antipsychotics, sodium valproate, etc.)

- Increased fluid intake (polydipsia) secondary to polyuria induced by lithium. Patients quench their thirst by consuming calorie-rich fluids.
- Weight gain may occur due to improved mood, leading to increased appetite and higher food intake.
- Lithium could contribute to weight gain by reducing the metabolic rate even without increased food consumption.
- Lithium, through its effect on noradrenergic activity in the hypothalamus, may lead to hyperglycemia, eventually leading to hyperinsulinemia, increased food intake, and weight gain.

Various endocrine and metabolic factors also contribute to weight gain due to lithium.

*Metabolic:*
- *Effect on carbohydrate metabolism:* Lithium exerts an insulin-like effect on carbohydrate metabolism by stimulating hexokinase and protein kinase, leading to increased glucose uptake into the cells. Thus, it enhances energy storage efficiency, leading to weight gain.[4]
- *Effect on lipid metabolism:* Lithium may cause increased utilization of glucose for the synthesis of phospholipids and triglycerides in blood, liver, and brain.[5]

*Endocrine:* Lithium's role in inducing hypothyroidism may further contribute to weight gain.[6]

## MANAGEMENT OF LITHIUM-INDUCED WEIGHT GAIN

Lithium-induced weight gain is multifactorial, as discussed in the previous section. Understanding the main factors contributing to weight gain with lithium can help clinicians in managing this metabolic side effect. Management strategies can be divided into prevention and treatment.

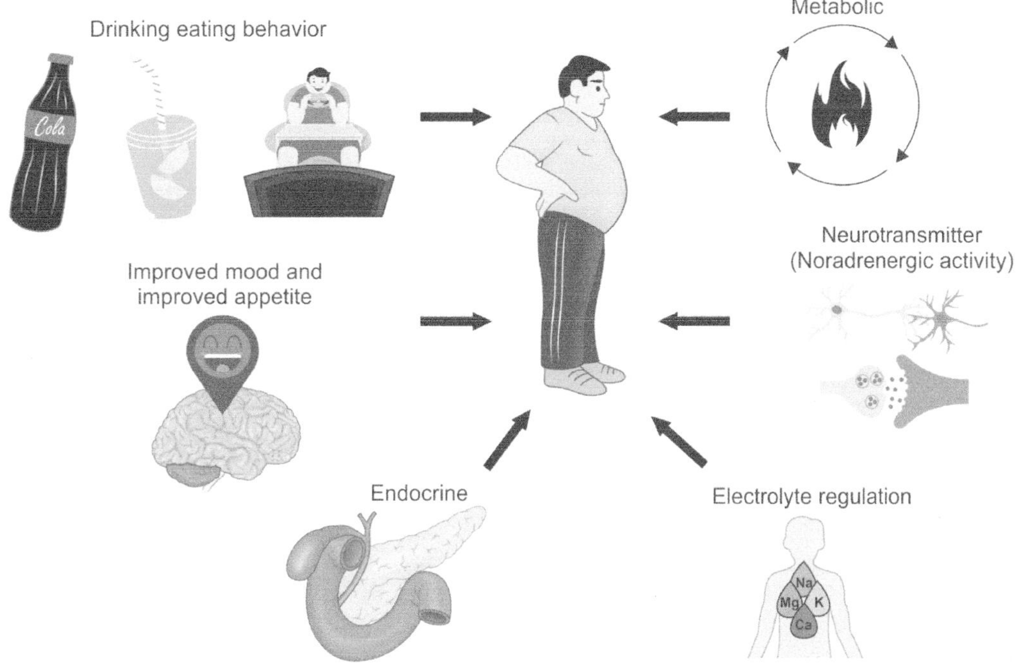


**Fig. 1:** Factors associated with lithium-induced weight gain.

## PREVENTION OF LITHIUM-INDUCED WEIGHT GAIN

- Discuss the likelihood of weight gain with patients and their relatives.
- Monitor weight and body mass index (BMI) at baseline, along with thyroid function test (TFT) and renal function test (RFT), before initiating lithium therapy.[7]
- Conduct follow-up monitoring of weight and BMI every 6 months (or more frequently at each follow-up visit), alongside monitoring renal and thyroid hormone parameters.[7]
- Early identification of weight gain or change in BMI is crucial.
- If not clinically indicated, avoiding irrational polypharmacy, especially with other psychotropics known to have pronounced metabolic side effects.
- Consider discontinuing antipsychotics coprescribed with lithium, particularly those having more metabolic side effects, once the acute phase of treatment (e.g., in the manic phase of bipolar disorder) is over, after conducting a proper risk-benefit analysis.
- When lithium is used in combination with another mood stabilizer that can also cause weight gain (e.g., sodium valproate), evaluate the risk-benefit ratio of discontinuing the second mood stabilizer (in this case, valproate).
- Provide psychoeducation to patients on lithium, advising them to avoid calorie-rich fluids to quench thirst induced by lithium. Encourage the adoption of a healthy dietary regimen and a routine of daily physical activity.[8]
- Manage comorbidities that can contribute to weight gain with lithium by addressing shared vulnerabilities, such as hypothyroidism, oedema, and renal failure (through water retention).

## MANAGEMENT OPTIONS FOR LITHIUM-INDUCED WEIGHT GAIN

The available literature emphasizes the outlined measures as the first line in preventing and managing lithium-induced weight gain. However, there is still no consensus on the optimal approach to managing weight gain associated with lithium use. Weight-loss agents like topiramate have been advocated as adjuncts to lithium when the above measures fail.[9] This recommendation also extends to metformin, an oral hypoglycemic agent,

**Flowchart 1:** Management of weight gain with lithium treatment.

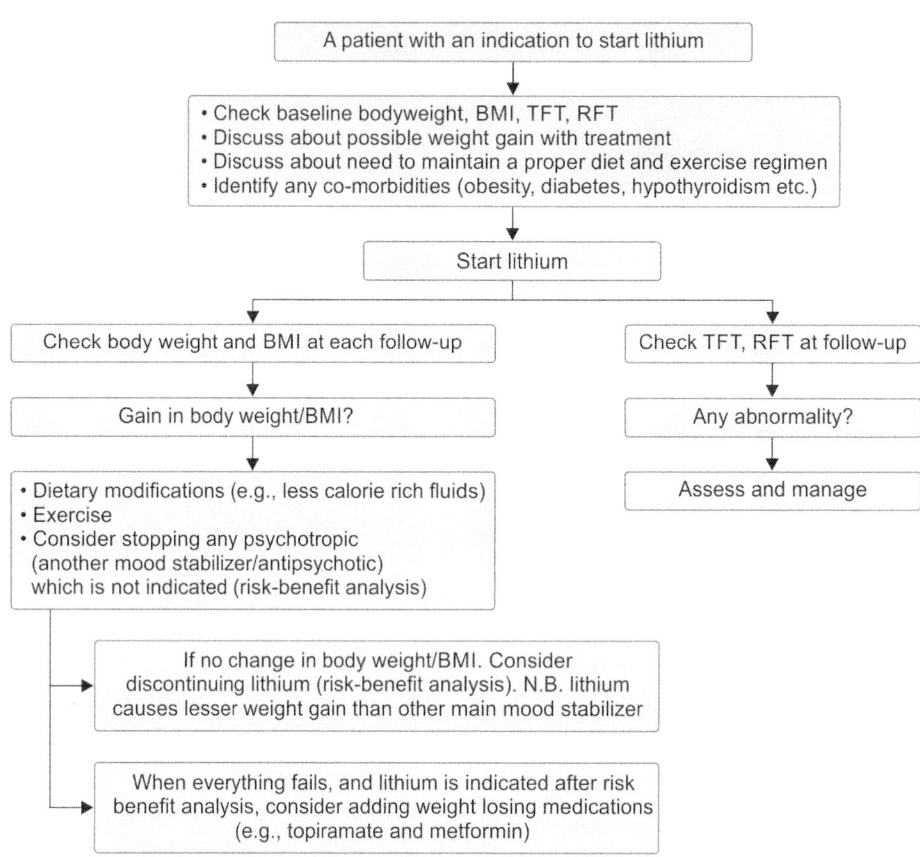


(BMI: body mass index; RFT: Renal function test; TFT: thyroid function test; NB: niobium)

which has also been used for weight gain with lithium treatment.[10] **Flowchart 1** discusses the management plan for addressing weight gain associated with lithium.

## REFERENCES

1. McKnight RF, Adida M, Budge K, Stockton S, Goodwin GM, Geddes JR. Lithium toxicity profile: a systematic review and meta-analysis. Lancet Lond Engl. 2012;379(9817):721-8.
2. Kerry RJ, Liebling LI, Owen G. Weight changes in lithium responders. Acta Psychiatr Scand. 1970;46(3):238-43.
3. Storlien LH, Higson FM, Gleeson RM, Smythe GA, Atrens DM. Effects of chronic lithium, amitriptyline and mianserin on glucoregulation, corticosterone and energy balance in the rat. Pharmacol Biochem Behav. 1985;22(1):119-25.
4. Vendsborg PB, Bech P, Rafaelsen OJ. Lithium treatment and weight gain. Acta Psychiatr Scand. 1976;53(2):139-47.
5. Krulík R, Janko L, Cerný M. Metabolism of lipids in lithium administered rats. Acta Univ Carol [Med] (Praha). 1971;17:533-40.
6. Shine B, McKnight RF, Leaver L, Geddes JR. Long-term effects of lithium on renal, thyroid, and parathyroid function: a retrospective analysis of laboratory data. Lancet. 2015;386(9992):461-8.
7. In: Taylor DM, Barnes TRE, Young AH (Eds). The Maudsley Prescribing Guidelines in Psychiatry, 14th edition. New Jersey: John Wiley & Sons; 2021.
8. Suwalska JKR, Aleksandra. Gastrointestinal, metabolic and body-weight changes during treatment with lithium. In: Suwalska JKR, Aleksandra (Eds). Lithium in Neuropsychiatry. New Delhi: CRC Press; 2013.
9. Roy Chengappa KN, Levine J, Rathore D, Parepally H, Atzert R. Long-term effects of topiramate on bipolar mood instability, weight change and glycemic control: a case-series. Eur Psychiatry J Assoc Eur Psychiatr. 2001;16(3):186-90.
10. Praharaj SK. Metformin for Lithium-induced Weight Gain: A Case Report. Clin Psychopharmacol Neurosci. 2016;14(1):101-3.

CHAPTER 49

# Management of Drug-induced Constipation

*Parag Shah, Heena Khanna*

## INTRODUCTION

Constipation is not a disease but a symptom, warranting attention from the treating psychiatrist. It is a widely prevalent symptom among psychiatric patients, with a reported two-year period prevalence of 36.3% in schizophrenia[1] and 57.7% in depression.[2] Unfortunately, only 18.5% of constipated psychiatric inpatients report the presence of constipation to their psychiatrists.[3] In addition, an incidence rate of 15 per 100 person-years has been observed in patients with severe mental illness (SMI).[4] The clinical consequences of constipation include the potential to cause or aggravate various common digestive symptoms, and it may even lead to severe complications such as fecal impaction, bowel perforation, paralytic ileus, and rarely death[5] **(Flowchart 1)**.

According to the Rome Criteria, there is constipation if patients who do not take laxatives report at least two of the following in any 12-week period during the previous 12 months:

- Fewer than three bowel movements (BMs) per week
- Hard stool in >25% of BMs
- A sense of incomplete evacuation in >25% of BMs.
- Excessive straining in >25% of BMs.
- A need for digital manipulation to facilitate evacuation.

However, in actual clinical practice, the symptoms and prevalence of constipation described by the patient may vary depending on how constipation is defined. To better understand the actual status of constipation, the Bristol Stool scale can be used **(Fig. 1)**.[6]

**Flowchart 1:** Causes of constipation in psychiatric patients.

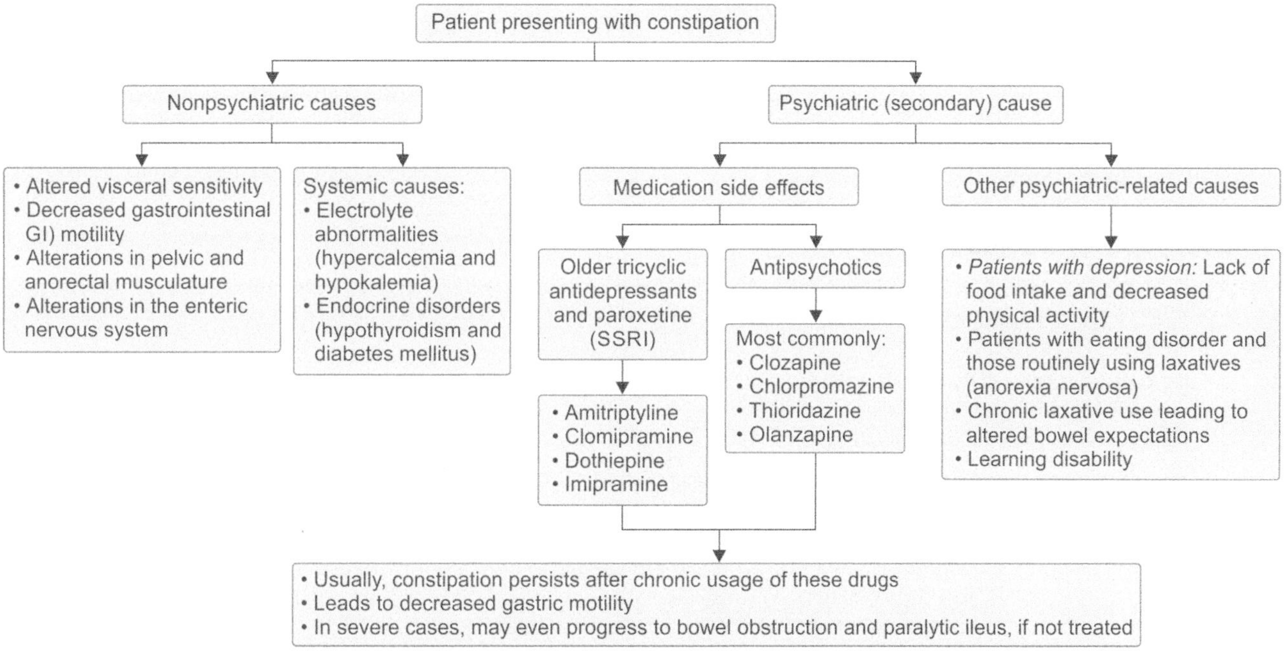

Patient presenting with constipation

- Nonpsychiatric causes
  - • Altered visceral sensitivity • Decreased gastrointestinal GI) motility • Alterations in pelvic and anorectal musculature • Alterations in the enteric nervous system
  - Systemic causes: • Electrolyte abnormalities (hypercalcemia and hypokalemia) • Endocrine disorders (hypothyroidism and diabetes mellitus)
- Psychiatric (secondary) cause
  - Medication side effects
    - Older tricyclic antidepressants and paroxetine (SSRI) → • Amitriptyline • Clomipramine • Dothiepine • Imipramine
    - Antipsychotics → Most commonly: • Clozapine • Chlorpromazine • Thioridazine • Olanzapine
    - → • Usually, constipation persists after chronic usage of these drugs • Leads to decreased gastric motility • In severe cases, may even progress to bowel obstruction and paralytic ileus, if not treated
  - Other psychiatric-related causes → • *Patients with depression:* Lack of food intake and decreased physical activity • Patients with eating disorder and those routinely using laxatives (anorexia nervosa) • Chronic laxative use leading to altered bowel expectations • Learning disability

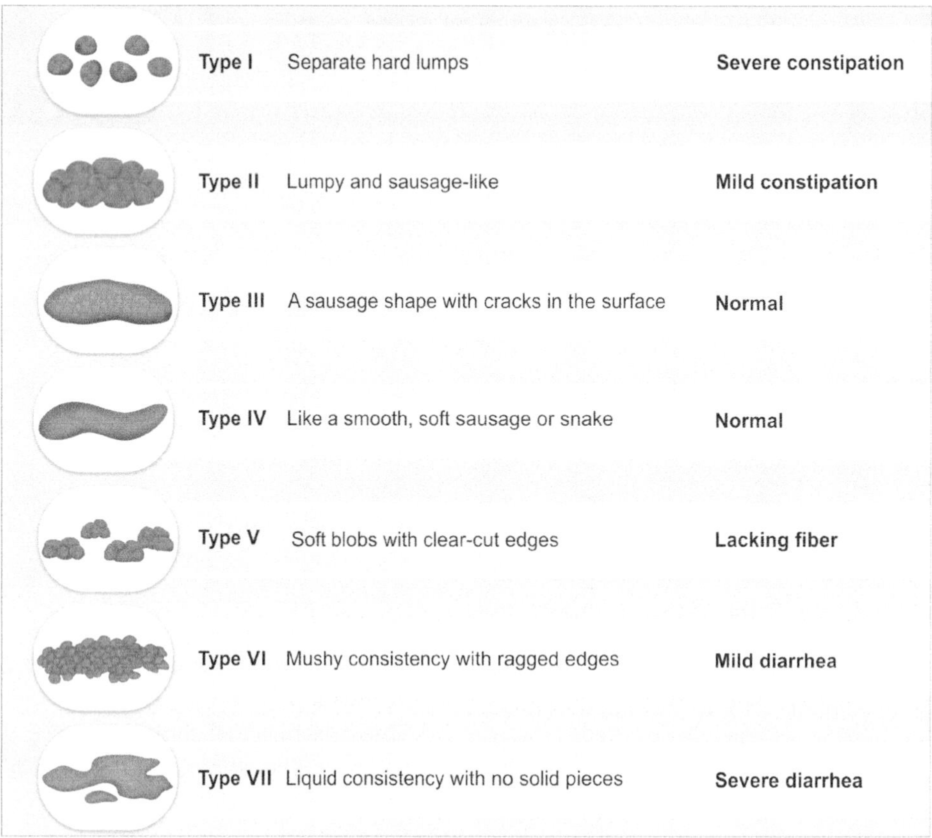


**Fig. 1:** Bristol Stool Scale.

## ALARMING SYMPTOMS

Any patients having the following symptoms should be referred to a specialist for endoscopic or clinical evaluation.

- Age ≥50 years.
- Family history of colon cancer or polyps.
- Family history of inflammatory bowel disease (ulcerative colitis or Crohn's disease).
- Rectal bleeding, anemia.
- Weight loss >5 kg
- New onset of chronic constipation without apparent cause in an elderly patient.
- Severe, persistent constipation, refractory to conservative management.

Overall, the rate of psychotropic drug-induced constipation has been found to be 11–12.5 %, with 4–7% of patients describing it as a bothersome side effect[7] **(Flowchart 2)**.

## GENERAL MEASURES (TABLE 1)[8]

**TABLE 1:** Nonpharmacological measures for drug-induced constipation.

| Step | Measures | |
|---|---|---|
| 1 | • Increase physical activity or daily walking<br>• Increase fluid intake (2 L/day)<br>• Increase dietary fiber intake (25–30 g/day) | |
| 2 | Fiber supplements | • When initial attempts at increasing physical activity, fluid, and dietary fibers fail to yield a response, fiber supplements are commonly used<br>• Advised to begin with a supplement that contains psyllium—such as Fiberall or Metamucil<br>• Other supplements containing methylcellulose, polycarbophil, or bran can be used<br>• Fiber supplements may cause increased gas and bloating, so start with low dose and gradually increase over several weeks to mitigate these side effects |

**Flowchart 2:** Approach to management of drug-induced constipation.[9]

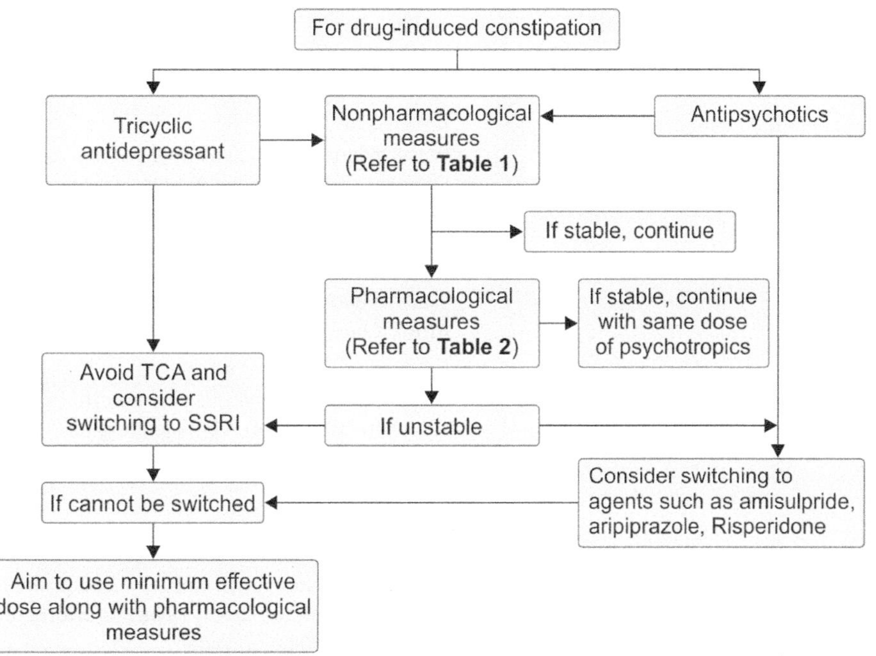


## SPECIFIC MEASURES (TABLE 2)[9]

**TABLE 2:** Pharmacological treatment of drug-induced constipation.

| ***Step*** | ***Measures*** | | |
|---|---|---|---|
| 1 | Over-the-counter laxative pills | If fiber supplements fail, try stimulant laxatives | |
| | | *Stimulant laxatives:* Stimulate the muscles of the gut lining and generally take 6–12 hours to work | *Examples include:*<br>• Senna, 7.5–15 mg once daily (usually at night), but higher doses may be prescribed under medical supervision (e.g., 45 mg in two to three divided doses; do not give >30 mg in a single dose)<br>• Bisacodyl, 10 mg once daily, increased up to 20 mg if necessary (usually at night)<br>• Sodium picosulfate, 5–10 mg once daily (usually at night) |
| | | *Bulk-forming laxatives:* Increase fecal mass and soften stool to stimulate a bowel motion. The onset of action is usually 48–72 hours | *Examples include:*<br>• Ispaghula husk (e.g., Fybogel), one sachet in water twice daily<br>• Methylcellulose, three to six tablets twice daily |
| | | *Emollient laxatives:* Stool softeners. The onset of action is usually 24–72 hours | *Examples include:*<br>Docusate sodium, up to 500 mg daily (as oral solution or capsule) in divided doses, adjusted according to response |

*Contd...*

*Contd...*

| Step | | | Measures |
|---|---|---|---|
| 2 | Over-the-counter laxative solutions/ osmotic laxatives | *Osmotic laxatives:* Draw water into the bowel to soften stool. The onset of action is usually 24–72 hours | *Examples include:*<br>• Lactulose, dose adjusted according to response, to 30–50 mL three times daily<br>• Polyethylene glycol (also known as macrogol and Movicol)<br>• Dose for chronic constipation (nonproprietary 'full-strength sachets' or Movicol oral powder), one to three sachets daily<br>• Dose for fecal impaction (nonproprietary 'full-strength sachets' or Movicol oral powder): four sachets on first day, then increased in steps of two sachets daily up to a maximum of eight sachets daily (drink daily dose in 6 hours) |
| 3 | Prescription laxatives | Lubiprostone | • Prostaglandin derivative<br>• Selective chloride channel activator that works only in the gut and results in net fluid excretion, leading to:<br>– Increased stool frequency<br>– Softens stool<br>– Decreased straining<br>– Helps with belly pain |
| | | Guanylate cyclase-C agonist | For people with no known cause for constipation or who have constipation that does not go away for a long time<br>• *Linaclotide:* 290 µg once daily<br>• *Plecanatide:* 3 mg once daily |
| | | Prucalopride | Class of serotonin receptor 5-HT4 agonist. Works by increasing gut peristalsis (2 mg once daily) |

## REFERENCES


1. De Hert M, Dockx L, Bernagie C, Peuskens B, Sweers K, Leucht S, et al. Prevalence and severity of antipsychotic related constipation in patients with schizophrenia: a retrospective descriptive study. BMC Gastroenterol. 2011;11(1):17.
2. Afridi MI, Siddiqui MA, Ansari A. Gastrointestinal somatization in males and females with depressive disorder. J Pak Med Assoc. 2009;59(10):675-9.
3. Koizumi T, Uchida H, Suzuki T, Sakurai H, Tsunoda K, Nishimoto M, et al. Oversight of constipation in inpatients with schizophrenia: A cross-sectional study. Gen Hosp Psychiatry. 2013;35(6):649-52.
4. Jessurun JG, van Harten PN, Egberts TCG, Pijl BJ, Wilting I, Tenback DE. The effect of psychotropic medications on the occurrence of constipation in hospitalized psychiatric patients. J Clin Psychopharmacol. 2013;33(4):587-90.
5. De Hert M, Hudyana H, Dockx L, Bernagie C, Sweers K, Tack J, et al. Second-generation antipsychotics and constipation: A review of the literature. Eur Psychiatry. 2011;26(1): 34-44.
6. Akasaka K, Akasaka F, Akasaka T, Okada K, Sadahiro S. Relationship between mental disorders, psychotropic drugs, and constipation in psychiatric outpatients. Medicine (Baltimore). 2022;101(37):e30369.
7. Kelly K, Posternak M, Alpert JE. Toward achieving optimal response: understanding and managing antidepressant side effects. Dialogues Clin Neurosci. 2008;10(4):409–18.
8. Winstead NS, Winstead DK. 5-Step Plan To Treat Constipation in Psychiatric Patients. Curr Psychiatr. 2008;7(5):29.
9. Pillinger T, Gaughran F, Taylor D. The Maudsley Practice Guidelines for Physical Health Conditions in Psychiatry. Hoboken: Wiley Blackwell, 2020.

# Management of Antipsychotic-Induced Constipation

*Aditya Somani, Anirban Saha, Chetan Anand*

## INTRODUCTION

- Antipsychotic drugs are crucial to the management of schizophrenia and acute psychosis and are commonly used in the management of bipolar disorders and other psychiatric conditions. Due to the chronic nature of the illnesses that are treated using antipsychotics, they are often used by patients for years.
- While the side-effects like metabolic derangements, QT interval prolongation, risk of cardiovascular conditions, elevations of prolactin level, sexual dysfunction, and drug-induced movement disorders have received a lot of attention, little attention has been given to a common and troublesome adverse reaction, *constipation*.[1]
- Constipation is a manifestation of decreased motility of the lower gastrointestinal tract, presenting symptoms like difficulty in passing stools, the need to strain while passing stools, passing hard stools, and reduced frequency of or incomplete defecation.[2]
- Prevalence of antipsychotic-induced constipation:
  - *For first-generation antipsychotics:* 5–40%
  - *Atypical antipsychotics (excluding clozapine):*
    - 2–30% in short-term
    - 4–15% in the long term
  - *Clozapine:* 9.4–80%
  - Some studies report it to be as common as 50%.[1]
  - The highest risk of constipation is seen with clozapine, followed by olanzapine, quetiapine, paliperidone, trifluoperazine, fluphenazine, and loxapine.

## IMPACT OF CONSTIPATION ON A PATIENT[1-4]

- Poor physical well-being, added psychological stress, and overall poor quality of life.
- This could worsen the mental state of patients with schizophrenia directly and indirectly through non-adherence to treatment.
- Require additional remedies/intervention and increased cost of treatment.
- Induce hemorrhoids, anal fissures, fecal impaction, or infections in the gut.
- It could lead to intestinal obstruction and ischemic bowel disease, resulting in serious medical complications such as septicemia, aspirational pneumonia, and intestinal perforation.
- Could lead to life-threatening paralytic ileus.[3]
- Mechanism of antipsychotic-induced constipation and contributing risk factors in patients of schizophrenia and other chronic psychiatric conditions **(Table 1)**:

**TABLE 1:** Mechanism and risk factors for antipsychotic-induced constipation.

| *Neurotransmitter-related mechanism* | *Additional contributing factors in patients with psychiatric illnesses* | *Other medical conditions* |
|---|---|---|
| Anticholinergic action (on muscarinic $M_1$ and $M_3$ receptors) | Lack of physical activity (due to negative symptoms, depression, or sedation) | • Aging<br>• Hypothyroidism<br>• Parkinson's disease |
| 5-hydroxytryptamine (5-$HT_3$ receptors) antagonism | Low-fiber diet and overall unhealthy diet | • Hypertension<br>• Diabetes mellitus |
| Histamine ($H_1$ receptor) antagonism | Inadequate water and fluid intake | Medications for medical conditions |
| | Decreased sensitivity to pain | |
| | Use of more than one antipsychotic | |
| | Use of anticholinergic drugs | |

## ASSESSMENT

- ROME IV criteria (two out of six mentioned below):[5]
  - Less than three bowel movements in a week
  - Straining during >25% of the time
  - Lumpy or hard stool >25% of the time
  - Sensation of anorectal obstruction >25% of the time
  - Sensation of incomplete evacuation >25% of the time
  - Manual maneuvers are required to aid defecation >25% of the time
- *Other tools:* Constipation Assessment Scale, Bristol Stool Form Scale

## GENERAL MEASURES

- Prevention of and general interventions for antipsychotic-induced constipation:
  - Regular screening and examination of the abdomen
  - Assessment of contributing medical risks **(Table 1)** and appropriate management or referral for them
  - Increased physical activity and exercise
  - Defecation training (deep relaxation)
  - Adequate fiber and fluid/water intake
  - Reducing the dose of antipsychotics, switching to low-risk agents, and avoiding polypharmacy
  - Avoiding the use of or reducing the dose of anticholinergic drugs

## MANAGEMENT

- There are no robust studies that have compared the various options to treat antipsychotic-induced constipation.[6] A protocol has been developed for clozapine, which shall be discussed in a separate chapter in this book.[7] The management options discussed below are based on empirical evidence and treatment approaches used in constipation due to other medical causes **(Table 2)**. The table mentions only the common and a couple of new drugs that are used by specialists in India to manage chronic constipation. **Flowchart 1** discusses the approach to assessing and managing constipation in a patient getting antipsychotic drugs.
- Red flag signs (suggest urgent intervention by a specialist)
  - Moderate to severe abdominal pain lasting for an hour or more.
  - Abdominal distension
  - Vomiting
  - Absent or high-pitched bowel sounds
  - Hemodynamic instability, metabolic acidosis, leukocytosis, or signs of sepsis

**TABLE 2:** Laxative agents for antipsychotic-induced constipation.

| *Category* | *Name of the agent* | *Dose and frequency* |
|---|---|---|
| Osmotic cathartics | Lactulose | 15–30 mL, could go up to 60 mL, once at bedtime |
| | Polyethylene glycol | 13.125 g, once at bedtime |
| Irritant laxatives | Bisacodyl | 5–15 mg, once at bedtime |
| Fiber | Psyllium husk (isabgul) | Two to three teaspoons daily<br>• Total daily fiber intake (dietary + supplement) must be 20–30 g<br>• Ensure adequate hydration<br>• Has a limited role in the treatment of antipsychotic-induced constipation |
| Novel drugs (prokinetic agents) | Prucalopride | 2 mg once daily |
| | Lubiprostone | 8 mcg twice daily, could go up to 24 μg twice daily |

**Flowchart 1:** Approach to a patient on anti-psychotic drugs experiencing constipation.

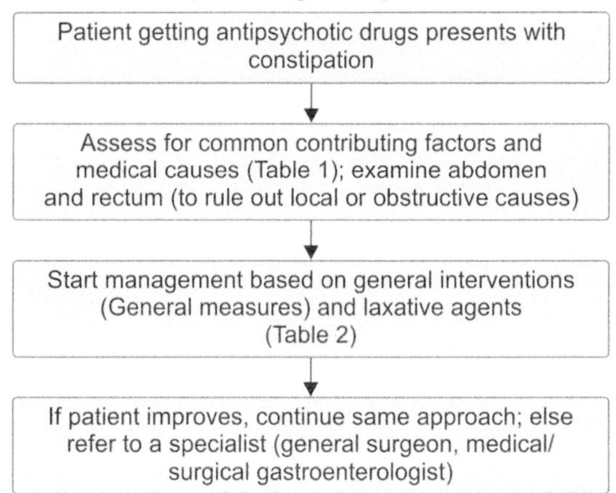


## REFERENCES

1. Xu Y, Amdanee N, Zhang X. Antipsychotic-induced constipation: A review of the pathogenesis, clinical diagnosis, and treatment. CNS Drugs. 2021;35(12):1265-74.
2. De Hert M, Hudyana H, Dockx L, Bernagie C, Sweers K, Tack J, et al. Second-generation antipsychotics and constipation: a review of the literature. Eur Psychiatry. 2011;26(1):34-44.

3. Cohen D, Bogers JP, van Dijk D, Bakker B, Schulte PF. Beyond white blood cell monitoring: screening in the initial phase of clozapine therapy. J Clin Psychiatry. 2012;73(10):1307-12.
4. Thomas N, Jain N, Connally F, Yeung JM, Pantelis C. Prucalopride in clozapine-induced constipation. Aust N Z J Psychiatry. 2018;52(8):804.
5. Jani B, Marsicano E. Constipation: Evaluation and management. Mo Med. 2018;115(3):236-40.
6. Every-Palmer S, Newton-Howes G, Clarke MJ. Pharmacological treatment for antipsychotic-related constipation. Cochrane Database Syst Rev. 2017;1(1):Cd011128.
7. Every-Palmer S, Ellis PM, Nowitz M, Stanley J, Grant E, Huthwaite M, et al. The Porirua Protocol in the treatment of clozapine-induced gastrointestinal hypomotility and constipation: A pre- and post-treatment study. CNS Drugs. 2017;31(1):75-85.

# Management of Clozapine-induced Constipation

*Srilakshmi Pingali*

## INTRODUCTION

Clozapine is a second-generation antipsychotic approved by the FDA for treatment-resistant schizophrenia. Its antipsychotic effects are due to its antagonism of serotonin ($5\text{-}HT_{2A}$) and dopamine ($D_1$, $D_2$, $D_3$, and $D_5$) receptors, as well as its antagonistic effect on adrenergic, cholinergic, and histaminergic receptors.

Clozapine-induced constipation is primarily due to its anticholinergic effect, which reduces gastrointestinal motility. Additionally, its serotonergic antagonism slows colonic transit, reduces gastro-colonic reflexes, increases colonic compliance, and reduces intestinal sensitivity to distension.

Constipation occurs in 30–60% of patients on clozapine,[1,2] making it twice as common as with other antipsychotics. Median colonic transit time in clozapine patients is 104.5 hours compared to 23 hours in those on other antipsychotics.[3]

## RISK FACTORS FOR CONSTIPATION WITH CLOZAPINE

- *Recent initiation of clozapine:* The risk is greatest during the first 4 months of treatment but can occur at any time.
- High dose or elevated plasma clozapine level
- Intercurrent illness
- History of bowel surgery
- Concurrent use of other drugs known to cause constipation, such as opioids and anticholinergic drugs (e.g., hyoscine hydrobromide, used for clozapine-induced hypersalivation).
- *Lifestyle issues:* Sedentary lifestyle and poor dietary habits
- Old age
- Obesity

## SYMPTOMS AND SIGNS

Constipation may be characterized by two or fewer spontaneous bowel movements per week, leading to hard stools, a sensation of incomplete evacuation, or straining. It may also cause abdominal pain, distention, nausea, or vomiting.

Self-reported symptoms of constipation may be unreliable, especially in patients with severe psychosis who may not clearly communicate discomfort. Physicians may underestimate symptoms due to the patient's flat affect. Additionally, drugs such as mood stabilizers that are used as add-on treatment may alter pain sensitivity.

Evaluation of constipation may require using scales in addition to history taking. Common scales include the eight-item Constipation Assessment Scale or the ROME IV instrument.[4]

## COMPLICATIONS

Clozapine-induced constipation may reflect serious gastrointestinal hypomotility, leading to complications such as intestinal obstruction, fecal impaction, megacolon, paralytic ileus, and intestinal ischemia or infarction, which may require hospitalization or surgery and can be fatal. The mortality rate from these complications is about 10–12/10,000, nearly three times higher than the rate for agranulocytosis.

## EVALUATION

Before initiating clozapine, obtain a detailed medical history to identify risk factors for constipation. This includes assessing current medications, lifestyle factors, and any comorbid medical or surgical conditions. A thorough physical examination should follow.

## PREVENTION

- *Psychoeducation:* Educate patients about the risk of constipation and the importance of reporting symptoms promptly.
- *Lifestyle modifications:* Encourage a healthy diet, adequate fluid intake, and regular physical activity.
- *Monitoring concomitant medications:* Avoid or minimize drugs that exacerbate constipation or reduce gastrointestinal motility.
- *Frequent constipation screening:* Screen for constipation regularly, such as weekly, for the first few months.
- *Abdominal examination:* Evaluate for signs of obstruction using auscultation, palpation, and percussion.
- *Prophylactic laxatives:* Consider preventive laxatives for high-risk patients while monitoring for overuse or adverse effects.

## TREATMENT

- Evaluate any patient with changes in bowel habits, abdominal pain, or fewer than three bowel movements per week.[2]
- Assess patients with elevated plasma clozapine levels for constipation.

The first step in treating clozapine-induced constipation is to taper down the clozapine dose. According to the American College of Gastroenterology, the first-line treatment includes stool softeners, followed by osmotic laxatives, and then stimulant laxatives. However, 20–50% of patients may still have symptoms despite these treatments. Newer laxatives such as lubiprostone and prucalopride may be considered for those who do not respond to first-line treatments **(Table 1)**. Often, a combination of laxatives is necessary. If bowel obstruction is suspected,

**TABLE 1:** Laxatives used in managing clozapine-induced constipation.[6]

| *Group of laxatives* | *Mechanism of action* | *Example* | *Dosage* | *Use in clozapine-induced constipation* |
|---|---|---|---|---|
| Bulk forming laxatives | Absorbs water in the intestine, swells, increases the water content of feces, softens, and facilitates colonic transit | Ispaghula | • 3–8 g in water/juice/milk<br>• Once or twice daily, acts in 1–3 days | Not used in clozapine induced constipation due to reduced gut motility<br>Used in the prevention of constipation |
| Stool softeners | Anionic detergent softens stool by net water accumulation, by acting on the intestinal mucosa. Emulsifies colonic contents and increases water penetration into feces to soften it | Docusates | 100–400 mg/day acts in 1–3 days | Can be used |
| Stimulant laxatives | Stimulate motor activity of the colon, accumulate water and electrolytes in the lumen by altering absorptive and secretory activity of mucosal cells | Bisacodyl | • 5–15 mg<br>• Acts in 6–8 hours | Can be used |
| Osmotic laxatives | Solutes that are not absorbed by the intestine retain water osmotically and distend the bowel, increasing peristalsis indirectly | Lactulose | • 10 g BD<br>• Acts in 1–3 days | Can be used |
| Newer laxatives Prucalopride (stimulant laxatives)[7] | 5-HT4 receptor agonist, which, when it acts on the receptors of the gastrointestinal system, leads to the release of acetylcholine, enhancing the motility of the gut | Prucalopride | 2 mg, acts in 2–3 days | Can be used |
| Lubiprostone (stimulant laxative) | A prostaglandin analog that increases the intestinal secretion | | 24 µg/day along with stool softeners and stimulant laxatives | Can be used, with limited evidence |

**Flowchart 1:** Stepwise approach to management of clozapine-induced constipation.

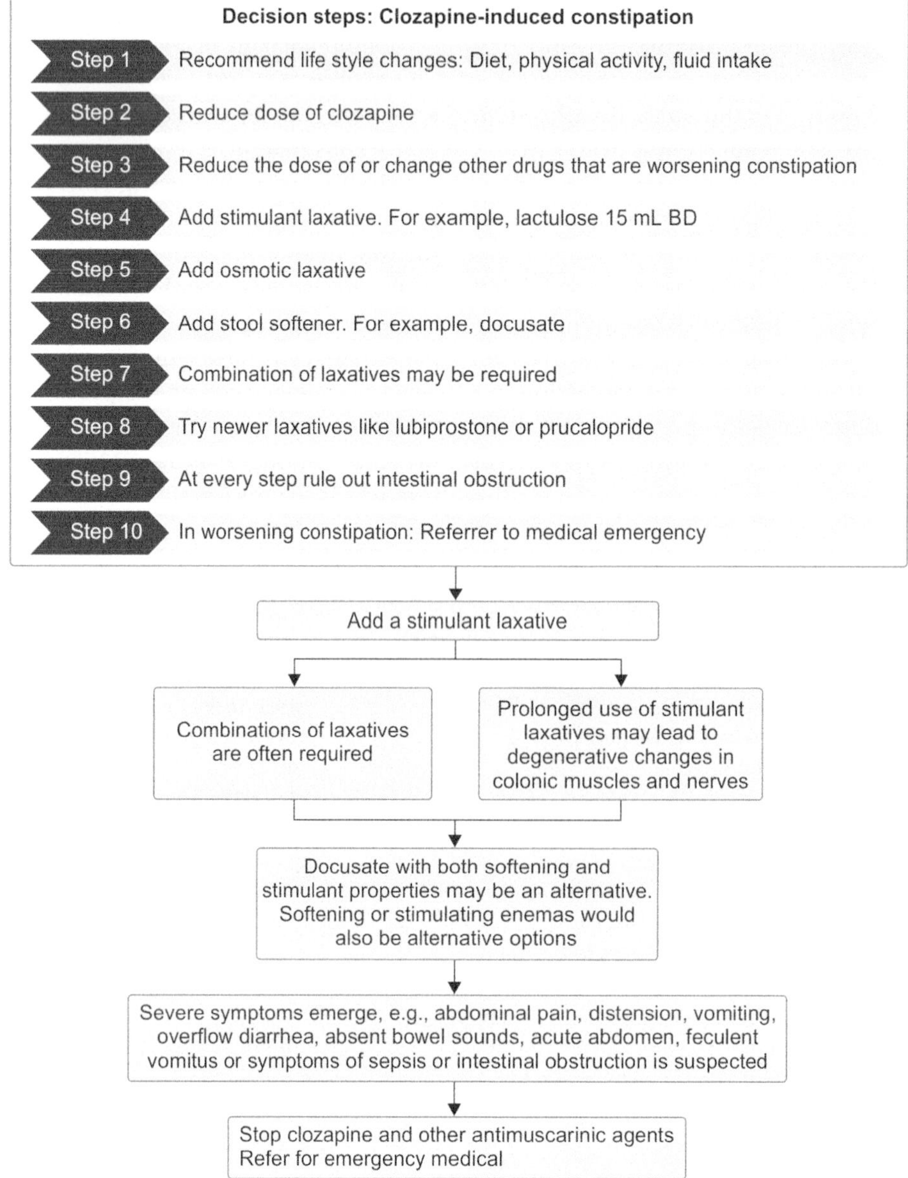


avoid stimulants or bulk-forming laxatives and refer the patient for urgent surgical evaluation.[5]

The decision chart to manage clozapine-induced constipation is summarized in **Flowchart 1**.[2]

## REFERENCES

1. Shirazi A, Stubbs B, Gomez L, Moore S, Gaughran F, Flanagan RJ, et al. Prevalence and Predictors of Clozapine-Associated Constipation: A Systematic Review and Meta-Analysis. Int J Mol Sci. 2016;17(6):863.
2. NHS Greater Glasgow & Clyde. Guidelines for the assessment and treatment of Clozapine Induced Constipation. [Online] Available from https://mypsych.nhsggc.org.uk/media/1801/mhs-mrg-038-guidelines-for-assessment-and-treatment-of-clozapine-induced-constipation.pdf [Last accessed June, 2025].
3. Damodaran I, Hui KO, Nordin ASA, Yee A, Gill JS, Francis B, et al. An Open-Label, Head to Head Comparison Study between Prucalopride and Lactulose for Clozapine Induced Constipation in Patients with Treatment Resistant Schizophrenia. Healthcare (Basel). 2020;8(4):533.

4. Rome Foundation. Appendix A: Rome IV Diagnostic Criteria for FGIDs. [Online] Available from https://theromefoundation.org/rome-iv/rome-iv-criteria/ [Last accessed June, 2025].
5. Correll CU, Agid O, Crespo-Facorro B, de Bartolomeis A, Fagiolini A, Seppälä N, et al. A Guideline and Checklist for Initiating and Managing Clozapine Treatment in Patients with Treatment-Resistant Schizophrenia. CNS Drugs. 2022;36(7):659-79.
6. Tomulescu S, Uittenhove K, Boukakiou R. Managing Recurrent Clozapine-Induced Constipation in a Patient with Resistant Schizophrenia. Case Rep Psychiatry. 2021;2021:9649334.
7. Tripathi KD (Ed). Essentials of medical pharmacology, 8th edition. New Delhi: Jaypee Brothers Medical Pvt Ltd; 2018.

# Management of Clozapine-induced Sialorrhea

*Sai Krishna Tikka, Shobit Garg, Mamidipally Sai Spoorthy*

## INTRODUCTION

Clozapine is the most common antipsychotic, and also the most common drug overall, to cause clinically significant sialorrhea. Clozapine-induced sialorrhea (CIS) is a troublesome side effect that leads to poor adherence and reduced quality of life, limiting the use of clozapine despite its unmatched efficacy.[1,2]

*Clinically significant sialorrhea:* When sialorrhea requires regularly clearing the mouth by spitting, swallowing excess saliva, wiping the corner of the mouth with a tissue, or using a "spit cup", it is termed "occult drooling" and is considered clinically significant.[3]

## PATHOPHYSIOLOGY

Although the exact pathophysiology of CIS is unclear, the proposed mechanisms are:[4]

- Agonistic action at $M_4$ muscarinic receptors, which regulate cholinergic and dopaminergic neurotransmission
- Antagonistic action at $\alpha_2$ adrenergic receptors
- Anticholinergic ($M_1$, $M_2$, $M_3$, and $M_5$ muscarinic) activity
- Circadian rhythm alteration causing increased salivation at night
- Decreased laryngeal peristalsis or inhibition of swallowing reflex.

## CLINICAL PRESENTATION (1, IN FLOWCHARTS 1 AND 2)

Sialorrhea can occur during the day (diurnal or daytime CIS), at night (nocturnal CIS), or throughout the day. Generally, it is present all day but is more severe at night. Patients often report waking up with a wet pillow, known as the "wet pillow" sign.[4]

### Clinical Sequelae[4]

- Wet pillows and clothing, which can be socially embarrassing and may cause a foul odor.
- Intermittent sensation of choking
- Sleep disturbances from waking up repeatedly due to choking
- Increased the risk of aspiration pneumonia from excess saliva
- Hoarseness of voice or dysphonia from saliva pooling near the vocal cords
- Chronic cough from saliva passing beyond the vocal cords
- Swelling and inflammation of the parotid gland (parotitis)
- Macerated skin around the chin and mouth, leading to cheilitis, and other skin infections from constant drooling
- "Symptomatic aerophagia", causing gas bloating, pain, and flatulence due to frequent swallowing.

The CIS is usually linked to minor complications, with life-threatening ones being rare. These complications are more common in the elderly, children, adolescents, and severely debilitated individuals.

### Relationship with Dose, Dosing, Duration, and Phase of Treatment

The CIS is probably dose related and associated with rapid dose titration. It is more severe in the early stages of treatment. While it may lessen over time, it can persist and remain problematic, especially nocturnal CIS.[4]

## MANAGEMENT

See **Flowcharts 1 and 2** for the management algorithms. While **Flowchart 1** presents a management algorithm

**Flowchart 1:** Management of CIS from severity of CIS point of view.

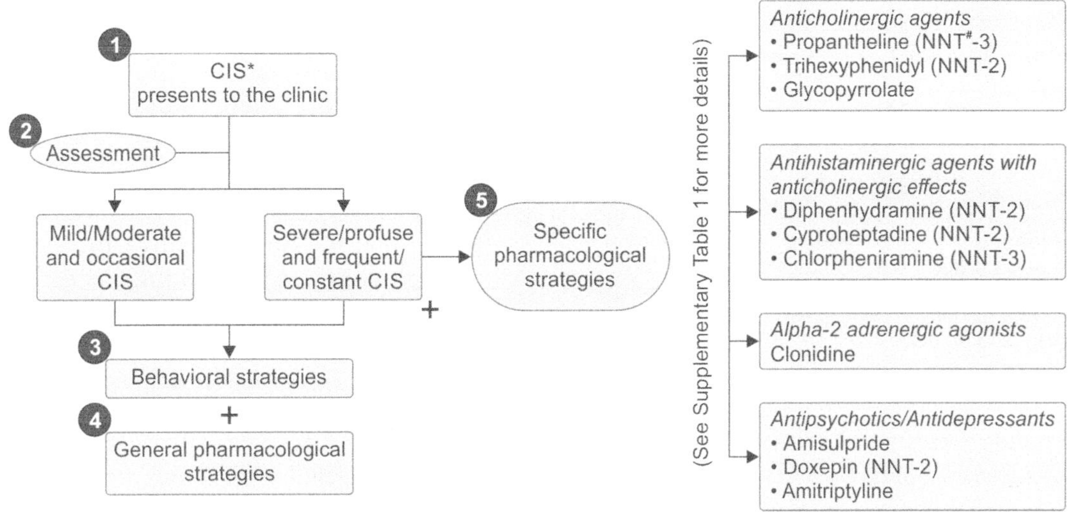


*Note:* *CIS: Clozapine-induced sialorrhea; #NNT: number needed to treat, 1,2,3,4,5 described in text.

**Flowchart 2:** Algorithm for management of clozapine-induced sialorrhea (CIS) from dosing and response point of view.

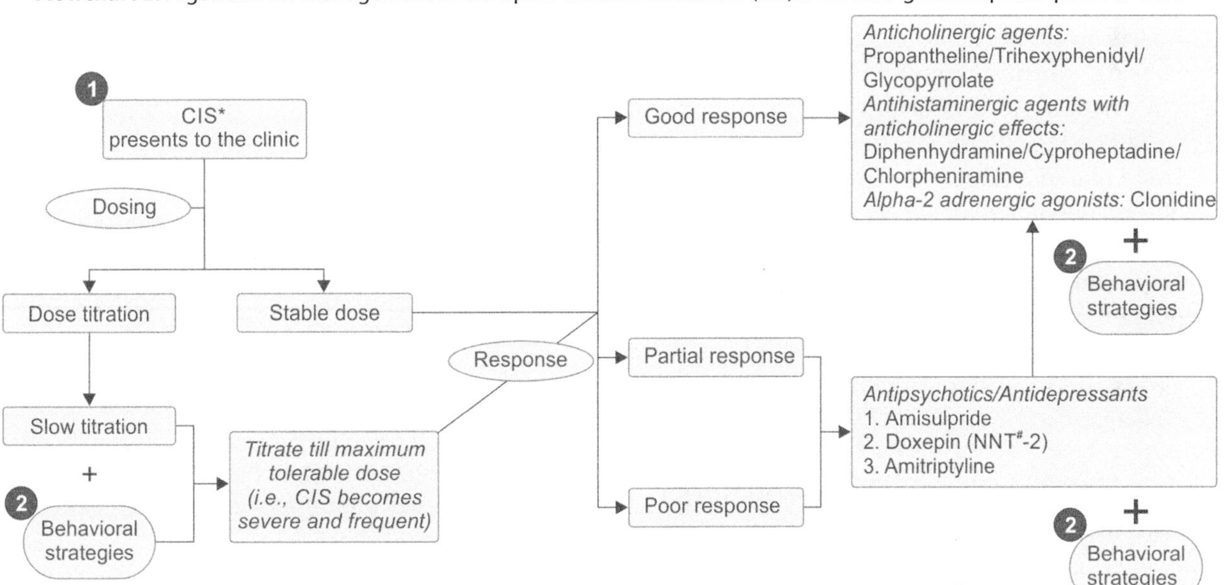


*Note:* *CIS: clozapine-induced sialorrhea; #NNT: number needed to treat; 1,2 described in text.

from a severity and frequency of CIS point of view, **Flowchart 2** presents management from the point of view of treatment response to clozapine and its dosing.

## Assessment[4] (2, in Flowchart 1)

Assessment in a case of CIS involves:

- Ascertaining the dose, duration, and phase relationship of sialorrhea to clozapine.
- Ruling out other potential causes of sialorrhea
- Measuring the severity and frequency of drooling
  - Some of the self-rated tools that can easily measure drooling on a Likert scale in clinical settings are **(Table 1)**:

**TABLE 1:** Self-rated tools to measure drooling severity and frequency.

| *Drooling Severity Scale (DSS)* | | *Drooling frequency* | |
|---|---|---|---|
| Never | Dry | Never | Never drools |
| Mild | Only wet lips | Occasional | Occasionally drools |
| Moderate | Wet on lips and chin | | |
| Severe | Clothing becomes wet | Frequent | Frequently drools |
| Profuse | Clothing, hands, tray, and objects become wet | Constant | Constantly drools |

- *Drooling Severity Scale (DSS):* A 5-point Likert scale (Never-Mild-Moderate-Severe-Profound) to assess drooling severity
- *Drooling frequency:* A 4-point Likert scale (Never-Occasional-Frequent-Constant) to assess drooling frequency
- *Teacher Drooling Scale (TDS):* A 5-point Likert scale (No-Infrequent-Occasional-Frequent-Constant) to assess drooling frequency in children

- Drool quotient (DQ) is based on semiquantitative observational method where the number of times drooling is present or absent is measured.
- Estimating the diameter of wet surface on bed/pillow or tissue paper placed over the pillow during sleep can be used as a rough yet simple guide to assess the severity of nocturnal CIS with some objectivity.

## Behavioral Interventions[4-7] (3, in Flowchart 1 and 2, in Flowchart 2)

- Proper education regarding CIS is important in every case to reduce fear and shame.
- To increase swallowing—chewing sugar-free gum
- To reduce the feeling of choking:
  - Swallowing two to three times without inhaling (by compression of nostrils)
  - Sleep with head propped up (for choking sensation during sleep)
- To prevent aspiration—maintaining lateral decubitus position
- To prevent pillow soaking—placing a towel over the pillows
- To prevent soiling of clothes—wearing chin-cups

## Pharmacological Interventions[4-9]

### *General Strategies (4, in Flowchart 1)*

- Avoid rapid dose titration
- If possible, reduction of clozapine dose may be tried. Measuring clozapine drug levels in the blood can guide this decision. If illness symptoms re-emerge, clozapine augmentation (especially with amisulpride) may be an alternative to reescalating the dose of clozapine and adding specific behavioral/pharmacological interventions for CIS.

### *Specific Strategies for Clozapine-induced Sialorrhea (5, in Flowcharts 1)*

- Specific pharmacological interventions are targeted based on pathophysiology of CIS as described earlier. Detailed descriptions of pharmacological agents studied so far in the treatment of CIS are presented in *supplementary* ***Table 2***.
- The specific drugs for CIS are primarily either anticholinergic that block muscarinic receptors or $\alpha2$ adrenergic agonists, both of which reduce salivary secretions (i.e., prevent "pooling").
- Among anticholinergic agents, highest evidence in the form of positive results from meta-analysis of randomized controlled trials (RCTs) is available for propantheline, benzhexol/trihexyphenidyl, and glycopyrrolate.
  - While most anticholinergic agents, including benzhexol, exaggerate the anticholinergic adverse effects of clozapine (e.g., constipation, urinary retention, blurring of vision, etc.), propantheline being a peripheral anticholinergic agents do not have central effects.
- Among $\alpha2$ adrenergic agonists, although not supported by meta-analysis, there is some positive evidence, especially from India for successful use of clonidine in CIS.
  - Treatment with $\alpha2$ adrenergic agonists increases the risk of orthostatic hypotension and falls and, requires regular blood pressure monitoring. Clonidine, in particular, may cause, or worsen depression/psychosis.
- Certain antihistaminergic drugs through their antimuscarinic actions are also used. In fact, diphenhydramine, cyproheptadine, and chlorpheniramine have positive evidence from meta-analysis of RCTs.

**TABLE 2:** Primary classes of drugs used for CIS, their specific indications, if any, level of evidence and Indian evidence, if any and possible adverse effects/precautions.

| | Dose | Specific indications | Level of evidence | Indian evidence | Adverse effects | Precautions |
|---|---|---|---|---|---|---|
| ***α2 adrenergic agonists*** | | | | | | |
| Clonidine | Weekly transdermal patch: 0.1–0.2 mg/day; Oral: 50–100 µg/day HS | – | Uncontrolled clinical trials and case series-positive evidence | Positive for oral clonidine | • Orthostatic hypotension and falls<br>• Cause or worsen depression/ psychosis<br>• Development of tolerance | Regular BP monitoring |
| Lofexidine | *Oral:* 0.2 mg twice daily | – | Positive evidence from case reports | Nil | Lack of adequate literature | Lack of adequate literature |
| Guanfacine | *Oral:* 1 mg/day | • May be preferred in cases of excess sedation<br>• Compared to clonidine has less sedation | Positive evidence from case reports | Nil | Lack of adequate literature | Lack of adequate literature |
| Guanabenz | Not studied for CIS, but theoretically hypothesized to be helpful | | | | | |
| *α*-methyldopa | | | | | | |
| Moxonidine | | | | | | |
| *Anticholinergic agents* | | | | | | |
| Propantheline | *Oral:* 30–120 mg/day | May be preferred in cases of already existing central anticholinergic effects | Positively supporting meta-analysis of RCTs | Nil | – | – |
| Hyoscine (scopolamine) | • *Oral:* 300 µg at night increased to<br>• 900 µg if required (in three divided doses)<br>• *72 hourly transdermal patch:* (1.5 mg/2.5 $cm^2$, 1 mg per 72 h) | Listed as first choice | Uncontrolled clinical trials-positive evidence | Nil | • Can cause cognitive impairment<br>• Patches can cause skin sensitivity | It is expensive compared to others |
| Pirenzepine | *Oral:* 25-100 mg per day, single or divided doses | May be preferred in cases of already existing central anticholinergic effects. As it does not cross blood-brain barrier, its chances are less | Conflicting evidence from uncontrolled clinical trials | Nil | Increase the anticholinergic adverse effects of clozapine (e.g., constipation, urinary retention, blurring of vision, etc.) | Should be used cautiously in narrow-angle glaucoma and prostatic hypertrophy |

*Contd...*

*Contd...*

| | *a2 adrenergic agonists* | | | | | |
|---|---|---|---|---|---|---|
| | ***Dose*** | ***Specific indications*** | ***Level of evidence*** | ***Indian evidence*** | ***Adverse effects*** | ***Precautions*** |
| Trihexyphenidyl (benzhexol) | *Oral:* 5–15 mg HS | – | Positive evidence from one RCT and other uncontrolled studies | Nil | Atropine can cause rebound sialorrhea in early morning hours | |
| Glycopyrrolate | *Oral:* 1–2 mg | – | Positive evidence from one RCT | Nil | | |
| Atropine | 1–2 drops of 1% atropine solution or eye drops sublingually at bedtime | | Case series/ report—positive evidence | Nil | | |
| Ipratropium bromide | Intranasal or sublingual—1–2 sprays (0.03%) bedtime | Those not responding to clonidine or benztropine | Positive evidence from case reports, but one negative RCT | Nil | | |
| Benztropine mesylate | *Oral:* 1–2 mg/day | – | Positive evidence from case reports | Nil | Lack of adequate literature | Lack of adequate literature |
| Biperiden | *Oral:* 6 mg/day | – | Positive evidence from case reports | Nil | Lack of adequate literature | Lack of adequate literature |
| Tiotropium bromide | Not studied for CIS, but theoretically hypothesized to be helpful | | | | | |
| *Antihistaminic agents* | | | | | | |
| Diphenhydramine | *Oral:* 25–200 mg/day | – | Positively supporting meta-analysis of RCTs | Nil | Excess sedation and risk of weight gain | – |
| Chlorpheniramine | *Oral:* 16–24 mg/day | – | Positively supporting meta-analysis of RCTs | Nil | | – |
| Astemizole | *Oral:* 10 mg | – | Conflicting evidence from 2 RCTs | Nil | | – |
| Cyproheptadine | *Oral:* 8–36 mg/day | | Positive evidence from one RCT | Nil | | – |

*Contd...*

*Contd...*

| *α2 adrenergic agonists* | | | | | | |
|---|---|---|---|---|---|---|
| | ***Dose*** | ***Specific indications*** | ***Level of evidence*** | ***Indian evidence*** | ***Adverse effects*** | ***Precautions*** |
| *Miscellaneous agents* | | | | | | |
| Amisulpride | *Oral:* 100–600 mg | Augment antipsychotic effects; allows clozapine dose reduction | Positive evidence from one RCT and uncontrolled studies/case reports | Yes–case reports | – | – |
| Metoclopramide | *Oral:* 10–30 mg/day | - | Positive evidence from one RCT | Nil | | |
| Doxepin | 50–100 mg | Depressive symptoms comorbid | Positive evidence from one RCT | Nil | – | – |
| Amitriptyline | *Oral:* 25–100 mg HS | Comorbid depressive and somatic symptoms | Positive evidence from uncontrolled studies/case reports | Nil | Anticholinergic adverse effects of clozapine (e.g., constipation, urinary retention, blurring of vision, etc.). Also, orthostasis, sedation, or lowering of the seizure threshold | – |
| Bupropion | *Oral:* 100–150 mg/day | Comorbid depressive symptoms and smoking cessation | Positive evidence from case reports | Nil | Lowering of the seizure threshold | – |
| Quetiapine | Not studied for CIS, but hypothesized to be helpful by allowing clozapine dose reduction | | | | | |
| Benztropine and terazosin | | | Positive evidence for combination compared to either alone from uncontrolled studies | Nil | – | – |
| Botulinum toxin injection | 150 IU injected into each parotid gland | | Positive evidence from case reports | Nil | – | – |
| Oxybutynin | 5–10 mg/day | – | Positive evidence from case reports | Nil | – | – |
| β-adrenoreceptor blockers (e.g., propranolol) | Not studied for CIS, but theoretically hypothesized to be helpful | | | | | |

(CIS: clozapine-induced sialorrhea; RCT: randomized controlled trial)

- Certain antipsychotics, especially amisulpride, have also been found to alleviate CIS (positive evidence from meta-analysis of RCTs). It also helps augment antipsychotic effects of clozapine and also allow clozapine dose reduction, which further helps reduce CIS.
- There are some other miscellaneous drugs that can also be tried, if the primary agents are not indicated/ available. Doxepin, an antidepressant, has also gathered positive evidence from meta-analysis of RCTs. Some studies, even from India, have shown effectiveness of amitriptyline in the treatment of CIS.

## REFERENCES


1. Sanagustin D, Martin-Subero M, Hogg B, Fortea L, Gardoki I, Guinart D, et al. Prevalence of clozapine-induced sialorrhea and its effect on quality of life. Psychopharmacology (Berl). 2023;240(1):203-11.
2. Maher S, Cunningham A, O'Callaghan N, Byrne F, Mc Donald C, McInerney S, et al. Clozapine-induced hypersalivation: an estimate of prevalence, severity and impact on quality of life. Ther Adv Psychopharmacol. 2016;6(3):178-84.
3. Freudenreich O. Drug-induced sialorrhea. Drugs Today (Barc). 2005;41(6):411-8.
4. Praharaj SK, Arora M, Gandotra S. Clozapine-induced sialorrhea: pathophysiology and management strategies. Psychopharmacology (Berl). 2006;185(3):265-73.
5. Gupta S, Khastgir U, Croft M, Roshny S. Management of clozapine-induced sialorrhoea. BJPsych Advances. 2020;26(2):106-8.
6. Taylor DM, Barnes TRE, Young AH. Clozapine-induced hypersalivation. In: The Maudsley Prescribing Guidelines in Psychiatry, 13th edition. New York: John Wiley & Sons; 2018. pp 189-92.
7. Bird AM, Smith TL, Walton AE. Current treatment strategies for clozapine-induced sialorrhea. Ann Pharmacother. 2011;45(5):667-75.
8. Syed R, Au K, Cahill C, Duggan L, He Y, Udu V, et al. Pharmacological interventions for clozapine-induced hypersalivation. Cochrane Database Syst Rev. 2008;2008(3):CD005579.
9. Chen SY, Ravindran G, Zhang Q, Kisely S, Siskind D. Treatment Strategies for Clozapine-Induced Sialorrhea: A Systematic Review and Meta-analysis. CNS Drugs. 2019;33(3):225-38.

# Management of Clozapine-induced Tachycardia

*Barikar C Malathesh*

## INTRODUCTION

Clozapine is an atypical antipsychotic used in cases of schizophrenia where other antipsychotics fail to produce a therapeutic response, a situation observed in nearly one-third of patients.[1] Despite its superior efficacy, clozapine is reserved for such cases due to its significant side effects, which include hematological, cardiac, anticholinergic, and chronotropic effects. Hematological side effects include agranulocytosis, while cardiac side effects include cardiomyopathy and myocarditis.

## PATHOPHYSIOLOGY

Clozapine is an antagonist at cardiac muscarinic $M_2$ receptors, presynaptic $\alpha_2$ adrenoceptors, and indirectly activates $\beta$ adrenoceptors, thereby leading to tachycardia.[2,3]

## CLINICAL PRESENTATION

Generally, heart rate increases by 10–15 beats per minute after initiation of clozapine therapy. Clozapine-induced tachycardia often goes unnoticed by the patient but can increase long-term cardiac risk, including coronary artery disease and cardiomyopathy. While most patients develop tolerance to tachycardia, it may persist in some cases.[4]

## MONITORING

Serial pulse rate monitoring is essential when starting clozapine. If tachycardia is detected, other causes such as cardiomyopathy and myocarditis must be ruled out. If no other cause is identified, consider gradually increasing the clozapine dose and allowing 4–6 weeks for the patient to develop tolerance to the tachycardia. After this period, therapeutic drug monitoring can assess if serum levels are elevated.

## PHARMACOLOGICAL MANAGEMENT

Studies on pharmacological management of clozapine-induced tachycardia are limited.[5] Traditionally, beta-blockers are used to treat the tachycardia associated with clozapine use. Among β-blockers, cardioselective agents such as bisoprolol and atenolol are preferred due to their minimal impact on blood pressure. Atenolol can be prescribed at doses up to 25 mg/day.[6] While bisoprolol may be used at doses ranging from 2.5 mg/day to a maximum of 10 mg/day.[7]

Beta-blockers should be avoided in patients with orthostatic hypotension or bronchial asthma. In such cases, ivabradine may be considered. Ivabradine is a novel cardiac drug that selectively inhibits $I_f$ currents across cardiac pacemaker without affecting other cardiac functions, thereby minimizing the risk of hypotension. However, ivabradine is contraindicated in acute cardiac failure, acute myocardial infarction, and unstable angina. Consultation with a cardiologist is recommended before initiating ivabradine, which is typically started at 5 mg twice daily and may be increased to a maximum of 7.5 mg twice daily.[8]

If the above measures fail, consider reducing the clozapine dose or switching to an alternative antipsychotic.

**Table 1** shows the list of drugs used in the management of clozapine-induced tachycardia along with their dosage regime. Approach to manage clozapine-induced tachycardia is summarized in **Flowchart 1**.

**TABLE 1:** List of drugs used in the management of clozapine-induced tachycardia.

| *Drug name* | *Mechanism of action* | *Dosage* | *Specific population* | *Contraindications* |
|---|---|---|---|---|
| Bisoprolol | Selective β1 blocker | 2.5–10 mg/day oral | Slow titration in both renal and hepatic impairment | Complete heart block, severe asthma |
| Atenolol | Selective β1 blocker | 25 mg/day oral | • No dose adjustment in hepatic impairment<br>• In renal impairment adjust depending upon creatinine clearance | Complete heart block, severe asthma, and pheochromocytoma |
| Ivabradine | $I_f$ channel blocker | 5–15 mg/day in divided dose | No adjustment in renal impairment and mild-to-moderate hepatic impairment. | Severe hepatic impairment Conduction abnormality |

**Flowchart 1:** Algorithm for management of clozapine-induced tachycardia.

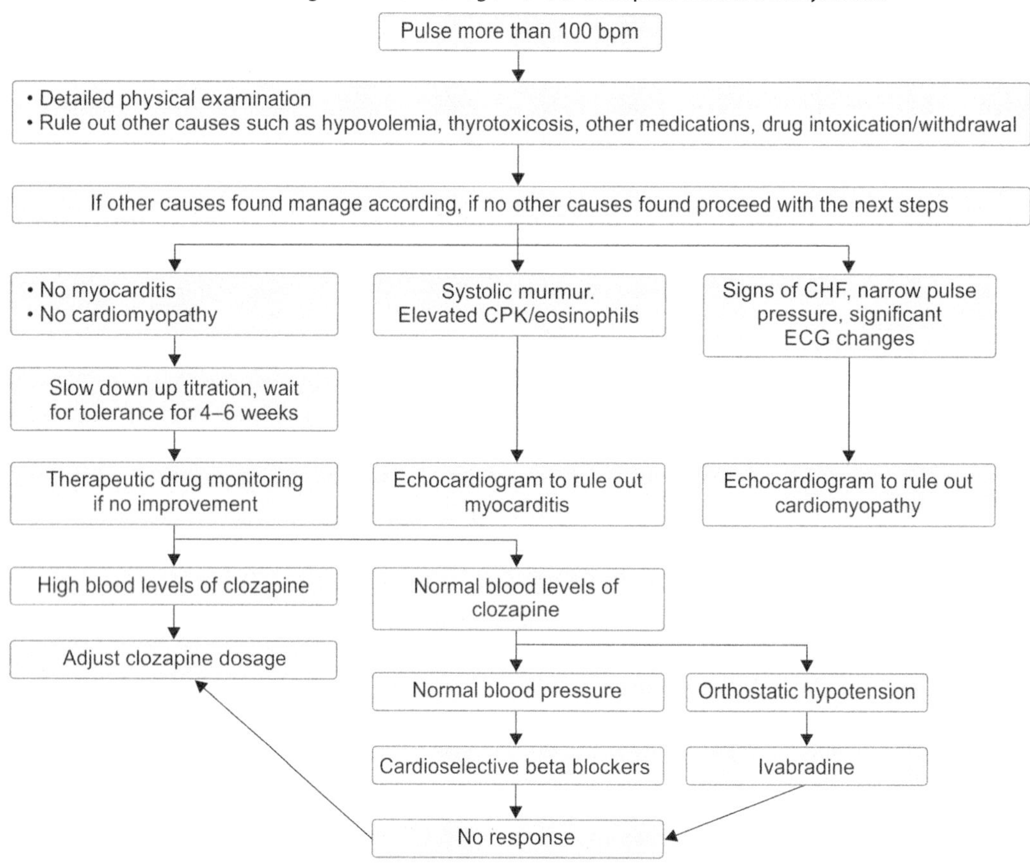


## REFERENCES


1. Leucht S, Cipriani A, Spineli L, Mavridis D, Örey D, Richter F, et al. Comparative efficacy and tolerability of 15 antipsychotic drugs in schizophrenia: a multiple-treatments meta-analysis. Lancet. 2013;382:951-62.
2. Merrill DB, Dec GW, Goff DC. Adverse Cardiac Effects Associated With Clozapine. J Clin Psychopharmacol. 2005;25:32.
3. Adeyemo S, Jegede O, Rabel P, Ahmed S, Tumenta T, Oladeji O, et al. Persistent Tachycardia in a Patient on Clozapine. Case Reports in Psychiatry. 2020;2020:6352175.
4. Safferman A, Lieberman JA, Kane JM, Szymanski S, Kinon B. Update on the Clinical Efficacy and Side Effects of Clozapine. Schizophr Bull. 1991;17:247-61.
5. Lally J, Docherty MJ, MacCabe JH. Pharmacological interventions for clozapine-induced sinus tachycardia. Cochrane Database Syst Rev. 2016;2016(6):CD011566.

6. Stryjer R, Timinsky I, Reznik I, Weizman A, Spivak B. Beta-adrenergic antagonists for the treatment of clozapine-induced sinus tachycardia: A retrospective study. Clin Neuropharmacol. 2009;32:290-2.
7. Nilsson BM, Edström O, Lindström L, Wernegren P, Bodén R. Tachycardia in patients treated with clozapine versus antipsychotic long-acting injections. Int Clin Psychopharmacol. 2017;32:219-24.
8. Lally J, Brook J, Dixon T, Gaughran F, Shergill S, Melikian N, et al. Ivabradine, a novel treatment for clozapine-induced sinus tachycardia: a case series. Ther Adv Psychopharmacol. 2014;4:117-22.

CHAPTER 54

# Management of Drug-induced Akathisia

*Sai Sreeja Vullanki, Snehil Gupta*

## INTRODUCTION

Akathisia, derived from the Greek term meaning "inability to sit", is a neuropsychiatric movement disorder characterized by both subjective and objective restlessness. The core symptoms include a subjective sense of mental uneasiness and dysphoria, characterized by a sense of restlessness that can lead to impulsive behaviors such as suicidality and aggression. When severe, an irresistible urge to move becomes prominent. The risk of akathisia associated with psychotropics ranges from 8–76%, with highest risk observed with first-generation antipsychotics (FGAs), such as haloperidol and trifluoperazine.[1] Among second-generation antipsychotics (SGAs), aripiprazole, cariprazine, lurasidone, and risperidone have a higher propensity to cause this adverse effect.

## SUBTYPES

- *Acute akathisia* occurs within days to weeks of initiating or increasing the dose of an antipsychotic.
- *Chronic akathisia*—persistent akathisia lasting >3 months.
- *Withdrawal akathisia* develops within 2–6 weeks of reducing dose or discontinuing an antipsychotic.
- *Tardive akathisia* typically occurs later, usually after 3 months of antipsychotic treatment, and can persist for years even after discontinuation of the offending antipsychotic. Its pathophysiology is similar to that of tardive dyskinesia.[2]

*Pseudoakathisia* refers to the appearance of objective signs of extreme restlessness in the absence of the subjective sense of restlessness.[2] However, it remains uncertain whether this presentation reflects chronic akathisia (where the patient may be unable to verbalize subjective dysphoria or where this component has faded over time), or if it represents a variant of tardive dyskinesia.[3]

## PATHOPHYSIOLOGY

Akathisia is caused by a relative imbalance in dopamine and norepinephrine/serotonin neurotransmission within the basal ganglia. Antipsychotics, which act as dopamine receptor (D2) blocking agents, reduce dopaminergic activity in the ventral striatum. This reduction leads to overactivation of noradrenergic neurons in the locus coeruleus and subsequent activation of the nucleus accumbens shell. This, in turn, results in overactivation of the limbic system and cortex, giving rise to purposeless movements and intense dysphoria in patients receiving these medications. The noradrenergic response can be attenuated with beta-blockers (e.g., propranolol) or $\alpha$-2 agonists (e.g., clonidine).[4,5]

However, the dopamine-noradrenergic system only partly explains the symptoms of akathisia, as not all patients respond to antiadrenergic medications. Evidence suggests that an imbalance in dopamine and serotonergic systems may also contribute to the symptoms of akathisia. Neurons in the ventral tegmental area receive inhibitory serotonergic inputs from the dorsal raphe nucleus. A hyperserotonergic state can reduce dopamine transmission in the basal ganglia, leading to symptoms of akathisia (e.g., selective serotonin receptor inhibitors can also cause akathisia). Therefore, drugs with 5-$HT_{2A}$ antagonistic properties, such as mirtazapine and mianserin, have been shown to improve akathisia.[5]

## PREDISPOSING FACTORS

Younger or older age, first-episode psychosis, no prior exposure to antipsychotics, the presence of affective disorders, the use of high-potency FGAs (e.g., haloperidol), high doses of antipsychotics, rapid dose escalation, abrupt drug discontinuation, and polypharmacy are significant predisposing factors for the development of drug-induced akathisia.[2,3] **Table 1** shows the various classes of drugs

**TABLE 1:** Drugs that can cause akathisia and their potential mechanism of action.

| *Class* | *Drugs* | *Pathways for akathisia* |
|---|---|---|
| Typical antipsychotics | Haloperidol, chlorpromazine, trifluoperazine, and flupentixol | Blockage of dopaminergic D2 receptors in basal ganglia |
| Atypical antipsychotics | Aripiprazole, cariprazine, lurasidone, olanzapine, risperidone, clozapine, quetiapine, and amisulpride | Blockage of 5-HT2 and D2 receptors/D2 partial agonism in the limbic system and basal ganglia |
| Antiemetics | Metoclopramide and prochlorperazine | Antagonism of mesocorticolimbic dopaminergic pathways |
| Mood stabilizers | Lithium | Activation of serotonergic neurotransmission |
| Selective serotonin reuptake inhibitors | Citalopram and fluoxetine | Enhancement of serotonergic activity → decrease in dopamine |
| • Serotonin-norepinephrine<br>• Reuptake inhibitors | Duloxetine and venlafaxine | Inhibitory effect on dopaminergic pathways in the basal ganglia |
| Calcium channel blockers | Cinnarizine and flunarizine | Reduce receptor hypersensitivity in the nigrostriatal system |
| Vesicular monoamine transporter two inhibitors | Reserpine, tetrabenazine, and valbenazine | Deplete synaptic dopamine neurotransmitter |

implicated in causation of akathisia along with their proposed causative pathways.

## CLINICAL FEATURES

- Subjectively, akathisia is often described as an unpleasant state of inner restlessness or intense dysphoria, associated with a desire or compulsion to move for partial relief.[3,6]
- Objectively, akathisia may present with the following signs:
  - Inability to sit, stand, or lie still
  - Fidgeting of hands and arms
  - Foot stamping when seated
  - Persistent leg movements, such as swinging, shuffling, or crossing and uncrossing legs
  - Continuous walking, pacing, or rocking from foot to foot[3,6]

These symptoms typically persist throughout the day but may completely dissipate during sleep. However, patients may experience frequent awakenings at night due to an irresistible urge to move.[6]

## DIFFERENTIAL DIAGNOSIS

Akathisia is often unrecognized or misdiagnosed. Medical conditions such as hyperthyroidism or substance withdrawal states (e.g., alcohol or benzodiazepine withdrawal) can produce restlessness that mimics akathisia.[7]

Similarly, excessive psychomotor agitation occurs in several psychiatric conditions, including bipolar mania, schizophrenia, depression, anxiety, posttraumatic stress disorder, tic and Tourette's disorder, and restless leg syndrome.[7]

## ASSESSMENT AND MANAGEMENT

Recognizing and treating akathisia early is crucial, as severe untreated akathisia accompanied by dysphoria can significantly increase the risk of suicidality, aggression, violence, and poor medication adherence.[8] One reliable indicator of akathisia is the onset of these symptoms following the administration of antipsychotics.

The *Barnes Akathisia Rating Scale* (BARS) is the most widely used assessment tool for evaluating both the subjective symptoms and objective signs of akathisia. This four-item scale includes a global assessment, where a score of 2 or higher indicates the presence of akathisia.[9]

Good clinical practice for minimizing the risk of akathisia includes administering the minimal effective dose of antipsychotics, avoiding rapid dose escalation, and eschewing antipsychotic polypharmacy.[3,8,10] Adequate psychoeducation for patients and caregiver can help identify akathisia early, facilitating timely consultation and mitigating potential distress caused by symptoms.

**Flowchart 1:** Treatment algorithm for drug-induced akathisia.

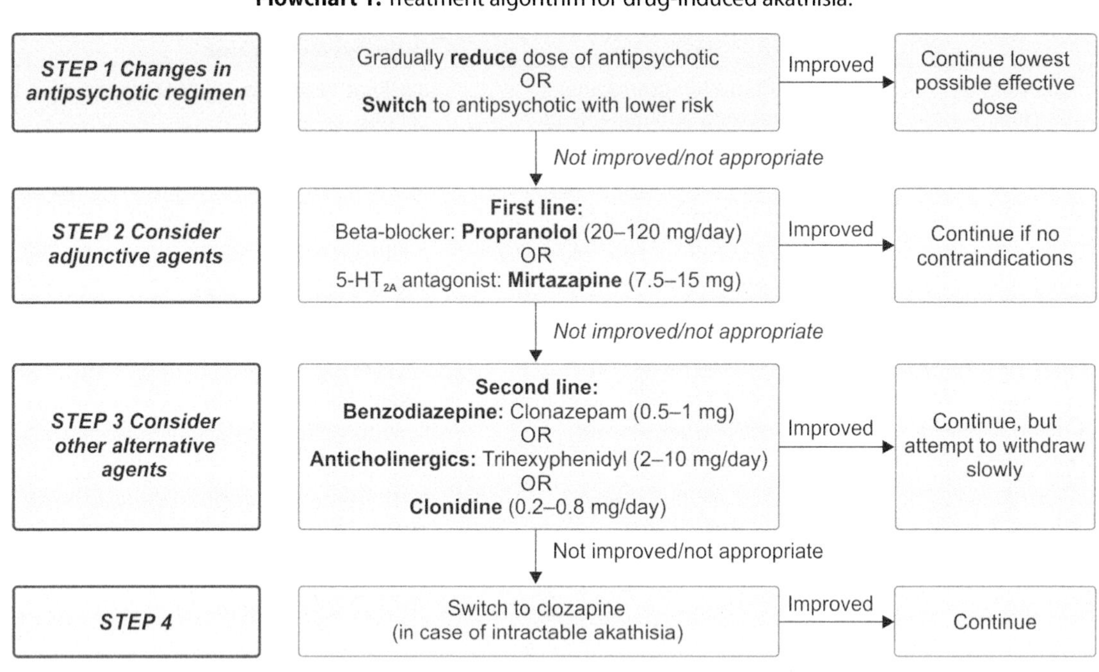


**TABLE 2:** Summary of pharmacological agents used to treat drug-induced akathisia.

| *Class* | *Drug* | *Mechanism of action* | *Dose (mg/d)* | *Side effects* | *Remarks* |
|---|---|---|---|---|---|
| Beta-blockers | Propranolol | Nonselective beta-blockade | 20–120 | Hypotension Contraindication—diabetes, bronchial asthma | First-line adjunctive treatment for a short term |
| Benzodiazepine | Clonazepam | GABA-A receptors agonist | 0.5–2 | Dependence, dizziness, and respiratory depression | It may help with mild subjective symptoms |
| Anticholinergics | Benztropine, biperiden, and trihexyphenidyl | Acetylcholine receptor antagonist | 1.5–8<br>2–6<br>2–10 | Confusion, dry mouth, constipation, and urinary retention | With concurrent extrapyramidal symptoms (EPS) |
| Central alpha agonist | Clonidine | α-2 receptors agonist | 0.2–0.8 | Hypotension, sedation | Limited evidence |
| Tetracyclic antidepressant | Mirtazapine | Antagonizes 5-$HT_{2A}$ receptors | 7.5–15 | Sedation, weight gain, dry mouth | If propranolol is contraindicated or intolerable |

Medication-induced akathisia is optimally managed by gradually reducing dose or switching to an antipsychotic with a lower potential for causing akathisia. Among SGAs, lurasidone, cariprazine, aripiprazole, and risperidone have the highest potential for akathisia, while olanzapine, iloperidone, quetiapine, and clozapine have less risk.[1] However, in clinical practice, switching antipsychotic regimens may not always be feasible due to the proven efficacy of the current medication, cost considerations, or other logistical factors **(Flowchart 1)**.[8]

Pharmacological agents such as beta-blockers (e.g., propranolol), antihistaminic/anticholinergic agents (e.g., benztropine and trihexyphenidyl), or benzodiazepines (e.g., clonazepam) are often used for managing akathisia, though evidence supporting their effectiveness is limited, particularly for long-term use **(Table 2)**. Other agents marketed for managing akathisia, such as mianserin, trazodone, cyproheptadine, vitamin B6, gabapentin, and pregabalin, lack robust evidence and require further research.[10]

## REFERENCES


1. Taylor, D. The Maudsley Prescribing Guidelines in Psychiatry, 14th edition. Philadelphia: Wiley; 2021.
2. Sachdev PS. Acute and tardive drug-induced Akathisia. In: Sethi KD (Ed). Drug-induced movement disorders. Boca Raton, FL: CRC Press; 2004. pp. 129-64.
3. Pringsheim T, Gardner D. The Assessment and Treatment of Antipsychotic-Induced Akathisia. Can J Psychiatry. 2018;63(11):719-29.
4. Lonnen A, Stahl S. The mechanism of drug-induced Akathisia. CNS Spectr. 2011;16:7-10.
5. Zareifopoulos N, Katsaraki M, Stratos P, Villiotou V, Skaltsa M, Dimitriou A, et al. Pathophysiology and management of Akathisia 70 years after the introduction of the chlorpromazine, the first antipsychotic. Eur Rev Med Pharmacol Sci. 2021;25(14):4746-56.
6. Poyurovsky M, Weizman A. Treatment of Antipsychotic-Induced Akathisia: Role of Serotonin 5-$HT_{2A}$ Receptor Antagonists. Drugs. 2020;80(9):871-82.
7. Tucci V. Psychiatric Emergencies for Clinicians: Management of Acute Drug-Induced Akathisia. J Emerg Med. 2020;58(6):922-6.
8. Salem H, Nagpal C, Pigott T, Teixeira AL. Revisiting Antipsychotic-induced Akathisia: Current Issues and Prospective Challenges. Curr Neuropharmacol. 2017;15(5):789-98.
9. Barnes TR. A rating scale for drug-induced Akathisia. Br J Psychiatry. 1989;154:672-6.
10. Thippaiah SM. Struggling to find Effective Pharmacologic Options for Akathisia? B-CALM! Psychopharmacol Bull. 2021;51(3):72-8.

# Management of Drug-induced Dyskinesia

*Karthick Subramanian, Suriya Kumar*

## INTRODUCTION

Tardive dyskinesia (TD) is a component of tardive syndrome, characterized by involuntary movements of the tongue (protrusion, twisting), jaw (chewing), lips (smacking and puckering), and trunk or extremities. It may also include choreiform, athetoid, and rhythmic movements. These movements are typically absent during sleep.[1,2]

## ONSET

The TD occurs after at least 2 months of exposure to a dopamine receptor-blocking agent (DRBA) (or 1 month if the patient is 60 years or older) while on medications, or within 4 weeks of withdrawal from an oral agent or within 8 weeks of discontinuing a long-acting injectable antipsychotic. Symptoms must persist for at least 4 weeks.[3]

## PATHOPHYSIOLOGY

Sustained blockade of dopamine receptors in the nigrostriatal pathway leads to receptor upregulation, making them "supersensitive" to dopamine, resulting in hyperkinetic involuntary movements.[4]

## EPIDEMIOLOGY

Tardive syndromes, including drug-induced dyskinesia (DID), are more common with first-generation antipsychotics (30%) compared to second-generation antipsychotics (21%).[5] Dyskinesia is associated with significant impairment in quality of life and can impose a considerable burden on caregivers.[6] Recent studies reveal increased levels of dopamine in the synapses of the striatum.[2] Women, children, and elderly individuals (age >50 years), those diagnosed with mood disorders, patients who experience acute extrapyramidal symptoms in the early phase of treatment, and individuals with brain damage are at a higher risk of developing TD.

## ASSESSMENT

Specific instruments for assessing dyskinetic movements include the Unified Dyskinesia Rating Scale (UDysRS),[7] the Rush Dyskinesia Rating Scale,[8] and the Clinical Dyskinesia Rating Scale (CDRS).[9] Other standard scales used to evaluate dyskinesia as part of abnormal involuntary movements are the Unified Parkinson's Disease Rating Scale (UPDRS),[10] the Movement Disorders Society-sponsored revision of the UPDRS (MDS-UPDRS),[11] and the Abnormal Involuntary Movement Scale (AIMS). The algorithm for the assessing and managing DID is depicted in **Flowchart 1**.

## LABORATORY ASSESSMENT

Various specialized apparatuses are available to measure the magnitude, velocity, and localization of dyskinetic movements. Surface electromyography (sEMG), wearable sensors, camera-based optical systems, and magnetic motion tracking systems are employed for identifying such characteristics.[12]

## PHARMACOLOGICAL MANAGEMENT

Vesicular monoamine transporter-2 (VMAT2) inhibitors, such as valbenazine and deutetrabenazine, are considered the first-line pharmacotherapy for TD.[13] Other treatment options have limitations, including small sample sizes in studies and limited or conflicting evidence.[13] **Table 1** outlines various treatment options for the management of DID.

**Flowchart 1:** Management of drug-induced dyskinesia.

Symptoms suggestive of tardive dyskinesia (TD)

↓

- Rule out other neurological movement disorders including oral-facial tics/bruxism in wakefulness/dental abnormalities
- Rule out functional neurological symptom disorder/persistent hallucinatory behavior

↓ If other causes ruled out

Stop anticholinergics if prescribed

↓ If TD persists

Reduce the dose of antipsychotic

If TD resolves → Continue the same drug and dosage

If TD persists → Switch to quetiapine or clozapin

↓ If TD persists

Consider

*Valbenazine:*
- Longer half-life (15–20 hours)
- Once daily dosing
- Narrow dosing range (40–80 mg/day)

*Deutetrabenazine:*
- Shorter half-life (9–20 hours)
- Twice daily dosing
- Wide dosing range (6–24 mg/day)

↓

Consider other agents/methods as mentioned in **Table 1**

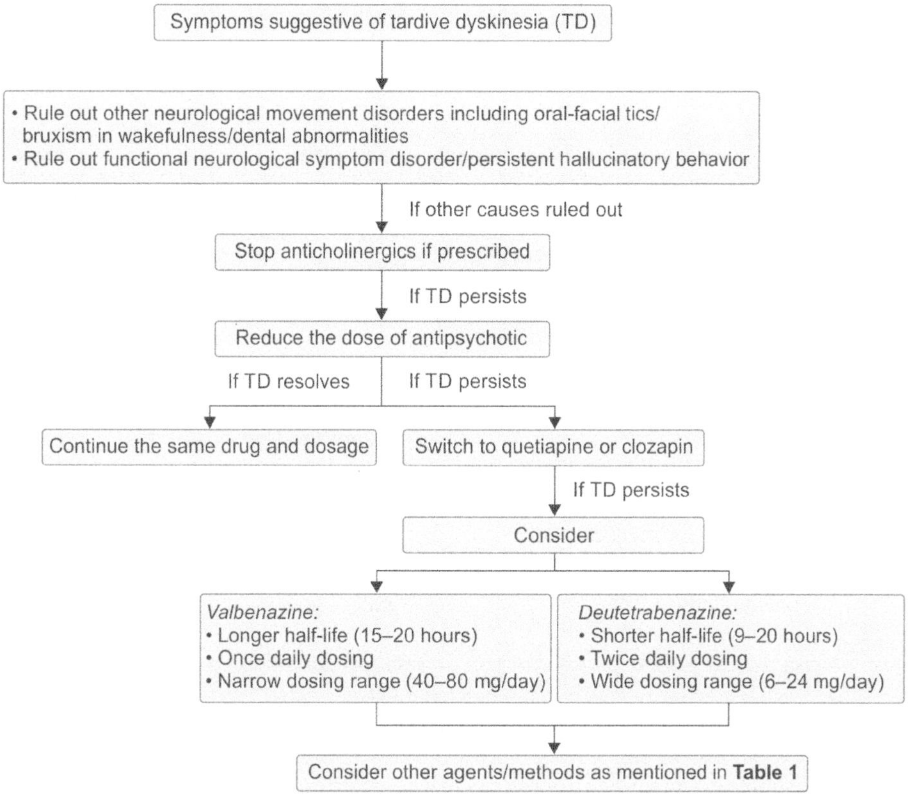

**TABLE 1:** Management options for drug-induced dyskinesia.[4,5]

| ***Class of drug*** | ***Agent name (dose range; dosage)*** | ***Mechanism of action*** | ***Side-effects*** |
|---|---|---|---|
| *First-line options* | | | |
| Vesicular monoamine transporter 2 (VMAT2) inhibitors | Tetrabenazine (12.5–150 mg/day; TID)<br>Valbenazine (40–80 mg/day; OD)<br>Deutetrabenazine (12–48 mg/day BID) | Blocks the sequestration of monoamines from cytosol back into vesicles leading to rapid degradation of monoamines | Depression, parkinsonism, akathisia |
| Atypical antipsychotic | Clozapine (up to 500mg/day) | Low affinity to striatal $D_2$ receptors | Sedation, drooling, agranulocytosis |
| *Second-line options* | | | |
| NMDA antagonist | Amantadine (100 mg three times a day) | Weak NMDA (N-methyl-D-aspartate) receptor antagonist | Insomnia, constipation, and dizziness |
| Benzodiazepines | Clonazepam (4–5 mg/day) | Increase GABA levels through $GABA_A$ receptors | Sedation and ataxia |
| Nutraceuticals | Gingko biloba extract (240 mg/day) | Antioxidant | None |
| *Third-line options* | | | |
| Antispasmodic agent | Baclofen (up to 120 mg/day) | Increase GABA levels through $GABA_A$ receptors | Dizziness, nausea, and insomnia |

*Contd...*

*Contd...*

| *Class of drug* | *Agent name (dose range; dosage)* | *Mechanism of action* | *Side-effects* |
|---|---|---|---|
| Antiepileptics | Levetiracetam (up to 3000 mg/day) | Inhibition of synaptic vesicle release; N-type calcium channel blockade | Sedation; headache; nasal; and congestion |
| Vitamins | Vitamin B6 (pyridoxine) (400 mg/day) | Antioxidant | None |
| Hormone | Melatonin (10–20 mg/day) | Antioxidant | None |
| Nootropics | Piracetam (4,800 mg/day) | N-type calcium channel blockade | Insomnia, anxiety, weight gain |
| Beta-blocker | Propranolol (up to 80 mg/day) | | Light-headedness, nightmares |
| Z-drugs | Zolpidem (10–20 mg/day) | Binds to GABA-benzodiazepine receptor complex | Sedation |
| Antiepileptic | Zonisamide | Sodium and T-type calcium channel blocker | Loss of appetite, weight loss, dizziness, and headache |
| *Surgical options* | | | |
| Deep brain stimulation | Deep brain stimulation of the globus pallidus interna (GPi) | Enhanced stimulation of the GPi reduces severity of dyskinesia | Falls, equipment-related complications |

(GABA: gamma-aminobutyric acid)

## REFERENCES


1. Boland R, Verdiun M, Ruiz P. Kaplan & Sadock's synopsis of psychiatry. Philadelphia: Lippincott Williams & Wilkins; 2021.
2. Damier P. Drug-induced dyskinesias. Curr Opin Neurol. 2009;22(4):394.
3. Sadock BJ, Sadock VA, MD DPR. Kaplan and Sadock's Comprehensive Textbook of Psychiatry—50th Anniversary Edition, Tenth edition. Philadelphia: Lippincott Williams and Wilkins; 2017. pp. 4997.
4. Factor SA. Management of tardive syndrome: Medications and surgical treatments. Neurother J Am Soc Exp Neurother. 2020;17(4):1694-712.
5. Factor SA, Burkhard PR, Caroff S, Friedman JH, Marras C, Tinazzi M, et al. Recent developments in drug-induced movement disorders: a mixed picture. Lancet Neurol. 2019;18(9):880-90.
6. Daneault JF, Vergara-Diaz G, Lee SI. Clinical management of drug-induced dyskinesia in Parkinson's disease: why current approaches may need to be changed to optimise quality of life. EMJ. 2016;1(4):62-9.
7. Goetz CG, Nutt JG, Stebbins GT. The unified dyskinesia rating scale: presentation and clinimetric profile. Mov Disord Off J Mov Disord Soc. 2008;23(16): 2398-403.
8. Goetz C, Stebbins G, Shale H, Lang A, Chernik D, Chmura T, et al. Utility of an objective dyskinesia rating scale for Parkinson's disease: inter-and intrarater reliability assessment. Mov Disord. 1994;9(4):390-4.
9. Hagell P, Widner H. Clinical rating of dyskinesias in Parkinson's disease: use and reliability of a new rating scale. Mov Disord Off J Mov Disord Soc. 1999;14(3):448-55.
10. Fahn S, Elton RL. Unified Parkinsons Rating Scale. Recent developments in Parkinsons disease. Florham Park: Macmillan Healthcare Information; 1987. pp. 153-63.
11. Goetz CG, Tilley BC, Shaftman SR, Stebbins GT, Fahn S, Martinez-Martin P, et al. Movement Disorder Society-sponsored revision of the Unified Parkinson's Disease Rating Scale (MDS-UPDRS): scale presentation and clinimetric testing results. Mov Disord Off J Mov Disord Soc. 2008;23(15):2129-70.
12. Carignan B, Daneault JF, Duval C. Assessing drug-induced dyskinesia in the clinic, the laboratory and the natural environment of patients. J Park Dis. 2011;1(4):329-37.
13. Widschwendter CG, Hofer A. Antipsychotic-induced tardive dyskinesia: update on epidemiology and management. Curr Opin Psychiatry. 2019;32(3):179-84.

CHAPTER 56

# Management of Drug-induced Hyperprolactinemia

*Shobit Garg, Shaily Mittal, Sai Krishna Tikka*

## INTRODUCTION

Hyperprolactinemia is the most common pituitary hormone hypersecretion syndrome in both men and women. It is defined as serum prolactin levels >25 ng/mL (>530 mIU/mL) in nonpregnant females and >20 ng/mL (>424 mIU/mL) in males. One of the most common causes of hyperprolactinemia is *drug-induced*.[1]

1 ng/mL = 21.2 mIU/mL, $T_{1/2}$ life of prolactin: 25–50 minutes

## CLINICAL PEARLS IN APPROACH TO HYPERPROLACTINEMIA (FLOWCHART 1)

A1: Why baseline prolactin levels?

- In the absence of a baseline prolactin value, attributing an elevated prolactin level to the offending drug can be challenging.
- Blood samples should be collected before administering any doses of antipsychotic (AP), as even a single dose can raise prolactin levels.
- If the baseline prolactin level is elevated and no dose of the prolactin-raising drug was taken, stress could be a plausible explanation. Stress may increase prolactin levels to as high as 42 ng/mL in women and 33 ng/mL in men.[1]

*Important:* If serum prolactin concentration is only slightly elevated (21–40 ng/mL), then the test should be repeated on a fasting sample before considering hyperprolactinemia.

A2: When can we skip baseline prolactin monitoring?

- In women over the age of 50 and men over 65 (elevated prolactin levels have no additional health consequences on bone health beyond these ages)
- *Measuring baseline prolactin levels is mandatory in children and adolescent population before initiating psychotropic medications.*[2]

B1: What are the causes of prolactin elevation other than drug-induced?

- *Physiological causes:* Stress, venipuncture stress, exercise, coitus, pregnancy (up to 600 ng/mL at term), nipple stimulation and lactation (up to 300 ng/mL), and seizures.

**Flowchart 1:** The clinical approach to hyperprolactinemia.

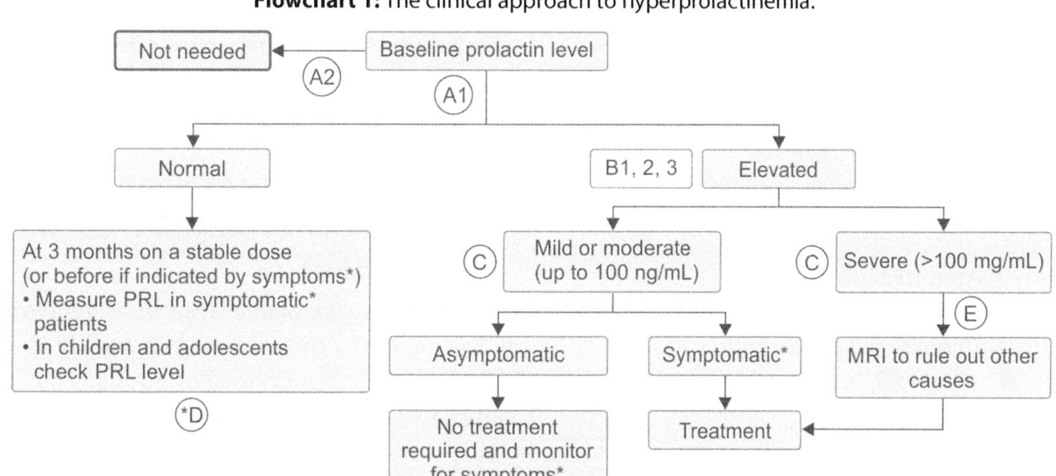

- *Pathological causes:* Hypothyroidism, polycystic ovary syndrome, chronic renal failure, liver cirrhosis, prolactinoma (ranging from mild elevation to 50,000 ng/mL), chest wall lesions (e.g., breast surgery, nipple rings, etc.), breast stimulation, macroprolactinoma, etc.
- *Macroprolactinemia:* Also referred to as "big prolactin", represents large circulating aggregates of prolactin and antibodies, approximately 150 kD in size. It is a benign, asymptomatic condition that does not require treatment but can be misdiagnosed as prolactin hypersecretion. To avoid misdiagnosis, clinicians can use polyethylene glycol (PEG) serum precipitation as a screening method.[1,3]

B2: What are the causes of prolactin elevation due to drugs other than psychotropics?

- *Prokinetics:* Metoclopramide and domperidone
- *Estrogen-containing oral contraceptives*
- *Antihypertensives:* Verapamil and α-methyldopa
- *Opiates:* Morphine and heroin (transient rise in prolactin levels for a few hours following the dose)
- *H2-receptor blocker agents:* Cimetidine (?) and ranitidine (?)[1,3]

B3: "3-day" Protocol

This approach is applicable when prolactin is elevated due to AP but no baseline prolactin values are available. If clinically feasible, withholding the current AP for a minimum of 3 days can help determine whether hyperprolactinemia is drug-induced, as prolactin levels should decrease in such cases.[2]

C: Severity of Hyperprolactinemia

- *Mild*: Up to 50 ng/mL
- *Moderate*: 50–100 ng/mL
- *Severe*: >100 ng/mL[3]

Drugs-induced hyperprolactinemia is largely *dose-dependent.* Most drugs do not typically elevate prolactin levels beyond 100 ng/mL; however, risperidone can cause elevations as high as 300–400 ng/mL.[3]

D: Symptoms of Hyperprolactinemia

- *Premenopausal women*:
  - *Mild hyperprolactinemia:* Infertility
  - *Moderate hyperprolactinemia:* Either amenorrhea or oligomenorrhea
  - *Severe hyperprolactinemia:* Amenorrhea, hypogonadism, gynecomastia, galactorrhea

  Females with amenorrhea due to hyperprolactinemia have lower bone mineral density compared to those with normal menses and hyperprolactinemia.[1-3]
- *Postmenopausal women* are already hypogonadal (hypoestrogenic); therefore, hyperprolactinemia does not significantly alter their hormonal status. Also, galactorrhea is very rare in this population.[1-3]
- *Men*:
  - *Hypogonadotropic hypogonadism:* Hyperprolactinemia causes decreased testosterone levels, resulting in short-term symptoms such as reduced energy and libido. Long-term effects include decreased muscle mass, reduced body hair, and osteoporosis.
  - *Erectile dysfunction:* This is caused by mechanisms unrelated to hypogonadism.
  - *Infertility:* Although uncommon, infertility due to hyperprolactinemia can occur in males, accounting for approximately 4% of cases.
  - *Galactorrhea:* This condition may develop in males but is less common compared to females.[1-3]
- *Children:* Hyperprolactinemia can delay puberty in children and adolescents.
- *Long-term complications*: Osteoporosis—amenorrhoeic women and men with low testosterone are at a higher risk of osteoporosis. While normalization of prolactin prevents further bone loss, bone mineral density typically *never returns to normal.*[1-3]

E: When is magnetic resonance imaging (MRI) recommended?

*An MRI of the pituitary with contrast* is indicated in cases of severe elevation of serum prolactin levels (>100 mg/mL), in those presenting with symptoms suggestive of raised intracranial pressure effects (e.g., visual field disturbances and headaches), and when high prolactin levels cannot be easily attributed to AP medication.[3]

## CLINICAL PEARLS IN APPROACH TO HYPERPROLACTINEMIA TREATMENT (FLOWCHART 2)

F: *Adjunctive aripiprazole:* Aripiprazole is typically started at 2.5 mg and titrated over 4–8 weekly intervals until reaching a maximum dose of 10 mg. Poor response to adjunctive aripiprazole has been specifically observed with amisulpride-induced hyperprolactinemia. Importantly, the goal of adjunctive aripiprazole is not to

**Flowchart 2:** Algorithm of the clinical approach to hyperprolactinemia treatment.

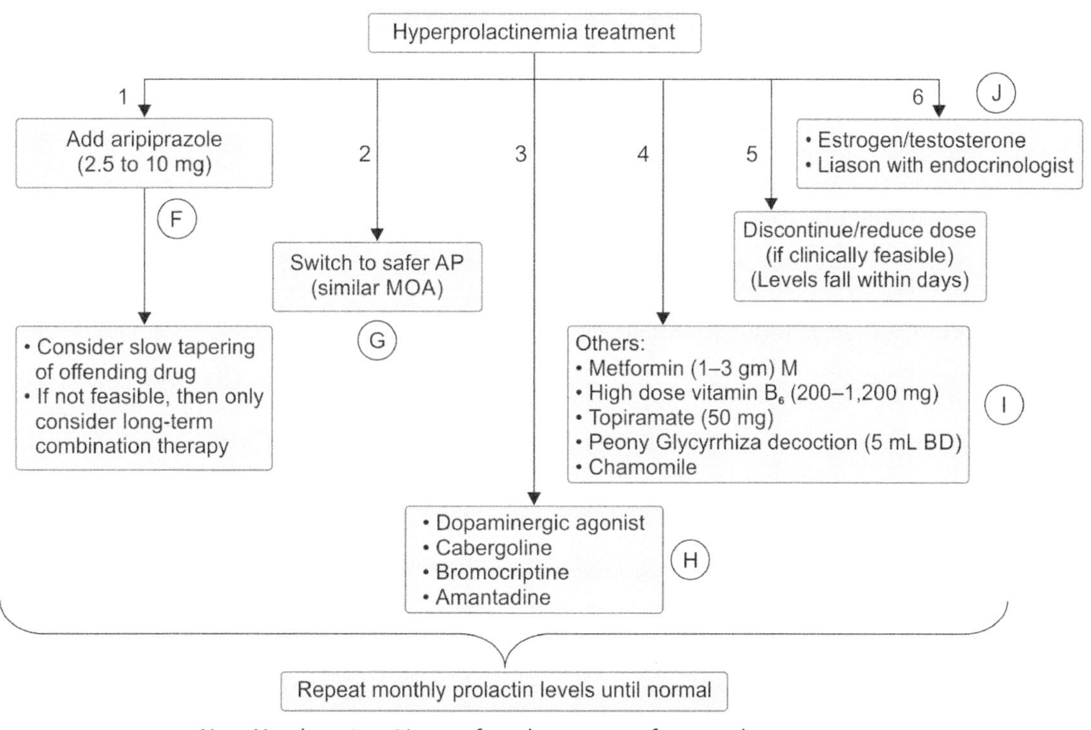


*Note:* Numbers 1 to 6 is a preferred sequence of approach to treatment.
(AP: antipsychotics, MOA: mechanism of action)

normalize prolactin levels, but to reduce them sufficiently to restore normal menses and sexual function. A decrease in prolactin could result in the return of fertility even before menses resume, so contraceptive advice may be needed. Better responses are seen with prolactin levels >50 ng/mL. Headache and somnolence are the most common side effects reported in the trials. Adjunctive aripiprazole received an A-grade recommendation in a consensus paper by Montejo et al.[4]

G: Hyperprolactinemia sparing and nonsparing antipsychotics are described in **Table 1**.

High-risk prolactin elevating APs are to be avoided in the following situations.

- Age before 25 years, i.e., before peak bone mass
- Young women
- Patients with osteoporosis
- Patients with hormone-dependent breast cancer

Switching to AP with a lower risk of hyperprolactinemia were assigned grade A, B, or C recommendations (depending on the specific agent) in a consensus paper by Montejo et al.[4]

**TABLE 1:** Describing antipsychotics based on their effects on prolactin levels.[5-7]

| *Prolactin sparing* | *Prolactin elevating (low risk)* | *Prolactin elevating (high risk)* |
|---|---|---|
| Quetiapine | Lurasidone* | Amisulpride |
| Aripiprazole | Ziprasidone | Risperidone |
| Clozapine | Olanzapine | Paliperidone |
| Cariprazine | Asenapine[@] | Sulpiride |
| Iloperidone | | FGA |

*Note:** Dose related; [@]Data limited
(FGA: first-generation antipsychotics)

H: *Dopaminergic agonist (DA):* They carry a potential risk of inducing psychosis or worsening preexisting psychosis, although this has not been clearly established by studies.

- *Cabergoline:* This is the most common DA used in hyperprolactinemia due to prolactinomas. Dose ranges from 0.125 mg weekly to 1 mg twice weekly, with a maximum dose of 1.5 mg twice weekly. Prolactin levels typically normalize within 3 months. Cardiac valvular abnormalities are among the more serious adverse events reported.

- *Bromocriptine:* This is preferred in pregnancy. Dose is 2.5 mg twice daily until prolactin normalizes, with a maximum dose of 15–20 mg/day. Nausea and vomiting are the most frequent side effects. Bromocriptine has better cardiac safety profile compared to cabergoline.[3]

The DAs should be avoided in cases of uncontrolled hypertension. The addition of DA received a B-grade recommendation in a consensus paper by Montejo et al.[4]

I: Other strategies to mitigate long-term risk of reduced bone mineral density or osteoporosis should be addressed, including smoking cessation, reducing sedentary lifestyle, correcting vitamin D deficiency (with supplements of 800–1,000 IU/day), and limiting alcohol intake. Calcium supplementation (500–1,000 mg/day) is recommended for patients with a calcium deficient diet, defined as consuming fewer than 4–5 daily serving of dairy products (equivalent to 1 liter of milk).[7,8]

J: Use of estrogen or testosterone in patients with long-term hypogonadism or low bone mass due to hyperprolactinemia should be considered in *liaison with an endocrinologist*. Additionally, phosphodiesterase inhibitors can be initiated to treat erectile dysfunction secondary to hyperprolactinemia.[3,7,8]

## REFERENCES

1. Vilar L, Vilar CF, Lyra R, Freitas MDC. Pitfalls in the Diagnostic Evaluation of Hyperprolactinemia. Neuroendocrinology. 2019;109(1):7-19.
2. Antipsychotic-induced hyperprolactinaemia. Trust guideline for identification, monitoring and management. Oxford: National Health Trust; 2015.
3. Melmed S, Casanueva FF, Hoffman AR, Kleinberg DL, Montori VM, Schlechte JA, et al.; Endocrine Society. Diagnosis and treatment of hyperprolactinemia: an Endocrine Society clinical practice guideline. J Clin Endocrinol Metab. 2011;96(2):273-88.
4. Montejo ÁL, Arango C, Bernardo M, Carrasco JL, Crespo-Facorro B, Cruz JJ, et al. Multidisciplinary consensus on the therapeutic recommendations for iatrogenic hyperprolactinemia secondary to antipsychotics. Front Neuroendocrinol. 2017;45:25-34.
5. Taylor DM, Barnes TRE, Young AH. The Maudsley Prescribing Guidelines in Psychiatry, 13th edition. Philadelphia: John Wiley & Sons; 2018.
6. Castle DJ, Galletly CA, Dark F, Humberstone V, Morgan VA, Killackey E, et al. The 2016 Royal Australian and New Zealand College of Psychiatrists guidelines for the management of schizophrenia and related disorders. Med J Aust. 2017;206(11):501-5.
7. Hasan A, Falkai P, Wobrock T, Lieberman J, Glenthoj B, Gattaz WF, et al.; World Federation of Societies of Biological Psychiatry (WFSBP) Task Force on Treatment Guidelines for Schizophrenia. World Federation of Societies of Biological Psychiatry (WFSBP) Guidelines for Biological Treatment of Schizophrenia, part 1: update 2012 on the acute treatment of schizophrenia and the management of treatment resistance. World J Biol Psychiatry. 2012;13(5):318-78.
8. Rusgis MM, Alabbasi AY, Nelson LA. Guidance on the treatment of antipsychotic-induced hyperprolactinemia when switching the antipsychotic is not an option. Am J Health Syst Pharm. 2021;78(10):862-71.

# Management of Drug-induced Sedation

Rajesh Gopalakrishnan, Jibi Achamma Jacob

## INTRODUCTION

Sedation is a common and generally dose-dependent side effect associated with the two major classes of psychotropic medications—(1) antipsychotic drug (APD) and (2) antidepressant drug (ADD). While considered a side effect, it may alleviate depressive and psychotic symptoms, normalize disrupted sleep patterns, and help in managing agitated, disruptive, or violent patients.

## MECHANISM AND DRUGS IMPLIED

The neurobiology of sedation caused by psychotropic medications is often linked to histaminergic ($H_1$) or 5-$HT_{2A}$ receptor antagonism and adrenergic blocking properties. Tolerance to sedation typically develops over time. Several risk factors increase the likelihood of sedation, including extremes of age, rapid dose escalation, higher doses, comorbid medical illnesses, substance use, irrational polypharmacy, and the concurrent use of sedatives such as benzodiazepines or zolpidem.[1]

**Table 1** lists the relative sedative effects of commonly used psychotropic medications.[1-3] Sedation may occur with both first-generation antipsychotics (FGAs) and second-generation antipsychotics (SGAs), though it is presumed to be more with FGAs. Among antidepressants, tricyclic antidepressants (TCAs) cause more sedation than all other classes of ADDs. Conventional mood stabilizers are also associated with dose-dependent sedation, with sodium valproate showing the highest propensity for this effect.[2]

While daytime drowsiness may be due to the sedating effect of medication, it may also result from poor sleep quality due to the underlying disease process or from an aggravation of underlying sleep disorder by the prescribed medication. It is essential to differentiate sedation from fatigue, another common side effect of psychotropic medication. Sedation must also be distinguished from negative symptoms such as avolition, cognitive impairment, and depressive symptoms, in patients with schizophrenia.[1]

## CONSEQUENCES

Severe sedation, especially in outpatient settings, can disrupt patients' functioning, impair their quality of life, reduce educational and occupational performance, result in neglect of self or others, and contribute to poor adherence. Sedation increases the risk of falls, injuries, and accidents, particularly in the elderly. Therefore, accurate assessment and appropriate treatment of sedation are essential components of long-term care to mitigate these risks and improve outcomes.

## ASSESSMENT

- Take a detailed history of the current sleep pattern using a sleep diary to rule out comorbid parasomnias. Check for loud snoring, periods of apnea, restlessness in lower limbs, etc.[4,5]
- Assess psychiatric or medical comorbidities such as depression, hypothyroidism, obstructive sleep apnea, or medication related side effects.
- A detailed review of the patient's medication list will help determine if synergistic action of coadministered medications or drug interactions that alter the metabolism of psychotropics is responsible for sedation.
- Assess for comorbid substance use (nicotine, alcohol, or other substances), as ongoing use can impair night-time sleep and cause daytime sleepiness.

## MANAGEMENT

General strategies for the management of sedation with psychotropic medications include the following **(Flowchart 1)**:

- Select the antipsychotic/antidepressant based on effectiveness and attempt to match the patient's symptom profile with the adverse effects of the medication.

**TABLE 1:** Sedative effects of antipsychotics, antidepressants and mood stabilizers.[1,2,9]

| *Antipsychotic medications* | *Sedation potential* | *Antidepressants* | *Sedation potential* |
|---|---|---|---|
| • *FGAs:* | | • *TCAs:* | |
| – Chlorpromazine | +++ | – Amitriptyline | +++ |
| – Haloperidol | + | – Clomipramine | +++ |
| – Trifluoperazine | + | – Dosulepin | +++ |
| – Fluphenazine | + | – Imipramine | ++ |
| – Zuclopenthixol | ++ | • *SSRIs:* | |
| – Pimozide | + | – Fluoxetine | – |
| – Sulpiride | – | – Sertraline | – |
| • *SGAs:* | | – Paroxetine | + |
| – Olanzapine | ++ | – Citalopram | – |
| – Risperidone | + | – Escitalopram | – |
| – Quetiapine | ++ | – Vilazodone | – |
| – Clozapine | +++ | – Vortioxetine | – |
| – Paliperidone | + | – Fluvoxamine | + |
| – Ziprasidone | + | • *Others:* | |
| – Lurasidone | + | – Agomelatine | + |
| – Cariprazine | – | – Mirtazapine | +++ |
| – Amisulpride | – | – Trazodone | +++ |
| – Aripiprazole | – | – Venlafaxine | – |
| – Iloperidone | – | – Bupropion | – |
| ***Mood stabilizers*** | ***Sedation potential*** | | |
| Lithium | + | | |
| Sodium valproate | ++ | | |
| Carbamazepine | + | | |
| Lamotrigine | +/– | | |

(FGAs: first-generation antipsychotics; SGAs: second-generation antipsychotics; TCAs: tricyclic antidepressants; SSRIs: selective serotonin reuptake inhibitors, +: low potential; ++: moderate potential; +++: high potential, –: very low potential; +/–: seen in a few patients)

**Flowchart 1:** Flowchart to manage sedation with psychotropic medications.

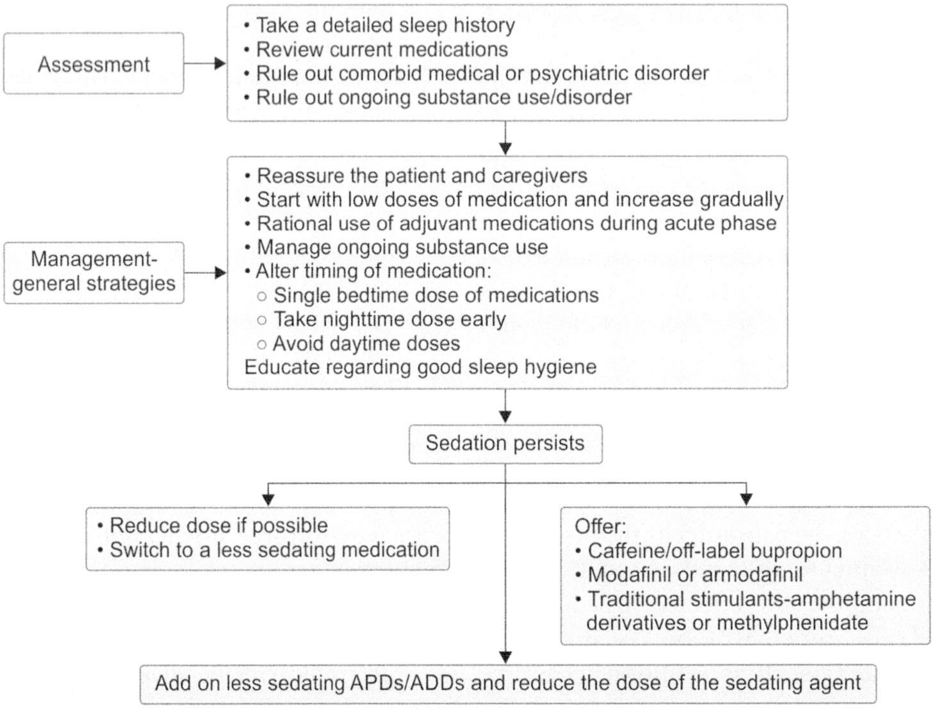

Assessment →
- Take a detailed sleep history
- Review current medications
- Rule out comorbid medical or psychiatric disorder
- Rule out ongoing substance use/disorder

↓

Management-general strategies →
- Reassure the patient and caregivers
- Start with low doses of medication and increase gradually
- Rational use of adjuvant medications during acute phase
- Manage ongoing substance use
- Alter timing of medication:
  - Single bedtime dose of medications
  - Take nighttime dose early
  - Avoid daytime doses

Educate regarding good sleep hygiene

↓

Sedation persists

↓

- Reduce dose if possible
- Switch to a less sedating medication

Offer:
- Caffeine/off-label bupropion
- Modafinil or armodafinil
- Traditional stimulants-amphetamine derivatives or methylphenidate

↓

Add on less sedating APDs/ADDs and reduce the dose of the sedating agent

- Reassure the patient and caregivers that excessive sedation will wear off within the first few weeks; this will help allay their anxiety.
- Start the drug at a low dose and slowly increase to the minimum effective dose. Short-term use of adjuvant medications, such as short-acting benzodiazepines for agitation and insomnia, can help reduce the need for higher doses of APDs during the acute phase.
- Comorbid substance use (nicotine, alcohol, or other substances) if present needs to be managed appropriately.
- Single bedtime dosing of medications, avoiding daytime doses of sedating medications, and taking the night dose earlier in the evening can be helpful.
- Education on good sleep hygiene is necessary, as adequate nighttime sleep can help minimize medication-related daytime sedation. Strategies include avoiding or reducing alcohol, nicotine, and caffeine consumption, especially after late afternoon, creating a relaxing bedtime routine, and avoiding phones, television, or other electronic devices in bed. Patients should be encouraged to maintain regular sleep habits and avoid daytime naps. An active daytime schedule with regular physical exercise may also help improve sleep.

### Specific Strategies to Reduce Sedation

- Consider gradually reducing the patient's medication dose if possible, while closely monitoring for worsening symptoms.
- Consider switching the patient to a less sedating antipsychotic, such as aripiprazole, brexipiprazole, or cariprazine, or antidepressant such as selective serotonin reuptake inhibitors, serotonin noradrenaline reuptake inhibitors, or bupropion.
- Explore other strategies to reduce oral dose effectively without affecting serum levels and efficacy. For example, using fluvoxamine 50–100 mg/day can reduce the metabolism of clozapine, thereby achieving higher serum levels at lower doses, resulting in less sedation. Adding less sedating APDs such as aripiprazole or cariprazine as adjuncts to clozapine could help avoid increasing the clozapine dose.[6]
- Strategies to improve the patient's alertness (in situations where dose reduction or change in APD is not an option):
    - Offer caffeine or off-label bupropion (75–100 mg once in the morning or up to twice daily). The evidence for these strategies is anecdotal.[3]
    - Consider prescribing medications such as modafinil (200–400 mg in the morning) or armodafinil (150–250 mg in the morning). There is some evidence that sedation in patients with mood disorder tends to improve with these medications, but there is no evidence of beneficial effects for this strategy in patients with schizophrenia.[4-7]
    - Traditional stimulants such as amphetamine derivatives or methylphenidate have been tried, but there is even less evidence and greater risks than in strategy above. Risks include tolerance, addiction, worsening of psychosis, and cardiovascular side-effects.[3,7]
    - Newer medications such as pitolisant and solriamfetol have been found to be beneficial in patients with comorbid narcolepsy and psychosis. These may have a role in managing medication-related sedation in the future.[5,8]

## REFERENCES

1. Taylor DM, Barnes TRE, Young AH. Schizophrenia and related psychoses. The Maudsley Prescribing Guidelines in Psychiatry, 14th edition. New Delhi: Wiley India Pvt. Ltd; 2021. pp 3-244.
2. Taylor DM, Barnes TRE, Young AH. Depression and anxiety disorders. The Maudsley Prescribing Guidelines in Psychiatry. 14th edition. New Delhi: Wiley India Pvt. Ltd; 2021. pp 305-448.
3. Miller DD. Sedation with antipsychotics: Manage, don't accept adverse 'calming' effect. Curr Psychiatr. 2007;6(8):39-51
4. Chervin RD. (2023). Approach to the patient with excessive daytime sleepiness. UpToDate. [online] Available from https://www.uptodate.com/contents/approach-to-the-patient-with-excessive-daytime-sleepiness [Last accessed June, 2025].
5. Murray BJ. (2021). Excessive daytime sleepiness due to medical disorders and medications. [online] Available from https://www.uptodate.com/contents/excessive-daytime-sleepiness-due-to-medical-disorders-and-medications [Last accessed June, 2025].
6. Gupta S, Parkinson S. Management of sedation due to clozapine. BJPsych Adv. 2022;1-2.
7. Fang F, Sun H, Wang Z, Ren M, Calabrese JR, Gao K. Antipsychotic Drug-Induced Somnolence: Incidence, Mechanisms, and Management. CNS Drugs. 2016; 30(9):845-67.
8. Dondé C, Polosan M, Guzun R. Pitolisant for treating narcolepsy comorbid with schizophrenia. J Clin Psychopharmacol. 2020;40(5):504-6.
9. Aiken C. Sedation: The Ups and Downs of a Side Effect. Psychiatric Times. 2021;38(4).

# Index

Page numbers followed by *b* refer to box, *f* refer to figure, *fc* refer to flowchart, and *t* refer to table

## T



## U



## V



## W



## Y



## Z